Antimicrobial Peptides

2ND EDITION

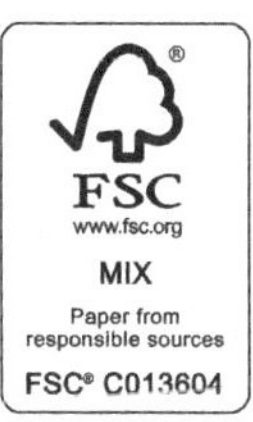

Antimicrobial Peptides

Discovery, Design and Novel Therapeutic Strategies

2ND EDITION

Edited by

Guangshun Wang

University of Nebraska Medical Center, Omaha, Nebraska, USA

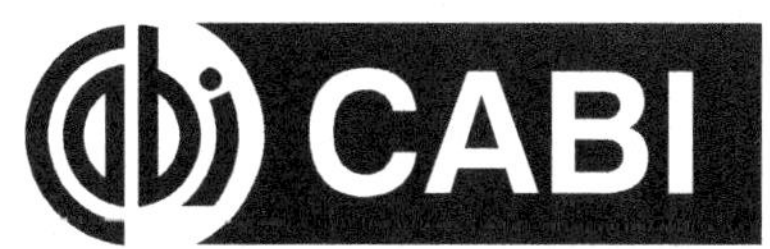

CABI is a trading name of CAB International

CABI	CABI
Nosworthy Way	745 Atlantic Avenue
Wallingford	8th Floor
Oxfordshire OX10 8DE	Boston, MA 02111
UK	USA
Tel: +44 (0)1491 832111	Tel: +1 (617)682-9015
Fax: +44 (0)1491 833508	E-mail: cabi-nao@cabi.org
E-mail: info@cabi.org	
Website: www.cabi.org	

British Library Cataloguing-in-Publication Data

A catalogue record for this book is available from the British Library.

Library of Congress Cataloging-in-Publication Data

Names: Wang, Guangshun.
Title: Antimicrobial peptides : discovery, design and novel therapeutic strategies / editor, Guangshun Wang.
Other titles: Antimicrobial peptides (Wang)
Description: 2nd edition. | Wallingford, Oxfordshire, UK ; Boston, MA : CABI, [2017] | Includes bibliographical references and index.
Identifiers: LCCN 2017016223 (print) | LCCN 2017018723 (ebook) | ISBN 9781786390400 (ePDF) | ISBN 9781786390417 (ePub) | ISBN 9781786390394 (hbk: alk. paper)
Subjects: | MESH: Antimicrobial Cationic Peptides | Anti-Infective Agents |Immunity, Innate | Drug Design
Classification: LCC RS431.P37 (ebook) | LCC RS431.P37 (print) | NLM QU 68 |DDC 615/.1--dc23
LC record available at *https://lccn.loc.gov/2017016223*

ISBN: 978 1 78639 039 4 (hardback)
            978 1 78639 040 0 (e-book)
            978 1 78639 041 7 (e-pub)

Commissioning editor: Rachael Russell
Editorial assistant: Emma McCann
Production editor: Alan Worth

Typeset by Typeset by AMA DataSet Ltd, Preston, UK
Printed and bound in the UK by CPI Group (UK) Ltd, Croydon, CR0 4YY

Contents

PART IV: MECHANISMS OF ACTION: BIOPHYSICS AND STRUCTURAL BIOLOGY

Contributors

Benincasa, Monica, Department of Life Sciences, University of Trieste, via Giorgieri 5, 34127 Trieste, Italy.

Bozelli, José Carlos Junior, Department of Biochemistry and Biomedical Sciences, McMaster University, Health Sciences Centre, Hamilton, Ontario, L8S 4K1, Canada.

Chowdhury, Mobaswar H., Department of Oral Biology, University of Florida College of Dentistry, Box 100424, Gainesville, FL 32610, USA.

Cotter, Paul D., Teagasc Food Research Centre, Moorepark, Fermoy, Co. Cork, Ireland; and APC Microbiome Institute, Cork, Ireland. Email: Paul.Cotter@teagasc.ie

D'Este, Francesca, Department of Medicine, University of Udine, Piazzale Kolbe, 4, 33100 Udine, Italy.

Diamond, Gill, Department of Oral Biology, University of Florida, Box 100424, Gainesville, FL 32610, USA. Email: GDiamond@dental.ufl.edu

Epand, Richard M., Department of Biochemistry and Biomedical Sciences, McMaster University, Health Sciences Centre, Hamilton, Ontario, L8S 4K1, Canada. Email: epand@mcmaster.ca

Ganguli-Indra, Gitali, Department of Pharmaceutical Sciences, College of Pharmacy, Oregon State University, 325 Pharmacy Building, Corvallis, OR 97331, USA. Email: Gitali.indra@oregonstate.edu

Gennaro, Renato, Department of Life Sciences, University of Trieste, via Giorgieri 5, 34127 Trieste, Italy.

Gombart, Adrian F., Linus Pauling Institute, Oregon State University, 307 Linus Pauling Science Center, Corvallis, OR 97331, USA. Email: adrian.gombart@oregonstate.edu

Hancock, Robert E.W., Department of Microbiology and Immunology, University of British Columbia, Room 232, 2259 Lower Mall Research Station, Vancouver, British Columbia, Canada, V6T 1Z4. Email: bob@hancocklab.com

Healy, Brian, Teagasc Food Research Centre, Moorepark, Fermoy, Co. Cork, Ireland; and APC Microbiome Institute, Cork, Ireland.

Indra, Arup K., Department of Pharmaceutical Sciences, College of Pharmacy, Oregon State University, 325 Pharmacy Building, Corvallis, OR 97331, USA. Email: arup.indra@oregonstate.edu

Mangoni, Maria Luisa, Department of Biochemical Sciences, La Sapienza University, via degli Apuli, 9-00185 Rome, Italy.

Mardirossian, Mario, Department of Life Sciences, University of Trieste, via Giorgieri 5, 34127 Trieste, Italy.

Mishra, Biswajit, Department of Pathology and Microbiology, University of Nebraska Medical Center, Omaha, NE 68198-6495, USA. Email: biswajit.mishra@unmc.edu

Reiling, Scott, Department of Pathology and Microbiology, University of Nebraska Medical Center, Omaha, NE 68198-6495, USA.

Runti, Giulia, Department of Life Sciences, University of Trieste, via Giorgieri 5, 34127 Trieste, Italy.

Ryan, Lisa Kathleen, Division of Infectious Diseases and Global Medicine, Department of Medicine, University of Florida College of Medicine, Box 100277, Gainesville, FL 32610, USA.

Schreier, Shirley, Laboratory of Structural Biology, Department of Biochemistry, Institute of Chemistry, University of São Paulo (USP), São Paulo, São Paulo, C.P. 26077, 05513-970, Brazil.

Scocchi, Marco, Department of Life Sciences, University of Trieste, via L. Giorgieri 5, 34127 Trieste, Italy. Email: mscocchi@units.it

Segev-Zarko, Li-av, Department of Biomolecular Sciences, The Weizmann Institute of Science, Rehovot, 76100, Israel.

Shai, Yechiel, Department of Biomolecular Sciences, The Weizmann Institute of Science, Rehovot, 76100, Israel. Email: yechiel.shai@weizmann.ac.il

Skerlavaj, Barbara, Department of Medicine, University of Udine, Piazzale Kolbe, 4, 33100 Udine, Italy.

Starr, Charles G., Department of Biochemistry SL43, Tulane University Health Sciences Center, New Orleans, LA, USA.

Tossi, Alessandro, Department of Life Sciences, University of Trieste, via Giorgieri 5, 34127 Trieste, Italy. Email: atossi@units.it

Van Hoek, Monique L., School of Systems Biology, George Mason University, Manassas, VA 20110, USA. Email: mvanhoek@gmu.edu

Wang, Guangshun, Department of Pathology and Microbiology, University of Nebraska Medical Center, Omaha, NE 68198-6495, USA. Email: gwang@unmc.edu

Wimley, William C., Department of Biochemistry SL43, Tulane University Health Sciences Center, 1430 Tulane Avenue, New Orleans, LA 70112-2699, USA. Email: wwimley@tulane.edu

Wuerth, Kelli C., Centre for Microbial Diseases and Immunity Research, Department of Microbiology and Immunology, University of British Columbia, Vancouver, Canada. Email: kelliw22@gmail.com

Xie, Jingwei, Department of Surgery-Transplant and Holland Regenerative Medicine Program, University of Nebraska Medical Center, Omaha, NE 68198-5965, USA. Email: jingwei.xie@unmc.edu

Zasloff, Michael, Transplant Institute, Georgetown University Medical Center, Medical/Dental Building NW210, 3900 Reservoir Road NW, Washington, DC 20007, USA. Email: maz5@georgetown.edu

Preface

In 1903, Niels Finsen received his Nobel Prize in medicine for the use of light therapy for tuberculosis (TB). In the 20th century, scientists found a connection between this light therapy and antimicrobial peptides (AMPs). Light can induce the hydroxylation of vitamin D in the skin and the subsequent association of 1,25-dihydroxylated vitamin D with its receptor induces the expression of the only human cathelicidin gene. The mature form called LL-37 is responsible for bacterial killing. The three-dimensional structure of human LL-37 in complex with bacterial membrane components has been elucidated, and is shown on the cover of this book. It consists of a cationic amphipathic helix ideal for recognizing anionic bacterial membranes. The known functions of human cathelicidin LL-37 continue to expand. It is now clear that LL-37 has a number of roles beyond direct killing of bacteria, viruses, fungi and parasites. It is also involved in immune modulation, apoptosis and wound healing, as well as diseases such as cancer and Type 1 diabetes. Meanwhile, the number of identified naturally occurring AMPs spanning the gamut from prokaryotes to eukaryotes has grown considerably since the publication of the first edition of this book in 2010. This second edition, which consists of 5 parts and 14 chapters, documents progress made in the field of AMPs, covering both antimicrobial and immune modulation aspects of such molecules.

It has been proposed that the serendipitous discovery of lysozyme by Sir Alexander Fleming was the beginning of both the antimicrobial peptide field and the study of innate immunity. Since then, AMPs have been identified in all the three life domains: bacteria, archaea and eukaryota. Chapter 1 highlights selected AMPs based on the discovery timeline website of the Antimicrobial Peptide Database (http://aps.unmc.edu/AP/timeline.php). As interest in such molecules grows, it is becoming clear that the beneficial effects of AMPs are not limited to antimicrobial effects. An emphasis on the immune modulation aspect led to the use of the term 'host defence peptides'. It appears that there is no limit to the potential functional roles of AMPs and a general term may be appropriate. In Chapter 1, a natural term 'innate immune peptide' is introduced to cover a variety of the functions of these peptides, currently known or to be discovered.

Although AMPs are diverse, they can be organized into four classes, irrespective of biological sources, activity or three-dimensional structure (Chapter 1). The four universal classes of AMPs are discussed in this book. A new Chapter 2 by Dr Alessandro Tossi deals with the structure and function of various cathelicidins, many of which are linear peptides

(Class L). Chapters 3 and 4 deal with sidechain-linked AMPs (Class S). The new Chapter 3 by Dr Monique van Hoek highlights a variety of disulfide-linked defensins, while Dr Paul Cotter describes bacterial lantibiotics with multiple thioether bonds (e.g. the food preservative nisin) in Chapter 4. Class P peptides contain a covalent bond between peptide sidechain and backbone. Typical examples are bacterial lassos (e.g. microcin J25) where the tail can go through the loop. Such peptides with known antimicrobial activity are tabulated in Chapter 10. The fourth class of AMPs (Class O) is characterized by a circular polypeptide chain formed by a peptide bond between the N- and C-termini of the polypeptide chain. Because of the protease stability of Class P and Class O peptides, they are important templates for drug development. Indeed, currently in-use peptide antibiotics such as daptomycin and colistin, as well as the recently discovered teixobactin (Chapter 1), are all Class P AMPs. In addition, both lassos and cyclotides have been utilized to graft peptide antigens as a potential therapy for cancer or human immunodeficiency virus type-1 (HIV-1) diseases (Chapter 10).

The book then widens its scope, from considering natural AMPs to examining synthetic peptides such as those obtained from combinatorial libraries as described by Dr William Wimley (Chapter 5), and predicted and designer peptides as summarized by me in Chapter 6. Synthetic peptides are designed and made by researchers based on certain rules. A large-scale library screening offers one useful approach to identification of potential useful templates. It is anticipated that the applications of AMP prediction methods to genomes and proteomes will substantially increase the total number of characterized natural AMPs in the future.

With natural or designed AMPs in hand, a subsequent in-depth understanding of the mechanisms of action of these peptides is essential for drug development. Consequently, Chapters 7–10 cover biophysical and structural characterization of antimicrobial peptides. In Chapter 7, Dr Yechiel Shai and his co-authors summarize mechanistic studies of antibacterial, antifungal, anticancer and antibiofilm peptides. Subsequently in Chapter 8, Dr Richard Epand and his team describe the role of biological membranes for peptide action and prediction. While many peptides, e.g. magainin 2 and LL-37, are known to target bacterial membranes, some can enter cells and associate with intracellular targets. It seems that membrane-targeting peptides can work by multiple mechanisms, including membrane permeation, polarization and pore formation. Their competitive nature is also evident, leading to lipid clustering and domain formation or replacement of surface-binding proteins. Similarly, intracellular targeting is more complex than originally thought. For instance, heat-shock proteins were initially proposed as a target for proline-rich peptides. However, more recent studies have uncovered ribosome binding, shining new light on the molecular basis of the peptide action. In Chapter 9, Dr Marco Scocchi provides a comprehensive view on non-membrane targets of AMPs. Structural determination sheds further light on how such peptides recognize membranes or non-membrane targets at atomic resolution. Because disulfide-free linear AMPs are usually random coils in aqueous solution, structures of membrane-targeting peptides are frequently determined by Nuclear Magnetic Resonance (NMR) spectroscopy using a membrane-mimicking system. These structures have enabled a view of the active form of AMPs when bound to bacterial membranes or ribosomes. In Chapter 10, I illustrate the application of multidimensional NMR and X-ray crystallography to studies of the structure, dynamics and interactions of AMPs with various targets. In addition, high-quality structures of AMPs provide a basis for structure-based peptide design.

With over 2700 naturally occurring AMPs discovered and characterized to date, it is likely that future research will focus mainly on understanding these molecules and seeking novel strategies for their applications to benefit humans, animals, agriculture and our ecosystems. One important approach is to combine new AMPs with existing antimicrobial agents. In Chapter 11, Dr Gill Diamond and his colleagues systematically discuss synergy between AMPs and other antimicrobial agents, such as antibiotics and nanoparticles. To overcome the shortcomings of natural AMPs, peptide analogues, including peptoids, β-peptides and small molecular mimics, are also used in synergistic studies. Combination therapy can reduce the peptide quantity needed for patient treatment, and helps extend the lifetime of existing antibiotics. The difficulty in eliminating established biofilms is well documented and, therefore, biofilm prevention strategies are preferred. One possible use would be to immobilize AMPs onto surfaces to prevent biofilm formation on implanted medical devices. In Chapter 12, Dr Biswajit Mishra and colleagues have summarized the immobilization chemistry, physics and biological aspects of immobilized AMPs. This chapter can be a useful starting point for newcomers who will further develop the technology for practical applications. Another strategy is to express AMPs at a target site at the required time. In Chapter 13, Dr Adrian Gombart and his collaborators have described expression of LL-37 under healthy and diseased conditions and the exciting use of nanofibers to deliver vitamin D or other chemicals that can induce the expression of AMPs. Finally, Dr Robert Hancock and his student provide an expert view on host defence peptides in immune modulation and their novel therapeutic strategies, including the use of peptides in clinical trials (Chapter 14).

This second edition of *Antimicrobial Peptides: Discovery, Design and Novel Therapeutic Strategies* has maintained the high standards of the first thanks to the enthusiasm and outstanding contributions of all the authors and anonymous reviewers who are experts in the field. As editor, I thank them all for finding time to make their great contributions to this book. Continuing a tradition set in the first edition, the anonymous review of the chapters written by my colleagues and me was handled by chapter editors: Drs Michael Zasloff, Richard Epand, Amram Mor and Monique van Hoek. I owe them a debt for their kind assistance. I am also grateful to Dr Zasloff for contributing a succinct introduction to the new edition that emphasizes the need for in-depth research in the field. My thanks are also extended to the editors from CABI who made the publication of this book a reality. Last, but not least, I thank my family and colleagues for their support, patience and understanding while I was writing and editing this book. It is our hope that this book will be useful to undergraduates, graduate students, postdoctoral fellows, research faculty, principal investigators, educators, clinicians and others (academia or industry) who are interested in the education, research, development, and applications of antimicrobial peptides and their analogues.

Guangshun Wang
University of Nebraska Medical Center
June 2017

Introduction to the Second Edition

The proliferation and prevalence of antibiotic resistant pathogens continue to increase unabated. The development of new antibiotics has not kept up to meet the challenge. The medical community has repeatedly warned of the impending threat to their management of infectious diseases. Antimicrobial peptides represent a solution, but a solution not yet realized. For this reason, research activity in antimicrobial peptides remains intense. Over the past six years since the publication of the first edition of this book, more than 50,000 relevant articles have appeared in the PubMed database. Many new molecules are being discovered as the search extends into previously unstudied plants and animals. As the numbers of new chemical entities increase, the diversity of mechanisms by which antimicrobial peptides can kill microbes has continued to grow as well. Structural modifications that influence antimicrobial activity and specificity, as revealed by natural variation or by rational design continue to inform us of how to best design a human therapeutic. We have come to better understand the biological contexts in which antimicrobial peptides are utilized in the organisms from which they were discovered, providing insights into the design of the innate immune system. These studies continue to highlight the reality that antimicrobial peptides generally serve multiple functions in the context of infection and injury, and do so by interacting with the other systems involved in wound repair and immunity. These insights have helped expand the potential utility of antimicrobial peptides as anti-infective agents that could in principle act synergistically with other divisions of our immune system. This new edition of *Antimicrobial Peptides: Discovery, Design and Novel Therapeutic Strategies* helps capture the excitement and intense research activity that has taken place since the prior publication.

Michael Zasloff
MedStar Georgetown Transplant Institute
Washington, DC
Maz5@georgetown.edu

1 Discovery, Classification and Functional Diversity of Antimicrobial Peptides

Guangshun Wang*

Department of Pathology and Microbiology, College of Medicine, University of Nebraska Medical Center, Omaha, NE 68198-6495, USA

Abstract

Antimicrobial peptides and proteins (AMPs), first discovered in 1922, have attracted much research attention since the 1980s. These innate immune molecules are universal and over 2700 have been discovered in all life forms, ranging from bacteria to humans. AMPs can have antibacterial, antiviral, antifungal and antiparasitic activities. The term 'host defence peptide' emphasizes immune modulatory functions such as chemotactic, apoptotic and wound healing properties. With further expansion in the known AMP functions beyond host defence, a natural and general term, 'innate immune peptides', may be used to cover antimicrobial, immune modulation and other functional roles of these molecules. Efforts have also been made in unifying nomenclature and classification of AMPs. While AMPs are normally named based on peptide properties, source organisms, or a combination of both, they can be classified based on source kingdoms, peptide chemical and physical properties, biological functions and mechanisms of action. Importantly, bacterial AMPs, including nisin, gramicidin A, gramicidin S, polymyxin and daptomycin, have been successfully utilized either clinically or as food preservatives. The multiple functions of AMPs provide a basis for developing other potential applications in the future.

Antimicrobial peptides and proteins, biopolymers of amino acids, are universal defence molecules of innate immune systems. In invertebrates, they are the major innate defence molecules of innate immunity, whereas in vertebrates they serve as both effectors in the innate immune system and modulators in the adaptive immune system (Epand and Vogel, 1999; Tossi and Sandri, 2002; Zasloff, 2002; Boman, 2003; Brogden *et al.*, 2005; Zanetti, 2005; Amiche *et al.*, 2008; Conlon, 2008; Gallo, 2013; Nuri *et al.*, 2015; Wang *et al.*, 2015; Hancock *et al.*, 2016). The diversity of AMPs in terms of sequence, structure and function continues to expand. Broadly, AMPs include gene-encoded antimicrobial peptides (<100 amino acids), antimicrobial proteins, and non-gene encoded peptide antibiotics. This chapter provides an overview on peptide discovery, nomenclature, classification and functional diversity. Section 1.1 highlights the discovery of important AMPs with a focus on those that have already found medical and industrial applications. Section 1.2 summarizes the main methods for peptide nomenclature. Section 1.3 discusses the

---

* Corresponding author e-mail: gwang@unmc.edu

classification of AMPs, including a unified and systematic classification, which is independent of peptide biological source, activity and three-dimensional structure. Finally, Section 1.4 describes a variety of functional roles of these innate immune peptides.

1.1 A Brief Timeline of Discovery

The majority of natural antimicrobial peptides are isolated chromatographically from bacteria, fungi, plants and animals. Table 1.1 lists selected AMPs based on the year of discovery. Prior to the 1980s, the first wave of AMP research led to the discovery of several non-gene encoded peptide antibiotics. The second wave, started in the 1980s, stimulated the research interest in innate immunity and mechanisms of action of gene-encoded AMPs as potential antimicrobials. Subsequently, other functional properties of AMPs, such as immune modulation, have been reported since around 2000. Due to limited space, I highlight here only a few examples of AMPs that have been used successfully, either clinically or in the food industry. A more detailed list can be consulted at the website for the antimicrobial peptide database (APD) provided in the footnote of Table 1.1.

The human lysozyme, discovered in 1922 by Sir Alexander Fleming, is now recognized as the first antimicrobial protein (Robert Lehrer, personal communication, 2013) and the beginning of innate immunity (Gallo, 2013). The discovery of lysozyme did not stir up much interest at that time, perhaps due to the subsequent discovery of penicillin in 1928 (ACS, 2016). Lysozyme inhibits bacteria by cleaving saccharides on the cell wall. This small protein may be used topically as its size makes it unsuitable for systemic use (Berman *et al.*, 2000).

Bacterial nisin was the first of the lantibiotics and it has been thoroughly studied. Rogers (1928) initially noticed its ability to inhibit bacteria. After many years of study, its chemical structure was discovered to contain multiple thioether rings (Gross and Morell, 1971). Nisin is the only bacteriocin approved by the US Food and Drug Administration (FDA) as a food preservative. It is used to preserve meat and dairy products (<12.5 mg/kg food) in over 50 countries. Nisin has an inhibitory effect on food-borne pathogens such as Gram-positive *Listeria monocytogenes* through attack on the cell wall. Nisin also inhibits Gram-negative pathogens such as *Escherichia coli* and *Salmonella* spp. when used in combination with chelators or heat treatment (Gharsallaoui *et al.*, 2016). In addition, pediocin PA-1 is also available commercially as a food preservative (Henderson *et al.*, 1992; Makhloufi *et al.*, 2013).

Dubos (1939) discovered gramicidin from a soil bacterium *Bacillus brevis*. Gramicidin A consists of alternating L and D-amino acids. The N-terminus of this peptide is formylated. In addition, essentially all amino acids are hydrophobic. Such sequence features are vital for the formation of a head-to-head dimer as a membrane channel (Urry, 1971). This is the first peptide antibiotic used clinically as a topical treatment.

Gramicidin S was isolated from bacteria and used to treat infectious wounds (Gauss and Brazhnikova, 1944). This small peptide is cyclic via a peptide bond formation between the termini (Synge, 1945). It deters both Gram-positive and Gram-negative bacteria. Gramicidin S is still used in topical ointments and eye drops (Greenwood, 2008).

Polymyxin E (colistin) is also a bacteriocin still in use clinically as the last resort to treat infections caused by Gram-negative pathogens. It has a cyclic peptide structure followed by a lipid tail (Stansly *et al.*, 1947). Daptomycin has a similar overall peptide design. With a net negative charge, daptomycin (cubicin) needs the presence of Ca^{2+} to show its full activity (Eliopoulos *et al.*, 1986). This lipopeptide was approved by the FDA in 2003 to treat Gram-positive bacterial infections.

Alamethicin is a peptide antibiotic isolated from the fungus *Trichoderma viride*. It is the founding member of the peptaibol

Table 1.1. Discovery timeline of important antimicrobial peptides.[a]

Year	Peptide discovered	Important facts	APD ID[b]
1922	Human lysozyme	The discovery of this first antimicrobial protein signals the start of innate immunity.	2257
1928	Bacterial nisin A	The first lantibiotic approved by the European Union in 1983 and US FDA in 1988 as a food preservative.	205
1939	Gramicidin A	The first D-amino acid-containing linear peptide that forms ion channels in membranes and is used clinically.	499
1944	Gramicidin S	The first circular peptide antibiotic used clinically in the Soviet Union to treat wounds.	2243
1947	Polymyxin	The last resort to treat resistant Gram-negative bacteria.	2204
1967	Alamethicin	The first fungal peptaibol proposed to form a barrel-stave pore.	2197
1973	Plant kalata B1	Used to assist in childbirth in Africa. Antibacterial activity and cyclic structure established in 1999.	729
1981	Insect cecropins	Initiated a new wave of the innate immunity research related to the discovery of the Toll signalling pathway in insects.	139
1985	Human α-defensins (HNP1)	The first α-defensins from mammals.	176
1986	Daptomycin (cubicin)	A lipopeptide approved by the FDA in 2003 as a peptide antibiotic to treat life-threatening infections caused by Gram-positive bacteria.	2203
1987	Frog magainins	A model amphibian peptide extensively studied and explored for clinical use.	144
1988	Human histatins	Histidine-rich AMP family.	798
	Bovine bactenecin	The first cathelicidin discovered.	8
1989	Insect apidaecins	The first proline-rich AMP; ribosomes have been a possible target since 2014.	6
1991	Cattle TAP	The first β-defensin.	235
1992	Pediocin PA-1	Class IIa bacteriocin used as a food preservative.	634
	Microcin J25	MccJ25 has an unusual lasso structure.	480
1996	Human cathelicidin LL-37	The best studied human cathelicidin; expression induced by light and vitamin D; connection with light therapy (Preface); immune modulation and other properties have also been investigated.	310
	Toad buforin II	A well-documented DNA-binding peptide.	308
1997	Tunicate styelin A	Highly modified AMPs from sea.	328
1998	Human granulysin	T cells also contain AMPs.	1161
1999	Monkey θ-defensins (RTD-1)	The only cyclic AMPs in non-human primates.	445
2000	Human thrombocidin	The first antimicrobial chemokine.	1373
2001	Fish piscidin 1	The first AMP from mast cells.	473
2002	Human RNase 7	The most abundant AMP in the human urinary tract.	2073
2004	Plant brazzein	A non-carbohydrate peptide sweetener (500–2000 times sweeter than sucrose) with antibacterial activity predicted based on the γ core motif.	1160
2005	Fungal plectasin	Extensively studied for potential medical use.	549
2010	Insect lucifensin	A key component of the long-sought antimicrobial factors of medicinal maggots of the blowfly *Lucilia sericata*.	1532
2012	Human KAMP-19	A glycine-rich AMP from human eyes. The first human AMP with a non-$\alpha\beta$ 3D structure.	2231
2014	Bacterial gageotetrin A	The shortest possible lipopeptide with two amino acids.	2381

Continued

Table 1.1. Continued.

Year	Peptide discovered	Important facts	APD ID[b]
2015	Bacterial teixobactin	The use of i-Chip technology to isolate new peptide antibiotic from an uncultivable bacterium. A potential new peptide antibiotic.	2249
	Bacterial cOB1	A sex pheromone inhibits multidrug-resistant *E. faecalis* V583 in the gut at a minimal inhibitory concentration (MIC) of 22 pg/ml.	2649

[a] Selected from the AMP discovery timeline at http://aps.unmc.edu/AP/timeline.php initially online in 2012. [b] Additional information for each peptide, including references, can be searched in the APD using the ID provided in the table (Wang *et al.*, 2016).

family. This peptide contains seven α-aminoisobutyric acids (Aib), which prefer a helical conformation. Alamethicin is active against Gram-positive bacteria and fungi. This is perhaps the only AMP with evidence to support a barrel-stave pore in membranes (Fox and Richards, 1982; Leitgeb *et al.*, 2007).

Plant kalata B1 was isolated from *Oldenlandia affinis*, the African herb used by women to assist in childbirth (Gran, 1973). This peptide is the prototype member for plant cyclotides. Its cyclic structure and antimicrobial activity was not established until 1999 (Tam *et al.*, 1999).

In the 1980s, Boman *et al.* discovered cecropins from the moth *Hyalophora cecropia* (Steiner *et al.*, 1981) and initiated a wave of innate immunity research, leading to the later discovery of the Toll signalling pathway by the Jules Hoffman laboratory (Lemaitre, 2004). Zasloff (1987) discovered magainins from the African clawed frog. These are linear peptides that adopt an amphipathic helical structure upon association with membranes. Meanwhile, Lehrer and his colleagues identified the first α-defensins from human neutrophils (Selsted *et al.*, 1985). Subsequently, the first β-defensin was discovered from cattle (Diamond *et al.*, 1991). The discovery of cyclic θ-defensins, a third type of defensins, was made by Tang *et al.* (1999). All of these defensins contain three pairs of disulfide bonds. Due to their small size and stability, there is substantial interest in developing therapeutic uses for θ-defensin miniproteins (Conibear and Craik, 2014).

In 1988, bovine bactenecin, the first member from the cathelicidin family, was identified (Romeo *et al.*, 1988). The word cathelicidin was coined from the well-conserved 'cathelin' domain of the precursor proteins (Zanetti, 2005). Based on a homologous gene search, the only human cathelicidin was discovered in 1995 (Gudmundsson *et al.*, 1996). Remarkably, the antimicrobial ability of human LL-37 can be linked to light therapy. Light induces hydroxylation of vitamin D, which then binds to the receptor, triggering the expression of the human cathelicidin LL-37 (3D structure on the book cover) that can kill tuberculosis (TB) (Zasloff, 2005). Since around 2000, human LL-37 has become a popular peptide for studying skin host defence and immune modulation (Lai and Gallo, 2009; Hancock *et al.*, 2016).

Lucifensin was discovered in 2010 from insects (Cerovský *et al.*, 2010). This defensin is probably a key antimicrobial element for traditional maggot therapy. Future research will verify whether this single compound is sufficient to achieve the insect treatment effects on certain types of wounds. Recent development experience with plectasin (Mygind *et al.*, 2005) may be useful to further enhance lucifensin.

In 2015, Lewis and co-workers discovered teixobactin, a new peptide antibiotic that did not develop resistance in a multiple passage experiment. They cultivated the bacteria (previously thought uncultivatable) via I-chip technology (Ling *et al.*, 2015). This bacteriocin may find medical use to combat Gram-positive pathogens in the near future.

In summary, all of the peptide antibiotics currently in use originate from bacteria (Table 1.1). These bacterial AMPs (bacteriocins) have preferred topologies owing to a head-tail backbone (e.g. gramicidin S) or sidechain-backbone connection (colistin and daptomycin). It is anticipated that other AMPs under development or clinical trials will reach the market (Zasloff, 2002). In addition, the induction of AMP expression, at a needed site and time, provides a new avenue for antimicrobial development (reviewed by Wang, 2014).

1.2 Nomenclature of Antimicrobial Peptides

Although various methods are employed to name a newly identified peptide, the most commonly used methods are listed below:

Source-based method

The most common approach is to derive the peptide name from the name of its source species. Usually, either the genus or the species name is taken. For example, sesquin is derived from *Vigna sesquipedalis* and palicourein is taken from *Palicourea condensata*. Sometimes, a combination of the scientific name is adopted. For instance, Hs-1 is derived from *Hypsiboas semilineatus*. In other cases, the peptide name is based on the common name of an organism (e.g. termicin from termites). Abbreviations of animal names are utilized to name homologous AMPs. The name of bBD-1 (bovine beta defensin-1) is analogous to hBD-1 (human beta defensin-1). Other animal-source abbreviations include p (pigs, e.g. PMAP-36), e (equine, e.g. e-CATH-1), s (sheep, e.g. SMAP-29), and oa (ovine, e.g. OaBac5). The sex of an organism is also implied in the name of insect andropin (male-specific). Sometimes, the names of organs or tissues are also used. Some examples are human neutrophil peptide-1 (HNP-1), liver-expressed antimicrobial peptide-2 (LEAP-2), dermcidin from skin, and human salvic from salivary glands.

Peptide-based method

AMPs are named based on a variety of peptide properties. Firstly, the name of magainin is derived from the Hebrew word for shield and that of defensin is derived from 'defence', implying the functional role of this family of peptides. Thanatin derives its name from the Greek word for death. Secondly, many AMPs are named after their amino acid sequences. Human histatins are rich in histidine residues, whereas PR-39 is a 39-residue peptide rich in proline and arginine residues. For plant cyclotides and cyclic dodecapeptide, 'cyclo' or 'cyclic' means polypeptide circularization. Thirdly, the word cathelicidin is coined from the well-conserved 'cathelin' domain of the precursor proteins (Zanetti, 2005). Therefore, cathelicidins represent a family of AMPs whose precursors share a common cathelin domain. Three antimicrobial peptides have been discovered from the precursor hCAP-18 (18-kDa human antimicrobial protein) encoded by the only human cathelicidin gene: LL-37 (a 37-aa peptide starting with two leucines), ALL-38 (Sorensen and Borregaard, 2005), and TLN-58 (Murakami *et al.*, 2016). Fourthly, peptide targets are also included in AMP names. For instance, AFP1 stands for antifungal protein 1. Sometimes, both the structure and activity of the peptide are implicit in the name. For example, in the name of θ-defensin, θ reflects the cyclic, cysteine-bridged structure and defensin the activity.

Source and peptide combined method

In many cases, source organisms and peptide features are combined to assign a unique name. For instance, Ib-AMP is abbreviated from *Impatiens balsamina* antimicrobial peptide. When there are multiple similar peptides, they are named by appending numbers (e.g., Ib-AMP1 to Ib-AMP4). Furthermore, the peptide part can also represent peptide family or peptide activity. While So-D1 is abbreviated from *Spinacia oleracea* defensin 1 (peptide family), Ee-CBP originates from *Euonymus europaeus* chitin-binding protein (activity).

Peptide discovery method

There are also approaches to naming that reflect the method of peptide discovery. For example, Combi-1 is one of the peptides obtained from combinatory library screening. DFTamP1 stands for the first anti-Staphylococcal peptide designed based on the database filtering technology.

1.3 Classification of Antimicrobial Peptides

This section describes classification of AMPs based on peptide source, synthesis machinery, and properties. Classification based on biological activity is described in Section 1.4.

1.3.1 Source kingdoms

AMP classification based on kingdoms or domains was first used in the Antimicrobial Peptide Database (Wang *et al.*, 2009). The five kingdoms proposed by Robert H. Whittaker in 1969 are Prokaryotae (bacteria and archaea, 276), Protista (protozoa and algae, 8), Fungi (fungi, 13), Plantae (plants, 335), and Animalia (animals, 2043). The count of AMPs in each kingdom is included in the parenthesis. A separation of bacteria from archaea enables a calculation of total AMPs in the three life domains (Woese *et al.*, 1990). Thus, there are 272 AMPs from bacteria, 4 from archaea and 2399 from the

eukarya domain in the current APD3 (Wang *et al.*, 2016).

It is evident that the majority of the currently known AMPs (77%) originate from the animal kingdom (Wang and Wang, 2004; Wang *et al.*, 2016). The diversity of animal AMPs requires further classification. Broadly, they belong to either invertebrates or vertebrates. Invertebrates include insects, spiders, molluscs, worms and crustaceans, whereas vertebrates comprise fish, amphibians, reptiles, birds and mammals. Interestingly, most of the vertebrate AMPs (~50% of animal AMPs) are found from amphibians, while most of the invertebrate AMPs (13% of animal AMPs) are derived from insects (Wang *et al.*, 2016). It is likely that the dominance of amphibian and insect AMPs in the animal kingdom (63%) is related to the inspiring discoveries made in the 1980s by Michael Zasloff and Hans Boman (see Section 1).

Classification of bacteriocins

Bacterial AMPs constitute another important part in the APD (10%). They share a general name of bacteriocins and their classification is summarized in Table 1.2. For Gram-positive bacteria, class I bacteriocins are lantibiotics characterized by the presence of thioether rings. Class II peptides are non-lantibiotics, which can be further classified into four sub-groups. While pediocin-like bacteriocins (e.g. leucocin A and divercin V41) are placed in class IIa, class IIb contains bacteriocins with two independent peptide chains (e.g. plantaricin JK and lactocin 705). Cyclic peptides are assigned

Table 1.2. Classification of bacteriocins.

Gram+ Bacteria	Definition	Gram− Bacteria	Definition
Class I	Lantibiotics	Class I	Microcins <5 kDa
Class II	Non-lantibiotics	Class II	Microcins (5–10 kDa)
IIa	Pediocin-like peptides	IIa	S-S bond-containing
IIb	Two-chain peptides	IIb	Linear
IIc	Circular peptides		
IId	Non-pediocin-like peptides		
Class III	Large proteins >10 kDa	Class III	Colicins >10 kDa

as class IIc. The remaining linear non-pediocin peptides are combined into class IId (e.g. entericin Q and MR10). Antimicrobial proteins (>10 kDa) are assigned as class III (Cotter *et al.*, 2005a). Large bacteriocins, such as lysostaphin, may also have clinical potential in controlling superbugs such as *S. aureus* (de Freire Bastos *et al.*, 2010). Also in Table 1.2, Gram-negative bacteria are classified in a similar manner (Duquesne *et al.*, 2007).

Recently, family names have been recommended for a variety of bacterial peptides (Arnison *et al.*, 2013). It can be useful to describe some lesser-known peptide families with established AMP members. A general name lantipeptide is introduced for all bacterial peptides with a lanthonine ring (i.e. thioether bond). Lantibiotics are lantipeptides with antimicrobial activity (e.g. nisin). In addition, linaridins refer to some related peptides (e.g. cypemycin) and their similarity to lantibiotics requires further investigation. Linear azol(in)-containing peptides such as microcin B17 and plantazolicin A have thiazole and methyloxazole heterocycles generated via post-translational modification. Many cyanobactins (e.g. Patellamide) are N- to C-macrocyclic peptides encoded by a precursor E. Thiopeptides (such as Micrococcin P1) contain a six-membered nitrogenous ring. Sublancin 168 and glycocin F are glycocins. Sactipeptides are a newly discovered peptide family with a unique covalent bond from the sidechain cysteine sulfur to the α-carbon of the backbone. Subtilosin A and thuricin CD are known examples. A recent classification (Alvarez-Sieiro *et al.*, 2016) has expanded the modified Class I bacteriocins by adding these peptides as new subclasses (LAPs, sactibiotics, glycocins, lasso peptides, cyclic peptides) together with lantibiotics. However, the classification of bacteriocins can be simplified based on the unified peptide classification scheme (Section 1.3.6).

Classification of fungal AMPs

There are two main classes of fungal AMPs. The first class is peptaibols from soil fungi of the genera *Trichoderma* and *Emericellopsis*. They consist usually of 15–20 amino acids with a high content of aminoisobutyric acid (Aib). In addition, the N-terminus generally contains an acetyl, while the C-terminus has a hydroxyl amino acid (ol). Therefore, they are given the family name peptaibols. The peptaibol database hosts 317 such peptides rich in non-standard amino acids (http://peptaibol.cryst.bbk. ac.uk/home.shtml). Other known fungal AMPs are defensin-like, usually containing multiple disulfide bonds. These AMPs, such as plectasin, micasin-1 and copsin, are collected in the APD database (http://aps. unmc.edu/AP).

Classification of plant AMPs

Plant AMPs have been a focused area of research for years, leading to over 335 such peptides (12%) in the APD. Based on sequence similarity and cysteine motifs (Egorov *et al.*, 2005), plant AMPs were classified into seven families. Table 1.3 provides an updated view of this classification where cyclotides and snakins are added as two new groups. In addition, the discovery and characterization of new members for MBP-like peptides led to a new family name, hairpin-like peptide. Unlike most of the plant AMPs, hairpin-like peptides possess a distinct structure, where the two helices are packed together and stabilized by disulfide bonds (Ryazantsev *et al.*, 2014).

Classification of animal AMPs

The classification of animal AMPs is complex. Some recommended families for amphibian AMPs are listed here: magainins, dermaseptins, brevinins, esculentins, japonicins, nigrocin-2, palustrins, ranacyclin, ranatuerins and temporin (Amiche *et al.*, 2008; Conlon, 2008). In insects, the well-known families are cecropins, defensins and proline-rich peptides (Bulet and Stocklin, 2005). In marine invertebrates, Otero-González *et al.* (2010) described AMPs from different phyla such as Porifera, Cnidaria, Mollusca, Annelida, Arthropoda, Echinodermata and Chordata. In mammals,

Table 1.3. Classification of plant antimicrobial peptides.[a]

Group	Plant peptides	Count	# of Cys	Examples
1	Defensins	78	4, 6 or 8	NaD1, PhD1, Rs-AFP1
2	Thionins[b]	13	4, 6 or 8	Tu-AMP1, Cp-thionin II
3	Lipid transfer proteins	3	2, 4 or 8	Cc-LTP1, LTP110
4	Hevein-like peptides	6	8 or 10	Pn-AMP1, WAMP-1
5	Knottin-type peptides	4	6	PAFP-S; Mj-AMP2
6	Glyine-rich peptides	5	0, 1 or 6	Shepherin I, Pg-AMP1
7	Hairpin-like peptides	3	4	MBP-1, EcAMP1
8	Cyclotides	160	6	Kalata B1, Cliotide 20
9	Snakin	6	12	Snakin-1; snaking-Z

[a]Obtained from the APD in July 2016. [b]Note that γ-thionins are included in defensins.

including humans, the major AMP families are defensins, cathelicidins and histatins (Zanetti, 2005). Other human AMP families are dermcidin, LEAP-1 (hepcidin), granulysin, chemokines and RNases (for a systematic review, refer to Wang, 2014).

1.3.2 Peptide synthesis machinery

Naturally occurring peptides can be classified into two classes: gene encoded and non-gene encoded AMPs. While gene-encoded AMPs are made by ribosomes, non-gene encoded peptides are synthesized by a multiple enzyme system. A total of 98% of AMPs in the APD are gene-encoded peptides. These peptides may be constitutively expressed or induced to keep the host healthy (Boman, 2003). Examples are human defensins and cathelicidin. A multiple enzyme system enables the incorporation of modified amino acids to make non-gene encoded peptides more drug-like. Examples are gramicidin, colistin and daptomycin (Section 1.1).

There are also synthetic and recombinant AMPs. Synthetic AMPs are made using the solid-phase peptide synthesis method (Merrifield, 1963), while recombinant AMPs are produced by bacteria, fungi or plants, which are transfected with a vector containing the AMP gene of interest (see first edition of this book: Wang, 2010). These technologies have greatly facilitated and accelerated the structure–activity relationship studies of AMPs.

1.3.3 Chemical modifications

Antimicrobial peptides can also be classified based on the type of chemical modification. A total of 24 types of chemical modifications for AMPs are annotated in the APD database, covering approximately 50% of AMPs (Wang *et al.*, 2016). Post-translational modifications modulate peptide properties. In the case of enterocin AS-48, a head–tail connection is required for peptide structure rather than bactericidal activity (Montalbán-López *et al.*, 2008). In contrast, the circular structure of kalata B1 is essential for activity. The same molecule may be modified differently depending on the functional context. Human cathelicidin LL-37 can be citrullinated, reducing its ability to neutralize endotoxin (Koziel *et al.*, 2014). It can also be ADP-ribosylated or carbamylated (Picchianti *et al.*, 2015; Koro *et al.*, 2016), thereby regulating its function *in vivo*. Some AMPs may be chemically modified at multiple sites. For instance, the sequence of styelin D from sea squirt is halogenated at Trp2 and hydroxylated at Arg, Lys and Tyr residues. Such modifications could be essential for the peptide to remain active even at high salt concentrations. Indeed, the native peptide is more active than a synthetic analogue without those modifications (Taylor *et al.*, 2000).

Understanding the mechanism of chemical modification of natural AMPs may provide unique tools for peptide engineering. Cotter *et al.* (2005b) found an enzyme that converts a dehydrated L-Ser to D-Ala. Such enzymes may be harnessed to incorporate D-amino acids into bacterially expressed polypeptides. The discovery of the broad substrate specificity of the nisin modification enzymes (Rink *et al.*, 2005) may open the door to enzyme-mediated introduction of thioether rings into a peptide template for required biological activity or structural stability (Chapter 4). Nature's chemical modifications have inspired strategies for engineering linear peptides (Wang, 2012).

1.3.4 Peptide charge, length and hydrophobic content

AMPs can be classified based on peptide length. Based on the APD database, the number of AMPs as a function of peptide length is plotted in Fig. 1.1A. The peak is located at 30 (i.e. 21–30 amino acids). The shortest lipopeptides contain only 2 amino acids, while the shortest peptide (no conjugation) contains only 5 amino acids. The longest peptide contains 100 amino acids due to an arbitrary definition for peptides (Wang, 2010). The majority of AMPs (~90%) consist of less than 50 amino acids.

AMPs can also be classified based on the hydrophobic content, which is the ratio between hydrophobic amino acids Ile, Val, Leu, Phe, Cys, Met, Ala and Trp (Kyte and Doolittle, 1982) and the total count of amino acids. Figure 1.1B shows peptide count in a defined hydrophobic range. The peak is located at 50%, with 78% of the AMPs possessing a hydrophobic content in the range of 30–60%. However, the hydrophobic contents of AMPs can vary from 0% to 100%. One can anticipate that those without hydrophobic amino acids will have little chance to bind to membranes, whereas those consisting of all hydrophobic amino acids (e.g. gramicidin) will have a long residence time in membranes.

Additionally, AMPs can be classified into cationic, neutral and anionic peptides. In the APD, the effect of chemical modification on the peptide net charge has been considered (Wang *et al.*, 2016). Figure 1.1C shows the number of AMPs as a function of net charge. The AMPs are distributed around the peak at +3. Of a total of 2722 AMPs, 87% are positively charged (73% in the range of +1 to +6), 7% are neutral, and 6% are negatively charged, leading to a full

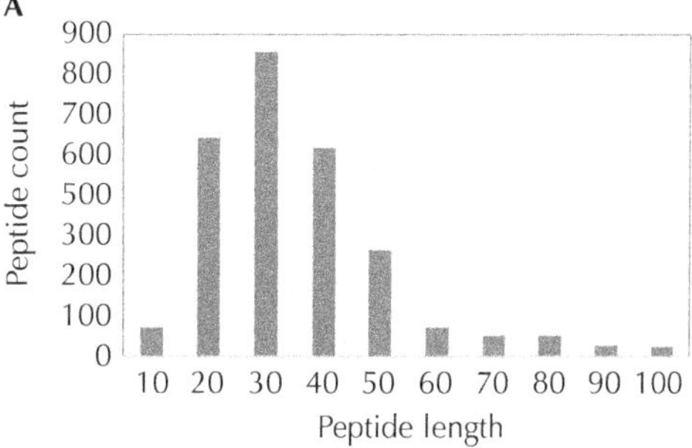

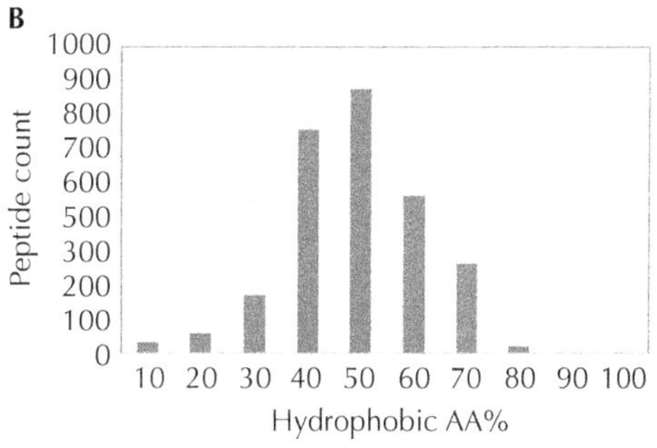

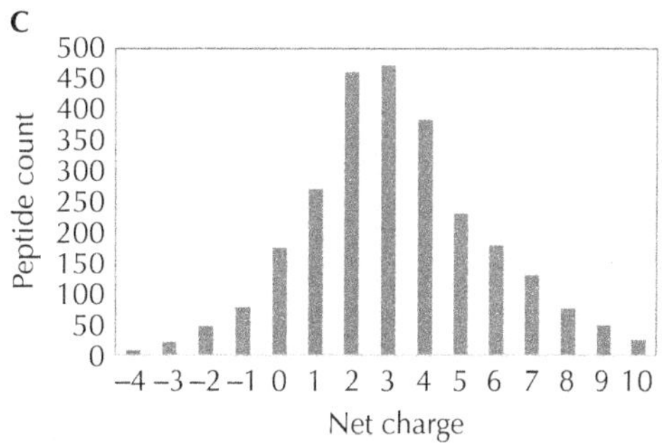

Fig. 1.1. Distribution of antimicrobial peptides in the APD3 versus peptide length (A), hydrophobic content (B), and net charge (C). A total of 2722 peptides are included in the analysis (Wang *et al.*, 2016). Although the peptide count increases from 1528 to 2722, these trends are the same as those observed previously (Wang, 2010).

spectrum of AMPs in terms of charge. There are a few outliers not depicted in this plot. Oncorhyncin II and OaBac11 are the most positively charged peptides with a net charge of +30, whereas cattle chrombacin is the most negatively charged AMP with a net charge of −12.

1.3.5 Three-dimensional structures

AMPs were initially classified into three classes: α, β, and rich in glycine, proline, tryptophan/arginine or histidine (Boman, 2003). Folded AMPs were also classified into four groups: α-helical peptides, β-sheet peptides, extended structures and loop peptides (Hancock and Sahl, 2006). In the first edition of this book, we proposed a unified structural classification for AMPs by modifying the scheme of Murzin *et al.* (1995). In our classification, AMPs are systematically classified into four families: α-helices, β-sheets, αβ structures and non-αβ structures, depending on whether there are α and β secondary structures in the three-dimensional structures determined experimentally (Wang, 2010). AMPs in the α-helical family are composed of α-helices, while those in the β-sheet family consist of at least two β-strands. The αβ family contains all AMPs that have both α and β secondary structures, regardless of whether they are packed or not. Finally, we define a non-αβ family that includes all AMPs that form neither α-helix or β-sheet structures. In humans, AMPs with α, β and αβ structures have all been found (Wang, 2014). Recently, a non-αβ structure has also been determined for a glycine-rich peptide KAMP-19 from human eyes (Lee *et al.*, 2016), thereby filling in a structural gap for human AMPs.

1.3.6 Unified peptide classification based on polypeptide chain bonding patterns

Polypeptide chains can be connected in different manners, generating a variety of molecular shapes (topologies). Based on the connection patterns, a unified and systematic peptide classification scheme has been proposed (Wang, 2015). In this scheme, peptides are classified into four general categories. The first unified class consists of linear peptides, which may consist of two linear polypeptides (class UCLL, or class L). Amino acids of peptides in this class may be chemically modified locally, but never between two different amino acids. The second unified class comprises peptides with sidechain-sidechain connections between different amino acids (UCSS, or class S) in the same chain or different chains. Examples are disulfide-bridged defensins and thioether bonded lantibiotics. The third unified class is made of peptides with a bond between the sidechain of one amino acid and the backbone of another amino acid (UCSB, or class P) usually within the same chain. Daptomycin and lassos belong to this class. Microcin J25, originally thought to form a head-to-tail peptide bond, consists of a ring structure between the backbone amide of residue Gly1 and the sidechain of Glu8 (Rosengren *et al.*, 2003). The last unified class (UCBB, or class O) contains circular peptides where the N- and C-termini of the polypeptide chain connected via a peptide bond (i.e., backbone–backbone connected peptides). Circular AMPs have been found in bacteria, plants and animals (Table 1.4). Circular peptides have the highest priority in this classification system followed by UCSB with UCLL the lowest. Peptides in each class can be further sorted into subclasses based on the number of chains and additional connections (Wang, 2015).

It is interesting to note that each unified class of AMPs possesses distinct sequence signatures (Table 1.4). For instance, each class contains a different set of frequently occurring amino acids (>9%). Both AMPs in UCSS and UCBB are rich in cysteines (C) owing to the multiple disulfide bonds in defensins or circular peptides and thioether bonds in the case of lantibiotics. Linear peptides are abundant in amino acids L, A, G and K, laying a basis for the formation of amphipathic helices as demonstrated experimentally (Wang *et al.*, 2009). Finally, the UCSB class has rather different abundant amino acids: V, A and G. The choice of such amino acids is likely to be determined by the polypeptide scaffold in each class. Only glycine is shared by all the classes as the abundant amino acid. The abundance in lysine (K) directly determines a higher averaged net charge for the UCLL and UCSS classes than the other two classes (Table 1.4).

1.3.7 Peptide binding targets and mechanisms of action

Broadly, AMPs can be classified into membrane targeting and non-membrane targeting. It is assumed that many membrane-targeting AMPs disrupt bacterial membranes by three major mechanisms: carpet, barrel-stave, and toroidal models (Ludtke *et al.*, 1996; Shai, 2002). Gramicidin A, alamethicin, and magainins target membranes. Non-membrane targeting peptides include all other AMPs that interfere with pathogen microbial function or survival by binding to intracelluar targets such as ribosomes and RNA polymerases (Wang *et al.*, 2015).

AMPs also associate with other non-membrane components on the cell surface. Class 2a pediocin-like bacteriocins associate with the C-subunit of the enzyme II mannose permease to achieve an inhibitory effect (Makhloufi *et al.*, 2013). SMAP-29 and hRNase 7 may bind to an outer membrane protein I (OprI) of *Pseudomonas*

aeruginosa for activity (Lin *et al.*, 2010). A total of 25 AMPs in the APD are known to bind lipid II, thereby blocking cell wall synthesis (Hasper *et al.*, 2006). For some plant AMPs such as Cy-AMP1, chitin-binding ability is critical for antifungal activity (Yokoyama *et al.*, 2009). Some defensins were shown to bind specifically to carbohydrate moieties of gp41 of HIV-1 and CD4 of T-cells to inhibit viral entry into human cells (Gallo *et al.*, 2006).

1.4 Functional Diversity and Terminology of Antimicrobial Peptides

1.4.1 Antimicrobial peptides

The term 'antimicrobial peptides' is the key word for the field and will likely remain so in the future (350,448 articles obtained from the PubMed as of Oct 15, 2016). The word 'antimicrobial' covers antibacterial, antiviral, antifungal and antiparasitic activities of AMPs. However, not all AMPs possess wide spectrum activity. Of the 2263 antibacterial peptides (Wang *et al.*, 2016), 853 peptides possess both antibacterial and antifungal activities. The peptide counts drop rapidly when three to four types of activities are searched simultaneously. There are 65 peptides with antibacterial, antifungal and antiviral activities, and only nine AMPs in the current APD have all of the four types of antimicrobial activities above. Although the drop in numbers may reflect peptide

Table 1.4. Four unified classes of peptides with different bonding patterns.[a]

Name	AMP count	Peptide length	Pho	Net charge	FOAA	Examples
Linear AMPs (UCLL; class L)	1513	21.8	49%	+2.25	L, A, G, K	Magainins; indolicidin; LL-37
Sidechain-linked AMPs (UCSS; class S)	985	37.7	43%	+3.99	C, G, K	α-Defensins; β-defensins; lantibiotics
Sidechain–backbone linked AMPs (UCSB; class P)	23	14.7	44%	+0.09	V, A, G	Daptomycin; microcin J25; colistin
Backbone-linked circular AMPs (UCBB; class O)	197	29.9	47%	+1.02	C, G	AS-48; cyclotides; θ-defensins

[a] Adapted from Wang *et al.* (2016). Pho = hydrophobic content; FOAA = frequently occurring amino acids (see the text). This is the first use of single letters as the name for each unified peptide class.

properties, it is also likely that not all the AMPs have been evaluated thoroughly. Indeed, some widely studied AMPs are among the short list of nine: amphibian magainin 2, dermseptin S1, dermseptin S4, insect melittin, human α-defensin HNP-1, cathelicidin LL-37, bovine BMAP-27, BMAP-28 and plant Kalata B2 (Selsted *et al.*, 1985; Zasloff, 2002; Zanetti, 2005; Amiche *et al.*, 2008; Nylén *et al.*, 2014; Fensterseifer *et al.*, 2015; Xhindoli *et al.*, 2016). It should be emphasized that medium conditions play an important role for *in vitro* assays and the type of animal models matters for *in vivo* studies. It is important to note that some polypeptide chains do not display antimicrobial activity when evaluated alone. For instance, bacterial enterocin L50 (Cintas *et al.*, 1998) and lichenicidin (Begley *et al.*, 2009) show an optimal activity when combined in a 1:1 molar ratio. In contrast to classic helical AMPs that inhibit bacteria at micromolar (µM) concentrations, bacteriocins frequently show narrow spectrum activity as well as very low MICs at nanomolar (nM) levels. Synergistic effects between different AMPs also appear to play an essential role in shaping host defence – one possible reason why so many AMPs are expressed in a species.

Antibacterial peptides

Antibacterial activity is the most common denominator for AMPs; 83% of the peptides in the APD possess such activity. This activity is usually attributed to the membrane targeting action of cationic peptides. As of September 2016, the net charge of the 2722 AMPs in the APD database is +3.2 on average (Fig. 1.1C). The positive charges are important for initial recognition of the negatively charged surfaces of bacteria. The hydrophobic component of the peptide (Fig. 1.1.B) is required for subsequent anchoring of the peptide to the membrane surface. The combination of positive charge and hydrophobicity explains the amphipathic nature of the majority of AMPs. In addition, 441 AMPs are active against only Gram-positive bacteria, whereas 221 peptides are only inhibitory to Gram-negative bacteria. Our database analysis revealed a higher net positive charge for those against Gram-negative bacteria than those against Gram-positive bacteria (Wang *et al.*, 2016).

Antifungal peptides

In the current APD database, 993 AMPs are antifungal (Wang *et al.*, 2016). Some plant AMPs are only known for antifungal activity. These peptides usually have multiple disulfide bridges to adopt a β-sheet structure. However, the α-helical hairpin structure has also been found for AMPs from the plant kingdom (Ryazantsev *et al.*, 2014).

Antiviral peptides

Including both enveloped and non-enveloped viruses, 177 AMPs are known to be antiviral. Over 100 are known to be HIV active. Human cathelicidin LL-37 showed activity against HIV-1, respiratory syncytial virus (RSV) and influenza viruses (Barlow *et al.*, 2011; Wang *et al.*, 2014; Hsieh and Hartshorn, 2016). It seems that the amphipathic nature of an AMP is also suited to interact with viral nucleic acids (DNA or RNA). This can be a useful feature in designing antiviral agents.

Cytotoxic effects

Most of the AMPs show selective activity against bacteria. The selectivity is proposed to come from their cationic nature, which enables the peptide to target anionic pathogens rather than host cells, which are rich in zwitterionic lipids and cholesterol in the membranes. However, some peptides appear to be poisonous, as they are highly haemolytic. Examples are those AMPs isolated from the venoms of spiders and scorpions (Wang and Wang, 2016). Haemolytic peptides have more hydrophobic amino acids than non-haemolytic AMPs (Wang, 2010). While human red blood cells are convenient for such assays, other types of human cells should also be used to better gauge the cytotoxicity of peptides. Ultimately, peptide cytotoxicity will be evaluated in proper animal models and during clinical trials.

Anticancer and spermicidal activity

There is also high interest in utilizing AMPs to neutralize cancer cells, which are transformed human cells. Anionic phosphatidylserines (PS) could be exposed on the surfaces of cancer cells. In addition, other acidic components such as O-glycosylated mucins can also be over-expressed on the cell surface (Gaspar *et al.*, 2013). Such features may make cancer cells sufficiently distinct from surrounding healthy cells that cationic AMPs can preferentially target them. This may be more challenging than the search for antibacterial peptides because the differences between eukaryotic cells are much smaller than those between prokaryotic and eukaryotic cells. However, novel anticancer therapies are urgently needed and AMPs could be considered as potential candidates. In addition, future work will validate whether the over-expression of certain AMPs serves as an early diagnostic biomarker for cancer (Wang, 2014).

A dozen AMPs are known to possess spermicidal effects, which may be useful to selectively eliminate sperm to avoid pregnancy. Human cathelicidin LL-37 is proposed as a promising peptide for this development (for a review, refer to Tanphaichitr *et al.*, 2016).

1.4.2　Host defence peptides

The term 'host defence peptide' was introduced to emphasize the immune modulatory role of AMPs (9755 articles obtained from the PubMed as of 15 October 2016). There is a hypothesis that such peptides may not kill microorganisms under physiological conditions where the concentration of the peptide is lower than the minimal inhibitory concentration (MIC). Instead, these peptides function primarily as immune modulating molecules. They modulate gene expression of monocytes or epithelial cells, chemoattract cells, induce chemokines and promote wound healing, angiogenesis and apoptosis (Murakami *et al.*, 2004; Hancock and Sahl, 2006;

Hancock *et al.*, 2016). Indeed, human defensins and cathelicidin LL-37 are known to have chemotactic effects (Taylor *et al.*, 2008). Interestingly, many chemokines such as CCL25 and CXCL14 also display a wide-spectrum antibacterial activity (Yang *et al.*, 2003; Maerki *et al.*, 2009; Wang, 2014). Thus, chemotaxis is an important property of AMPs that links the innate and adaptive immune systems (Zasloff, 2002).

1.4.3　Innate immune peptides

AMPs may also have functions beyond host defence. Under such circumstances, one may use a natural term 'innate immune peptides' (Wang, 2016) as they are key components of the innate immune system. For instance, β-defensins can modulate the melanocortin signalling and can determine the colours of dogs' coats (Candille *et al.*, 2007). In the male reproductive system, β-defensins play the dual role of anti-infection and sperm maturation (Dorin and Barratt, 2014). The functional roles of AMPs are known to be even wider, due to the discovery of anti-microbial properties for polypeptides initially known for other biological activities. For example, the discovery of the γ-core motif in cysteine-containing AMPs such as defensins led to testing the antimicrobial activity of plant brazzein (Young and Yeaman, 2004), the smallest sweetener protein about 1000-fold sweeter than sucrose (Hellekant and Danilova, 2005). The combination of this non-carbohydrate sweetener and antimicrobial activity makes brazzein an appealing candidate for oral hygiene. Some neuropeptides and hormones exhibit antimicrobial activity and participate in host defence as well (Brogden *et al.*, 2005). Remarkably, hormones can inhibit microbes at an ultra-low concentration. While α-MSH inhibits *C. albicans* at 1 fM to 1 pM (Cutuli *et al.*, 2000), commensal bacterium *Enterococcus faecalis* can secrete sex pheromone cOB1 to inhibit the growth of multidrug-resistant *E. faecalis* V583 in the gut also at pM (Gilmore *et al.*, 2015). Such extremely low inhibitory concentrations are attractive for developing novel antimicrobials because doing so requires very little material, thereby solving the cost issue for peptide production. This study also suggests a novel strategy for preventing invading pathogen infection by maintaining the commensal bacteria population.

1.5 Concluding Remarks

The discovery of lysozyme by Alexander Fleming in 1922 is regarded as the beginning of the antimicrobial peptide and protein field, as well as the birth of the science of innate immunity. Since the 1980s, there has been a rapid increase in AMP discovery, leading to the discovery of thousands of such molecules. These peptides are diverse in terms of source, amino acid sequence, 3D structure, activity and mechanism of action. The ever-expanding functional roles of AMPs led to the use of the term 'host defence peptides'. When required, a more general term, 'innate immune peptides' can also be utilized. In the first edition of this book, I stated that, 'We should emphasize that the classification issue of AMPs is not fully resolved due to incomplete information as well as diversity of the peptides'. To help meet this challenge, a source and activity independent classification has been proposed (Wang, 2015). This unified classification can be applied to all peptides, including AMPs. Bioinformatic analysis reveals that these classes of AMPs are distinct in terms of amino acid composition, peptide length and net charge (Table 1.4). Such results could guide us in designing AMPs with desirable properties. Meanwhile, a more complete understanding of the functional roles of innate immune peptides will generate new avenues for the discovery of novel therapeutic molecules. Finally, it is anticipated that the classic work on the discovery of novel AMPs from nature (especially unexplored species) will continue in response to the need for new antibiotics. We have reason to be optimistic because several bacteriocins are already in use, either clinically or as food preservatives (Table 1.1).

Acknowledgements

GW acknowledges the NIAID/NIH grants R01 AI105147 and R03 AI128230 during this study. This chapter is the author's contribution and does not reflect the view or policy of the funding agency.

Chapter editor: Richard Epand.

References

ACS (2016) *The Discovery and Development of Penicillin 1928–1945*. Available at: https://www.acs.org/content/acs/en/education/whatischemistry/landmarks/flemingpenicillin.html (accessed 1 August 2016).

Amiche, M., Ladram, A. and Nicolas, P. (2008) A consistent nomenclature of antimicrobial peptides isolated from frogs of the subfamily Phyllomedusinae. *Peptides* 29, 2074–2082.

Arnison, P.G., Bibb, M.J., Bierbaum, G., Bowers, A.A., Bugni, *et al.* (2013) Ribosomally synthesized and post-translationally modified peptide natural products: overview and recommendations for a universal nomenclature. *Natural Product Reports* 30, 108–160.

Alvarez-Sieiro, P., Montalban-Lopez, M., Mu, D. and Kuipers, O.P. (2016) Bacteriocins of lactic acid bacteria: extending the family. *Applied Microbiology and Biotechnology* 100, 2939–2951.

Barlow, P.G., Svoboda, P., Mackellar, A., Nash, A.A., York, I.A., *et al.* (2011) Antiviral activity and increased host defence against influenza infection elicited by the human cathelicidin LL-37. *PLoS One* 6, e25333.

Begley, M., Cotter, P.D., Hill, C. and Ross, R.P. (2009) Identification of a novel two-peptide lantibiotic, lichenicidin, following rational genome mining for LanM proteins. *Applied Microbiology and Biotechnology* 75, 5451–5460.

Berman, H.M., Westbrook, J., Feng, Z., Gilliland, G., Bhat, T.N., *et al.* (2000) The Protein Data Bank. *Nucleic Acids Research* 28, 235–242.

Boman, H.G. (2003) Antibacterial peptides: basic facts and emerging concepts. *Journal of Internal Medicine* 254, 197–215.

Brogden, K.A., Guthmiller, J.M., Salzet, M. and Zasloff, M. (2005) The nervous system and innate immunity: the neuropeptide connection. *Nature Immunology* 6, 558–564.

Bulet, P. and Stocklin, R. (2005) Insect antimicrobial peptides: structures, properties and gene regulation. *Protein and Peptide Letters* 12, 3–11.

Candille, S.I., Kaelin, C.B., Cattanach, B.M., Yu, B., Thompson, D.A., *et al.* (2007) A β-defensin mutation causes black coat color in domestic dogs. *Science* 318, 1418–1423.

Cerovský, V., Zdárek, J., Fucík, V., Monincová, L., Voburka, Z. and Bém, R. (2010) Lucifensin, the long-sought antimicrobial factor of medicinal maggots of the blowfly *Lucilia sericata*. *Cellular and Molecular Life Science* 67 455–466.

Cintas, L.M., Casaus, P., Holo, H., Hernandez, P.E., Nes, I.F. and Håvarstein, L.S. (1998) Enterocins L50A and L50B, two novel bacteriocins from *Enterococcus faecium* L50, are related to staphylococcal hemolysins. *Journal of Bacteriology* 180, 1988–1994.

Conibear, A.C. and Craik, D.J. (2014) The chemistry and biology of θ-defensins. *Angewandte Chemie International Edition* 53, 10612–10623.

Conlon, J.M. (2008) Reflections on a systematic nomenclature for antimicrobial peptides from the skins of frogs of the family Ranidae. *Peptides* 29, 1815–1819.

Cotter, P.D., Hill, C. and Ross, R.P. (2005a) Bacteriocins: developing innate immunity for food. *Nature Reviews Microbiology* 3, 777–788.

Cotter, P.D., O'Connor, P.M., Draper, L.A., Lawton, E.M., Deegan, L.H., Hill, C. and Ross, R.P. (2005b) Posttranslational conversion of L-serines to D-alanines is vital for optimal production and activity of the lantibiotic lacticin 3147. *Proceedings of the National Academy of Sciences of the USA* 102, 18584–18589.

Cutuli, M., Cristiani, S., Lipton, J.M., and Catania, A. (2000) Antimicrobial effects of alpha-MSH peptides. *Journal of Leukocyte Biology* 67, 233–239.

de Freire Bastos, M.C., Coutinho, B.G. and Coelho, M.L.V. (2010) Lysostaphin: a staphylococcal bacteriolysin with potential clinical applications. *Pharmaceuticals* 3, 1139–1161.

Diamond, G., Zasloff, M., Eck, H., Brasseur, M., Maloy, W.L. and Bevins, C.L. (1991) Tracheal antimicrobial peptide, a cysteine-rich peptide from mammalian tracheal mucosa: peptide isolation and cloning of a cDNA. *Proceedings of the National Academy of Sciences of the USA* 88, 3952–3956.

Dorin, J.R. and Barratt, C.L. (2014) Importance of β-defensins in sperm function. *Molecular Human Reproduction* 20, 821–826.

Dubos, R.J. (1939) Studies on a bactericidal agent extracted from a soil bacillus: I. Preparation of the agent. Its activity *in vitro*. *Journal of Experimental Medicine* 70, 1–10.

Duquesne, S., Destoumieux-Garzon, D., Peduzzi, J. and Rebuffat, S. (2007) Microcins, gene-encoded antibacterial peptides from enterobacteria. *Natural Product Reports* 24, 708–734.

Egorov, T.A., Odintsova, T.I., Pukhalsky, V.A. and Grishin, E.V. (2005) Diversity of wheat anti-microbial peptides. *Peptides* 26, 2064–2073.

Eliopoulos, G.M., Willey, S., Reiszner, E., Spitzer, P.G., Caputo, G. and Moellering, R.C. Jr. (1986) *In vitro* and *in vivo* activity of LY 146032, a new cyclic lipopeptide antibiotic. *Antimicrobial Agents and Chemotherapy* 30, 532–535.

Epand, R.M. and Vogel, H.J. (1999) Diversity of antimicrobial peptides and their mechanisms of action. *Biochimica et Biophysica Acta* 1462, 11–28.

Fensterseifer, I.C., Silva, O.N., Malik, U., Ravipati, A.S., Novaes, N.R., Miranda, P.R., Rodrigues, E.A., Moreno, S.E., Craik, D.J. and Franco, O.L. (2015) Effects of cyclotides against cutaneous infections caused by *Staphylococcus aureus*. *Peptides* 63, 38–42.

Fox, R.O., Jr. and Richards, F.M. (1982) A voltage-gated ion channel model inferred from the crystal structure of alamethicin at 1.5-Å resolution. *Nature* 300, 325–330.

Gallo, R.L. (2013) The birth of innate immunity. *Experimental Dermatology* 22, 517.

Gallo, S.A., Wang, W., Rawat, S.S., Jung, G., Waring, A.J., *et al.* (2006) Theta-defensins prevent HIV-1 Env-mediated fusion by binding gp41 and blocking 6-helix bundle formation. *Journal of Biological Chemistry* 281, 18787–18792.

Gaspar, D., Veiga, A.S. and Castanho, M.A. (2013) From antimicrobial to anticancer peptides. A review. *Frontiers in Microbiology* 4, 294.

Gause, G.F. and Brazhnikova, M.G. (1944) Gramicidin S and its use in the treatment of infected wounds. *Nature* 154, 703.

Gharsallaoui, A., Oulahal, N., Joly, C. and Degraeve, P. (2016) Nisin as a Food Preservative: Part 1: Physicochemical Properties, Antimicrobial Activity, and Main Uses. *Critical Reviews in Food Science and Nutrition* 56, 1262–1274.

Gilmore, M.S., Rauch, M., Ramsey, M.M., Himes, P.R., Varahan, S., *et al.* (2015) Pheromone killing of multidrug-resistant *Enterococcus faecalis* V583 by native commensal strains. *Proceedings of the National Academy of Sciences of the USA* 112, 7273–7278.

Gran, L. (1973) On the effect of a polypeptide isolated from 'Kalata-Kalata' (*Oldenlandia affinis* DC) on the oestrogen dominated uterus. *Acta Pharmacologica et Toxicologica* 33, 400–408.

Greenwood, D. (2008) *Antimicrobial Drugs: Chronicle of a Twentieth Century Medical Triumph.* Oxford University Press, Oxford, UK.

Gross, E. and Morell, J.L. (1971) The structure of nisin. *Journal of the American Chemical Society* 93, 4634-4635.

Gudmundsson, G.H., Agerberth, B., Odeberg, J., Bergman, T., Olsson, B. and Salcedo, R. (1996) The human gene FALL39 and processing of the cathelin precursor to the antibacterial peptide LL-37 in granulocytes. *European Journal of Biochemistry* 238, 325–332.

Hancock, R.E.W. and Sahl, H. (2006) Antimicrobial and host-defence peptides as new anti-infective therapeutic strategies. *Nature Biotechnology* 24, 1551–1557.

Hancock, R.E.W., Haney, E.F. and Gill, E.E. (2016) The immunology of host defence peptides: beyond antimicrobial activity. *Nature Reviews Immunology* 16, 321–334.

Hasper, H.E., Kramer, N.E., Smith, J.L., Hillman, J.D., Zachariah, C., *et al.* (2006) An alternative bactericidal mechanism of action for lantibiotic peptides that target lipid II. *Science* 313, 1636–1637.

Hellekant, G. and Danilova, V. (2005) Brazzein a small, sweet protein: discovery and physiological overview. *Chemical Senses* 30, i88–i89.

Henderson, J.T., Chopko, A.L. and van Wassenaar, P.D. (1992) Purification and primary structure of pediocin PA-1 produced by *Pediococcus acidilactici* PAC-1.0. *Archives of Biochemistry and Biophysics* 295, 5–12.

Hsieh, I.-N. and Hartshorn, K.L. (2016) The role of antimicrobial peptides in influenza virus infection and their potential as antiviral and immunomodulatory therapy. *Pharmaceuticals* 9, 53.

Koro, C., Hellvard, A., Delaleu, N., Binder, V., Scavenius, C., *et al.* (2016) Carbamylated LL-37 as a modulator of the immune response. *Innate Immunity* 22, 218–229.

Koziel, J., Bryzek, D., Sroka, A., Maresz, K., Glowczyk, I., *et al.* (2014) Citrullination alters immuno-modulatory function of LL-37 essential for prevention of endotoxin-induced sepsis. *Journal of Immunology* 192, 5363–5372.

Kyte, J. and Doolittle, R.F. (1982) A simple method for displaying the hydropathic character of a protein. *Journal of Molecular Biology* 157, 105–132.

Lai, Y. and Gallo, R.L. (2009) AMPed up immunity: how antimicrobial peptides have multiple roles in immune defence. *Trends in Immunology* 30, 131–141.

Lee, J.T., Wang, G., Tam, Y.T. and Tam, C. (2016) Membrane-active Epithelial Keratin 6A fragments (KAMPs) are unique human antimicrobial peptides with a non-αβ structure. *Frontiers in Microbiology* 7, 1799.

Leitgeb, B., Szekeres, A., Manczinger, L., Vágvölgyi, C. and Kredics, L. (2007) The history of alamethicin: a review of the most extensively studied peptaibol. *Chemistry and Biodiversity* 4, 1027–1051.

Lemaitre, B. (2004) The road to Toll. *Nature Reviews Immunology* 4, 521–527.

Lin, Y.M., Wu, S.J., Chang, T.W., Wang, C.F., Suen, C.S., *et al.* (2010) Outer membrane protein I of *Pseudomonas aeruginosa* is a target of cationic antimicrobial peptide/protein. *Journal of Biological Chemistry* 285, 8985–8994.

Ling, L.L., Schneider, T., Peoples, A.J., Spoering, A.L., Engels, I., *et al.* (2015) A new antibiotic kills pathogens without detectable resistance. *Nature* 517, 455–459.

Ludtke, S.J., He, K., Heller, W.T., Harroun, T.A., Yang, L. and Huang, H.W. (1996) Membrane pores induced by magainin. *Biochemistry* 35, 13723–13728.

Maerki, C., Meuter, S., Liebi, M., Mühlemann, K., Frederick, M.J., Yawalkar, N., Moser, B. and Wolf, M. (2009) Potent and broad-spectrum antimicrobial activity of CXCL14 suggests an immediate role in skin infections. *Journal of Immunology* 182, 507–514.

Makhloufi, K.M., Carré-Mlouka, A., Peduzzi, J., Lombard, C., van Reenen, C.A., Dicks, L.M. and Rebuffat, S. (2013) Characterization of leucocin B-KM432Bz from *Leuconostoc pseudomesenteroides* isolated from boza, and comparison of its efficiency to pediocin PA-1. *PLoS One* 8, e70484.

Merrifield, R.B. (1963) Solid phase peptide synthesis. I. The synthesis of a tetrapeptide. *Journal of the American Chemical Society* 85, 2149–2154.

Montalbán-López, M., Spolaore, B., Pinato, O., Martínez-Bueno, M., Valdivia, E., Maqueda. M. and Fontana, A. (2008) Characterization of linear forms of the circular enterocin AS-48 obtained by limited proteolysis. *FEBS Letters* 582, 3237–3242.

Murakami, M., Lopez-Garcia, B., Braff, M., Dorschner, R.A. and Gallo, R.L. (2004) Postsecretory processing generates multiple cathelicidins for enhanced topical antimicrobial defence. *Journal of Immunology* 172, 3070–3077.

Murakami, M., Kameda, K., Tsumoto, H., Tsuda, T., Masuda, K., *et al.* (2016) TLN-58, an additional hCAP18 processing form, found in the lesion vesicle of palmoplantar pustulosis in the skin. *Journal of Investigative Dermatology* 137, 322–331.

Murzin, A.G., Brenner, S.E., Hubbard, T. and Chothia, C. (1995) SCOP: a structural classification of protein database for the investigation of sequences and structures. *Journal of Molecular Biology* 247, 536–540.

Mygind, P.H., Fischer, R.L., Schnorr, K.M., Hansen, M.T., Sönksen, C.P., *et al.* (2005) Plectasin is a peptide antibiotic with therapeutic potential from a saprophytic fungus. *Nature* 437, 975–980.

Nuri, R., Shprung, T. and Shai, Y. (2015) Defensive remodeling: how bacterial surface properties and biofilm formation promote resistance to antimicrobial peptides. *Biochimica et Biophysica Acta* 1848, 3089–3100.

Nylén, F., Miraglia, E., Cederlund, A., Ottosson, H., Strömberg, R., Gudmundsson, G.H. and Agerberth, B. (2014) Boosting innate immunity: development and validation of a cell-based screening assay to identify LL-37 inducers. *Innate Immunity* 20, 364–376.

Otero-González, A.J., Simas Magalhães, B., Garcia-Villarino, M., López-Abarrategui, C., Amaro Sousa, D., Campos Dias, S. and Luiz Franco, O. (2010) Antimicrobial peptides from marine invertebrates as a new frontier for microbial infection control. *FASEB Journal* 24, 1320–1334.

Picchianti, M., Russo, C., Castagnini, M., Biagini, M., Soldaini, E. and Balducci, E. (2015) NAD-dependent ADP-ribosylation of the human antimicrobial and immune-modulatory peptide LL-37 by ADP-ribosyltransferase-1. *Innate Immunity* 21, 314–321.

Rink, R., Kuipers, A., de Boef, E., Leenhouts, K.J., Driessen, A.J., Moll, G.N. and Kuipers, O.P. (2005) Lantibiotic structures as guidelines for the design of peptides that can be modified by lantibiotic enzymes. *Biochemistry* 44, 8873–8882.

Rogers, L.A. (1928) The inhibiting effect of *Streptococcus lactis* on *Lactobacillus bulgaricus*. *Journal of Bacteriology* 16, 321–325.

Romeo, D., Skerlavaj, B., Bolognesi, M. and Gennaro, R. (1988) Structure and bactericidal activity of an antibiotic dodecapeptide purified from bovine neutrophils. *Journal of Biological Chemistry* 263, 9573–9575.

Rosengren, K.J., Clark, R.J., Daly, N.L., Göransson, U., Jones, A. and Craik, D.J. (2003) Microcin J25 has a threaded sidechain-to-backbone ring structure and not a head-to-tail cyclized backbone. *Journal of the American Chemical Society* 125, 12464–12474.

Ryazantsev, D.Y., Rogozhin, E.A., Dimitrieva, T.V., Drobyazina, P.E., Khadeeva, N.V., Egorov, T.A., Grishin, E.V. and Zavriev, S.K. (2014) A novel hairpin-like antimicrobial peptide from barnyard grass (*Echinochloa crusgalli* L.) seeds: structure-functional and molecular-genetics characterization. *Biochimie* 99, 63–70.

Selsted, M.E., Harwig, S.S., Ganz, T., Schilling, J.W. and Lehrer, R.I. (1985) Primary structures of three human neutrophil defensins. *Journal of Clinical Investigation* 76, 1436–1439.

Shai, Y. (2002) Mode of action of membrane active antimicrobial peptides. *Biopolymers* 66, 234-248.

Sorensen, O.E. and Borregaard, N. (2005) Cathelicidins – nature's attempt at combinatorial chemistry. *Combinatorial Chemistry & High Throughput Screening* 8, 273–280.

Stansly, P.G., Shepherd, R.G. and White, H.J. (1947) Polymyxin: a new chemotherapeutic agent. *Bulletin of the Johns Hopkins Hospital Journal* 81, 43–54.

Steiner, H., Hultmark, D., Engström, A., Bennich, H. and Boman, H.G. (1981) Sequence and specificity of two antibacterial proteins involved in insect immunity. *Nature* 292, 246–248.

Synge, R.L. (1945) 'Gramicidin S': over-all chemical characteristics and amino-acid composition. *Biochemical Journal* 39, 363–367.

Tam, J.P., Lu, Y.A., Yang. J.L. and Chiu, K.W. (1999) An unusual structural motif of antimicrobial peptides containing end-to-end macrocycle and cystine-knot disulfides. *Proceedings of the National Academy of Sciences of the USA* 96, 8913–8918.

Tang, Y.Q., Yuan, J., Osapay, G., Osapay, K., Tran, D., Miller, C.J., Ouellette, A.J. and Selsted, M.E. (1999) A cyclic antimicrobial peptide produced in primate leukocytes by the ligation of two truncated α-defensins. *Science* 286, 498–502.

Tanphaichitr, N., Srakaew, N., Alonzi, R., Kiattiburut, W., Kongmanas, K., *et al.* (2016) Potential use of antimicrobial peptides as vaginal spermicides/microbicides. *Pharmaceuticals* 9, 13.

Taylor, K., Clarke, D.J., McCullough, B., Chin, W., Seo, E., *et al.* (2008) Analysis and separation of residues important for the chemoattractant and antimicrobial activities of beta-defensin 3. *Journal of Biological Chemistry* 283, 6631–6639.

Taylor, S.W., Craig, A.G., Fischer, W.H., Park, M. and Lehrer, R.I. (2000) Styelin D, an extensively modified antimicrobial peptide from ascidian hemocytes. *Journal of Biological Chemistry* 275, 38417–38426.

Tossi, A. and Sandri, L. (2002) Molecular diversity in gene-encoded, cationic antimicrobial polypeptides. *Current Pharmaceutical Design* 8, 743–761.

Urry, D.W. (1971) The gramicidin A transmembrane channel: a proposed pi(L,D) helix. *Proceedings of the National Academy of Sciences of the USA* 68, 672–6.

Wang, G. (ed.) (2010) *Antimicrobial Peptides: Discovery Design and Novel Therapeutic Strategies.* CABI, Wallingford, UK.

Wang, G. (2012) Post-translational modifications of natural antimicrobial peptides and strategies for peptide engineering. *Current Biotechnology* 1, 72–79.

Wang, G. (2013) Database-guided discovery of potent peptides to combat HIV-1 or superbugs. *Pharmaceuticals* 6, 728–758.

Wang, G. (2014) Human antimicrobial peptides and proteins. *Pharmaceuticals* 7, 545–594.

Wang, G. (2015) Improved methods for classification, prediction, and design of antimicrobial peptides. *Methods in Molecular Biology* 1268, 43–66.

Wang, G. (2016) Structural analysis of amphibian, insect and plant host defense peptides inspires the design of novel therapeutic molecules. In Epand, R.M. (ed.) *Host Defense Peptides and Their Potential as Therapeutic Agents.* Springer, Switzerland, pp. 229–252.

Wang, G., Li, X. and Wang, Z. (2009) APD2: the updated antimicrobial peptide database and its application in peptide design. *Nucleic Acids Research* 37 (Database issue), D933–D937.

Wang, G., Mishra, B., Epand, R.F. and Epand, R.M. (2014) High-quality 3D structures shine light on antibacterial, anti-biofilm and antiviral activities of human cathelicidin LL-37 and its fragments. *Biochimica et Biophysica Acta* 1838, 2160–2172.

Wang, G., Mishra, B., Lau, K., Lushnikova, T., Golla, R. and Wang, X. (2015) Antimicrobial peptides in 2014. *Pharmaceuticals* 8, 123–150.

Wang, G., Li, X. and Wang, G. (2016) APD3: the antimicrobial peptide database as a tool for research and education. *Nucleic Acids Research* 44 (Database issue), D1087–D1093.

Wang, X. and Wang, G. (2016) Insights into antimicrobial peptides from spiders and scorpions. *Protein and Peptide Letters* 23, 707–721.

Wang, Z. and Wang, G. (2004) APD: the antimicrobial peptide database. *Nucleic Acids Research* 32 (Database issue), D590–592.

Woese, C.R., Kandler, O. and Wheelis, M.L. (1990) Towards a natural system of organisms: proposal for the domains Archaea, Bacteria, and Eucarya. *Proceedings of the National Academy of Sciences of the USA* 87, 4576–4579.

Xhindoli, D., Pacor, S., Benincasa, M., Scocchi, M., Gennaro, R. and Tossi, A. (2016) The human cathelicidin LL-37 – a pore-forming antibacterial peptide and host-cell modulator. *Biochimica et Biophysica Acta* 1858, 546–566.

Yang, D., Chen, Q., Hoover, D.M, Staley, P., Tucker, K.D., Lubkowski, J. and Oppenheim, J.J. (2003) Many chemokines including CCL20/MIP-3alpha display antimicrobial activity. *Journal of Leukocyte Biology* 74, 448–455.

Yokoyama, S., Lida, Y., Kawasaki, Y., Minami, Y., Waranabe, K. and Yagi, F. (2009) The chitin-binding capability of Cy-AMP1 from cycad is essential to antifungal activity. *Journal of Peptide Science* 15, 492–497.

Young, N.Y. and Yeaman, M.R. (2004) Multidimensional signatures in antimicrobial peptides. *Proceedings of the National Academy of Sciences of the USA* 101, 7363–7368.

Zanetti, M. (2005) The role of cathelicidins in the innate host defences of mammals. *Current Issues in Molecular Biology* 7, 179–196.

Zasloff, M. (1987) Magainins, a class of antimicrobial peptides from Xenopus skin: isolation, characterization of two active forms, and partial cDNA sequence of a precursor. *Proceedings of the National Academy of Sciences of the USA* 84, 5449–5453.

Zasloff, M. (2002) Antimicrobial peptides of multicellular organisms. *Nature* 415, 389–395.

Zasloff, M. (2005) Sunlight, vitamin D, and the innate immune defences of the human skin. *Journal of Investigative Dermatology* 125, xvi–xvii.

2 Structural and Functional Diversity of Cathelicidins

Alessandro Tossi[1],*, Barbara Skerlavaj[2], Francesca D'Este[2] and Renato Gennaro[1]

[1]Department of Life Sciences, University of Trieste, via Giorgieri 5, 34127 Trieste, Italy; [2]Department of Medicine, University of Udine, Piazzale Kolbe, 4, 33100 Udine, Italy

Abstract

Cathelicidins are a ubiquitous family of host defence peptides (HDPs) in vertebrate animals. Unlike other HDP families, they are defined by the common and relatively well conserved proregion rather than the mature active peptides, which are highly diverse and conform to at least five different structural groups. They seem to have followed a rather distinctive evolutionary path in their development. Cathelicidin-derived peptides play a relevant role in defending the host against microbial infection, by displaying both a broad-spectrum, direct antimicrobial activity and the capacity to modulate other host responses to infection and injury. Both types of effect depend on the structural type, which in turn affects the particular mode of action of each peptide. This chapter begins by briefly describing the discovery of cathelicidins before discussing their molecular diversity and considering their evolution. It then considers their expression and processing, the structure-dependence of the distinct modes of action shown by different members, and briefly touches on their pleiotropic roles in modulating host defence.

2.1 Introduction

Cathelicidins are a family of vertebrate host defence peptides (HDPs) characterized by a relatively well conserved proregion linked to a structurally highly variable C-terminal antimicrobial region. They form one of the principal vertebrate HDP families, another one being that of the defensins (Zasloff, 2002; Doss *et al.*, 2010; Antcheva *et al.*, 2013), and are a prime example of diversity in antimicrobial peptides (AMPs).

Since their discovery in the late 1980s, cathelicidin-derived peptides have demonstrated a remarkably wide functional repertoire, with direct antibiotic activities displayed against bacterial, fungal, viral and parasitic microorganisms. They can also help orchestrate other aspects of the immune response to infection, and modulate inflammation, limiting or enhancing it to aid in host defence depending on the context (Yang *et al.*, 2001; Ramanathan *et al.*, 2002; Lai and Gallo, 2009; Wu *et al.*, 2010; Chow *et al.*, 2013; Linde *et al.*, 2013). The term cathelicidin, *sensu stricto*, relates to the pro-form (Zanetti *et al.*, 1995), while the active HDPs are variously indicated by their provenance, size and sequence

* Corresponding author e-mail: atossi@units.it

features (e.g. CRAMP for Cathelin Related Antimicrobial Peptide, BMAP-28 for Bovine Myeloid Antimicrobial Peptide of 28 residues, and LL-37 from the first two sequence residues and length) (Zanetti, 2005). However, it has become customary to refer to the active HDPs as cathelicidins as well.

Over the past three decades, cathelicidins have been intensely studied due to their fundamental roles in vertebrate host defence, as well as their perceived potential as leads for novel anti-infective agents for biomedical, veterinary or biotechnological uses. Most cathelicidin peptides are linear and are therefore relatively easy to produce and modify by solid phase peptide synthesis, making them easier to explore as leads than the defensins, characterized by multiple disulfide bonds. They also tend to have more robust antimicrobial activities than defensins, being less susceptible to their environment (salt concentrations, medium or serum components) (Nagaoka *et al.*, 2000). Finally, they display a remarkable array of host-cell modulating activities as already mentioned.

This chapter will provide a brief overview of the discovery of cathelicidins – their evolution, diversity and expression, considerations on antimicrobial modes of action, their capacity to affect host cells leading to beneficial or cytotoxic effects, and their potential for the development of therapeutic agents. The literature on cathelicidins is vast, and this chapter provides only a flavour of all these topics. For a more complete understanding the reader is referred to the many excellent reviews on the family or on members of particular relevance (Zanetti *et al.*, 1995; Yang *et al.*, 2001; Gennaro *et al.*, 2002; Zaiou and Gallo, 2002; Sorensen and Borregaard, 2005; Tomasinsig and Zanetti, 2005; Zanetti, 2005; Jenssen *et al.*, 2007; Scocchi *et al.*, 2011; Mookherjee *et al.*, 2013).

2.2 Discovery of Cathelicidins

The first papers on cathelicidin peptides (not yet known as such at that time) were by the Trieste group in the late 1980s, and referred to apparently unrelated peptides of different sizes from granule extracts of bovine neutrophils, but with indications of a larger inactive precursor (Marzari *et al.*, 1988; Gennaro *et al.*, 1989; Romeo *et al.*, 1988; Frank *et al.*, 1990). It was subsequently determined that these peptides, generically called bactenecins, were synthesized in immature bone marrow cells of the myeloid lineage as prepro-forms and targeted to the so-called large granules of bovine neutrophils (Zanetti *et al.*, 1990). The active HDPs were released from the pro-form by the neutral serine protease elastase. It was proposed the pro-part might be required for sorting to granules and/or to keep the HDPs inactive until release (Zanetti *et al.*, 1991; Scocchi *et al.*, 1992).

Cloning studies then showed that the proregion had significant sequence identity to the pig cathepsin inhibitor cathelin (Ritonja *et al.*, 1989), and surprisingly that structurally quite diverse HDPs from different mammals all shared this homologous proregion (Zanetti *et al.*, 1995). These included the small bovine cyclic dodecapeptide (Storici *et al.*, 1992), long Pro-rich peptides from cow and pig (Zanetti *et al.*, 1995; Agerberth *et al.*, 1996), an amphipathic helical peptide from rabbit (Larrick *et al.*, 1991) and a bovine Trp-rich peptide (Del Sal *et al.*, 1992; Selsted *et al.*, 1992). There soon followed a spate of distinctive HDPs from other mammals, all linked to a cathelin-like domain (CLD), but only one human homologue was ever found, the helical peptide LL-37/hCap18 (Agerberth *et al.*, 1995; Cowland *et al.*, 1995; Larrick *et al.*, 1995). Many other cathelicidin HDPs have now been identified in mammalian and non-mammalian vertebrate species (see below and Table 2.1), several of which have been characterized for their antimicrobial and other roles in host defence. These HDPs can be very different in size, sequence, structure and physico-chemical features, but are all linked to a relatively well conserved, cathelin-like domain (CLD) in their pro-forms. Thus the family name '*cathelicidin*' – from peptides with a CLD, able to kill bacteria (Zanetti *et al.*, 1995).

Table 2.1. Sequence and structural types for selected cathelicidin HDPs from mammalian and non-mammalian vertebrates.

	Species (N°)[a]	Genes[b]	AMP[c]	Type[d]	Sequence[e]
Eutheria	*Primates (26)*	1			
	human		HssLL-37	α^0	LLGDFFRKSKEKIGKEFKRIVQRIKDFLRNLVPRTES (*)
	chimpanzee		PtrLL-37	α^0	LLGDFFRKSKEKIGKEFKRIVQRIKDFLRNLVPRTES
	rhesus		mmuRl-37	α^0	RLGNFFRKVKEKIGGGLKKVGQKIKDFLGNLVPRTAS
	Tree shrews & culogos (2)	1			
	tree shrew		predicted	α^0	KLTGLLRRGGEKLAEKFEKIGQKIKNFFRKLLPETES
	culogo		predicted	α^0	RLGGLIQRGGQKLGEKLERIGQRIKDFFRNLAPRTES
	Glires (15)	1			
	mouse		CRAMP	α^0	RLAGLLRKGGEKIGEKLKKIGQKIKNFFQKLVPQPEQ
	rabbit		CAP-18	α^0	GLRKRLRKFRNKIKEKLKKIGQKIQGLLPKLAPRTDY (*)
	naked molerat		predicted	α^0	RRTVGLSKFFRKARKKLGKGLQKIKNVLRKYLPRPQYAYA
	Carnivores (11)	1			
	dog		K9CATH	α^0	RLKELITTGGQKIGEKIRRIGQRIKDFFKNLQPREEKS
	seal		predicted	α^0	RLRDLIRRGRQKIGRRINRLGRRIQDILKNLQPGKVS
	bear		predicted	α^0	KAGHKIRGSIRRIGGRIWRIGKGIRDILKNLPPRPQV
	Perissodactyls (3)	3–4			
	horse		eCATH-3	α^0	KRFHSVGSLIQRHQQMIRDKSEATRHGIRIITRPKLLLAS
	rhinoceros		predicted	α^0	CFGGITDKFCDKIGKIRDKIGRIHDGIRDFIQHRIVLES
	Cetartiodactyls (10)	up to 10			
	cow		BMAP-34	α^0	GLFRRLRDSIRRGQQKILEKARRIGERIKDIFRG
	sheep		SMAP-34	α^0	GLFGRLRDSLQRGGQKILEKAERIGDRIKDIFRG
	pig		PMAP-37	α^0	GLLSRLRDFLSDRGRRLGEKIERIGQKIKDLSEFFQS
	Moles & hedgehogs (2)	1			
	mole		predicted	α^0	GRLRDLIKKGTQKIGRKLRKVGQQIKDFIRNLRPREEDS
	hedgehog		predicted	α^0	GKVGDFLKRGGQKIGEKIEKIGKRIKDFFQNLKPREEA
	shrew		predicted	α^0	RGLGGLIKKGVQKIGKGIGKIARKLHLLPFSLDTPGGT
	Bats (6)	multiple			
	myotis		predicted	α^0	LGERIKNAKKKVWEKIKSFGRRIKDFFRKPSPEVEP
	fruit bat		predicted	α^0	GLGGLLRLGGRKIGEGIEGLGRKIKGIFSSLRPRPES

Afrotehrians (6)	1			
elephant		predicted	α^0	GLRKFFRKSKEKLKKVGRKVGFFRDVLRRVPYLPGPRFSYAF
aardvark		predicted	α^0	FLGGLLQRGGKRIGEKIERIGQRIKDFFQNLAPRTEES
procavia		predicted	α^0	GLGERLWRGGKEIWGKIARAGQKIKDFFKNLPPRTAS
Xenarthrans (2)	1			
armadillo		predicted	α^0	GLIDRFREGARKIGEKLKRFKDIVLDFIRNLSPRTEP
sloth		predicted		PLHRRIPETSVDSLSELQTLQG-IEDLLTNLAPRTES
Cetartiodactyls (10)	up to 10			
cow		BMAP-28	α	GGLRSLGRKILRAWKKYG------PIIVPIIRI-am
		BMAP-27	α	GRFKRFRKKFKKLFKKL------ SPVIPLLH–am (*)
sheep		SMAP-29	α	RGLRRLGRKIAHGVKKYG-------PTVLRIIRIA-am
pig		PMAP-36	α	GRFRRLRKKTRKRLKKIGKVLKWIPPIVGSIPLGC–am
cow		indolicidin	WR	ILPWKWPWWPWRR (*)
pig		tritrpticin	WR	RRFPWWWPFLRR (*)
		PMAP-23	WR	RIIDLLWRVRRPQKPKFVTVWVR (*)
cow		dodecapep	β	RLC-RIVVIRVCR
sheep		dodecapep	β	RIC-RIIFLRVCR
pig		protegrin	β	RGGRLCYCRRRFCVCVGR-am
cow		Bac7	PR	RRIRPRPPRLPRPRPRPLPFPRPGPRPIPRPLPFPRPGPRPIPRPLPFPRPGPRPIPRPL (*)
sheep		OaBac7.5	PR	RRLRPRRPRLPRPRPRPRPRSLPLPRPQPRRIPRPILLPWRPPRPIPRPQPQPIPRWL
pig		PR-39	PR	RR-RPRPPYLPRPRPPPFFPPRLPPRIPPGFPPRFPPRFP
cow		Bac5	PR	RFRPPIRRPPIRPPFYPPFRPPIRPPIFPPIRPPFRPPLGPFPGRR
sheep		OaBac5	PR	RFRPPIRRPPIRPPFRPPFRPPVRPPIRPPFRPPFRPPIGPFPGRR
pig		prophenin	PR	RRPRLRRQAFPPPNVPGPRFPPPNFPGPRFPPPNFPGPRFPPPNFPGPRFPPPNFPGPPFPPPIFPGPWFPPPPPFRPPPFG PPRFPGRR
Metatheria *Marsupials (3)*	up to 12			
possum		predicted	α	MNDGFWYQLIRTFGNLIHQKYRKLLEAYRKLRDIFSG
wallaby		predicted	α	KSEGFLRRITRGFANLIYQKYRILQNVFRKLRNIFSRGRDDKE
tasmanian devil		predicted	α	KREDFLDQIIRDFRNFIYQKYRRLRDEFRKLRDILSG
possum		predicted	α	SRRTPLPKQKNGSKNRRFRIGGYTMISMKQPRVQKAPYMEAL

Continued

Table 2.1. Continued.

	Species (N°)[a]	Genes[b]	AMP[c]	Type[d]	Sequence[e]
	wallaby		predicted	α	SRRSPLPGRKKGSK--RHKPGSYSVIALGKPGVKKSPYMEAL
	tasmanian devil		predicted	α	SR-SPGLRSSVFFPLQPEKIKRIGLIRLIGKILRGLRRLG
	Monotremes (1)	up to 6	predicted	α	RRGLRKTLRKLKKKLKKFLPKSPRYFQVSKDF
			predicted	α	RRIKLIKNGVKKVKDILKNNNIIILPGSNEK
Amphibia	*Frogs & toads (8)*	2–3			
	bullfrog		Rc-Cath1	α	KKC-KFFCKVKKKIK--SIGFQIPIVSIPFK
	spiny frog		Ny-Cath-PY	α	RKC-NFLCKLKEKLR-TVITSHIDKVLRPQG (*)
	Large-headed frog		Lf- Cath2	α	GKC-NVLCQLKQKLRSIGSGSHIGSVVLPRG
	clawed frog		predicted	?	SEEESGSGEIIQDAKSRCRRPGSCTLIGRFNQRINRNQV
			predicted	?	SRTKRSTKTKKCKTSGCRFTGAGSAIAGVKPLQSIG
	clawed frog		predicted	GS	RRSRNGGRGGGGR-SGGRGGGGSRGGGSRGGGSRGGCSRGGGSRGGGGGRSGSGSSIAGGGG...
	sucker frog		Al-Cath	GS	RRSRRGRGGGGRRGGSGGRGGRGGGGRSGAGSSIAGVGSRGGGGGRHYA
	Salamander (3)	2			
	mexican salamander		predicted	?	RRSRQARQCVREKGRLKCKPPPRPGFASAVARTSKDKIV
	crocodile newt		predicted	?	RRPRQTRKCVRQNNKRVCK
Reptilia	*Snakes (15)*	2			
	cobra		Na-Cath	α	KRFKKFFKKLKNSVKKRAKKFFKKPKVIGVTFPF
	sea snake		Hc-Cath	α	KFFKRLLK----SVRRAVKKFRKKPRLIGLSTLL
	python		predicted	α	KRFKKFFRKIKK---GFRKIFKKTKIFIGGTIPI
	viper		predicted	?	RNGKVRKLLRKLKKILPGGGSIIAHAKPVRPFHMVAARVA
	Turtles (4)	2			
	painted turtle		predicted	?	RRSRSPRRSRWPRRWYLP-GSYTLIAHGGGKGKGKGSRLQMA
	softshell turtle		predicted	?	RRSRSPRRKWTWKPRRR--GSYTLISQGGNKGKHN--RLQMA
	green sea turtle		predicted	?	RRSIFRKLRRKIKKGLKKGIQH--LLAGGRQGLPQGGRPGMI
	painted turtle		predicted	?	RSRWRRFTRRAGGFIRKNRWNIISTALKWIG
	softshell turtle		predicted	?	RGRWGRFKRRAGRFIRRNRWQIISTGLKLIG
	green sea turtle		predicted	?	RGRWKRFWRGAGRFFRRHKEKIIRAAVDIVLS

	Lizards (2)	2			
	gekko		predicted	α	RSRWRRFWGKAKRGIKKHGVSIALAALRLRG
	anolis lizard		predicted	α	RSRWGRFWRGAKRFVKKHGVSIALAGLRFG
	Crocodilians (2)				
	alligator		predicted	?	RRSGWWNGHKRRRGSGTRRGRFSHIAHGGRKGHERIA
	Birds (19)	up to 4			
	chicken		Gg-Cath1	α	KRVWPLVIR---TVIAGYNLYRAIKKK (*)
	wild duck		Ap-Cath1	α	KRFWQLVPLAI-------KIYRAWKRR
	parrot		Ae-Cath3	α	KRFWPLLVTAIRTVAAGVGIFKSFKG
	chicken		Gg-cath2	α	GRFGRFLRKIRRFRPKVTIT—IQGSARFG
	wild duck			α	GRFGRFLGKIRHLRPRVRIRVKADATVSFG (*)
	penguin		predicted	?	GRTQTSRLMRLFARLREHFGGFFQCGKIWIRDKLNLKYPKA
	parrot		predicted	?	GSIRKSGVRNLFGRIKERFKGFFQCSKIWIRDKLNLKKPKS
	chicken		Gg-CathB1	?	PIRNWWIRIWEWLNGIRKRLRQRSPFYVRGHLNVTSTPQP
	turkey		Mg-CathB1	?	PIRNWWTRIREWWDGIRKRLRQRSPFYVRGRLNITSTPQP
Fish	*Ray-finned fish (10)*	2			
	trout		Rt-Cath1	GS	RRSKVRICSRGKNCVSRPGVGSIIG-RPGGGSLIGRPGGGSVIGRPGGGSPPGGGSFNDEF...
	salmon		As-Cath1	GS	RRSQARKCSRGNGGKIGSIRCRGGGTRLGGGSLIGRLRVALLLGVAPFLLDLSQINVMEIAFA
	cod		codCath	GS	RRSRSGRGS-GKGGRGGSRGSSGSRGSKGPSGSRGSSGSRGSKGSRGGRSGRGSTIAGNGNR...
	ayu		aCath	GS	RRSKSGKGS-GGSKGSGSKGSKGSKGSGSKGSGSKGGSRPGGGSSIAGGGSKGKGGTQTA
	trout		Rt-Cath2b	GS	RRGKDSGGPKMGRKYSK---GGWRGRPGSGSRPGFGSSIAGASGVNHVGTLTA
	salmon		As-Cath2	GS	RRGKPSGGSRGSKMGSKDSKGGWRGRPGSGSRPGFGSSIAGASGRDQGGTRNA
	Hagfish (1)	2	MgCath37	α	GWFKKAWRKVKHAGRRVLDTAKGVGRHYLNNWLNRYR-am (Trp may be monobrominated)
			MgCath29	α	GWFKKAWRKVKNAGRVLKGVGIHYGVGLI-am
	Lamprey (1)	?	predicted	?	GEPQDGNKKPRRRPGFMHIAGRPGKPDTKKDNPHSH

[a]Number of species in which cathelicidins have already been identified; [b]Estimated number of cathelicidin genes per species, based on current knowledge; [c]Common name given to the cathelicidin antimicrobial peptide if characterized, predicted indicates it has only been identified at the nucleotide level; [d]Structural type: α indicates generically helical peptides, $α^0$ indicates α-helical peptides encoded by orthologous CAMP genes in each species, β indicates hairpin peptides stabilized by cystine bridges, WR indicates Trp/Arg-rich peptides, PR indicates Pro/Arg-rich peptides, GS indicates Gly/Ser-rich peptides; e) conserved residues that are diagnostic for orthologous peptides are shaded grey.
The ending '–am' indicates that the peptide is C-terminally amidated.; (*) indicates that a solution structure has been determined, as shown in Fig. 2.2.

2.3 Evolution, Structural Diversity and Features of the Proregion

2.3.1 Evolution

Cathelicidins are quite widespread and ancient components of vertebrate innate immunity (see Table 2.1). They have been identified in species that diverged over 500 million years ago, ranging from the hagfish (a basal vertebrate), to ray-finned fish, amphibians, reptiles, birds and all mammals, including marsupials, glires, dogs and other carnivores, artiodactyls, perissodactyls and primates (Uzzell *et al.*, 2003; Zanetti, 2004; Tomasinsig and Zanetti, 2005; Zelezetsky *et al.*, 2006; Sang *et al.*, 2007; Maier *et al.*, 2008; Lu *et al.*, 2010; Wang *et al.*, 2011; Hao *et al.*, 2012; van Hoek, 2014; H. Yu *et al.*, 2015). No cathelicidins have yet been reported from invertebrates.

In a recent review, 148 database entries for cathelicidins were reported from 31 vertebrate species (Linde *et al.*, 2013). We have been keeping track of cathelicidins in protein and annotated or unassembled nucleotide sequence databases and have found evidence for them in over 150 vertebrate species to date, including lampreys (another basal vertebrate), numerous fish species, amphibian, reptile and avian species, as well as placental and non-placental mammals. Comparison of the HDP domains suggests that an orthologue of human LL-37 is present in all placental mammals, and indeed the gene encoding it – *CAMP* – is often the only one present (e.g. in primates, glires and other rodents, carnivores and several other orders, see Table 2.1). For some mammalian species, however, multiple cathelicidins may be present. In some orders (e.g. bats and perissodactyls) these are due to simple duplication and diversification of the *CAMP* gene, but for cetartiodactyls (e.g. cows, pigs and sheep), the structurally very diverse HDPs suggest a more complex evolutionary process.

The cathelicidin gene/genes in different species map to regions of conserved synteny, as shown by the *CAMP* gene locus in different mammals (Larrick *et al.*, 1996;

Huttner *et al.*, 1998; Sang *et al.*, 2007; Zhu, 2008). When there are several genes, these cluster in the same region (Castiglioni *et al.*, 1996; Scocchi *et al.*, 1997; Huttner *et al.*, 1998). All vertebrate cathelicidin genes are composed of four exons, of which the first three code for the preproregion and the fourth for the antimicrobial domain (see Fig. 2.1). Structure and sequence similarity places their products in the same superfamily as cystatins and kininogens. It has been suggested that they derive from a common ancestral protein, and that the cathelicidin gene acquired an extra fourth exon, which corresponds to the C-terminal antimicrobial peptide domain (Zhu, 2008). This probably initially coded a helical HDP, these being the most widespread (see Table 2.1). The gene then underwent duplication, as many vertebrates have multiple cathelicidins, and while the CLD sequences were conserved, the antimicrobial sequences seem to have been subjected to accelerated evolution leading to quite diverse HDPs. As only one gene is present in many orders of placental mammals, coding for a helical peptide, the common ancestor may have only had this type of gene. It then underwent several duplications, and in cetartiodactyls further diversifications seem to have occurred through exon reshuffling and/or post duplication sequence remodelling, resulting in insertion of novel sequences (Zhu and Gao, 2009), leading to structurally very diverse HDPs.

2.3.2 Structural diversity

Cathelicidin HDPs show a wide repertoire of sequences, sizes and structures, for some of which the NMR structures have been determined, as shown in Fig. 2.2. The most widely observed structure is that of an amphipathic α-helix, as found in hagfish, reptiles, amphibians, birds and mammals (see also Fig. 2.1), suggesting that this is the ancestral type (Zhu, 2008; Zhu and Gao, 2009). This conformation is also often found in AMPs that are unrelated to cathelicidins, and leads to a membranolytic antimicrobial

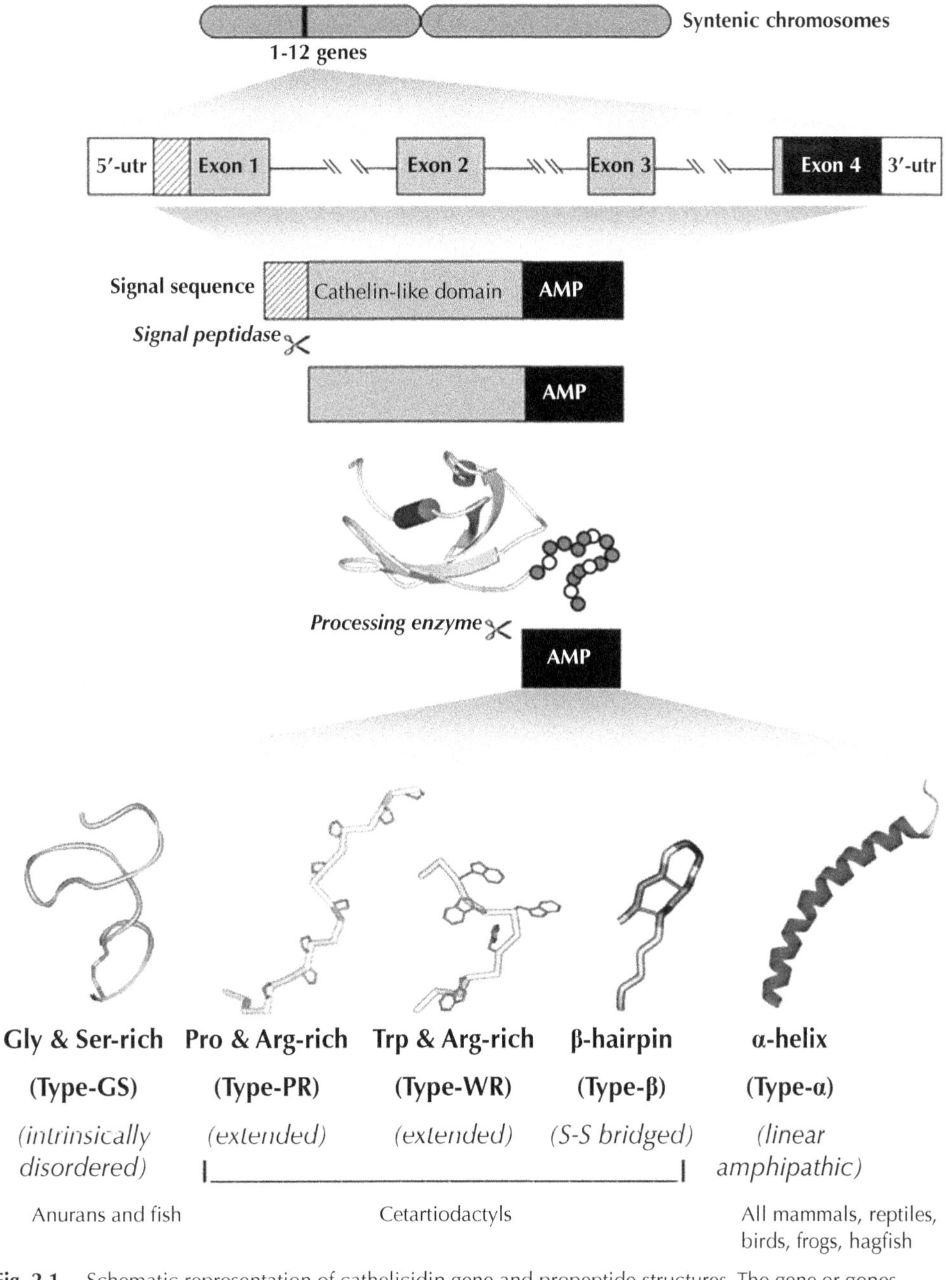

Fig. 2.1.　Schematic representation of cathelicidin gene and propeptide structures. The gene or genes encoding cathelicidin(s) are located on syntenic chromosomes and have 4 exons and 3 introns. Processing to the pro-form, with removal of the signal sequence, occurs before storage in leukocyte granules, or secretion by epithelial cells. Mature HDPs of different structural types are released by serine proteases (that differ depending on the organism and/or district) only after extracellular secretion. Some mammalian species express only one cathelicidin, which is invariably helical, others express multiple helical peptides, while cetartiodactyls cathelicidin HDPs can be helical, β-sheets, Pro/Arg-rich extended peptides or wedge-shaped Trp-rich peptides. Non-mammalian species generally express multiple cathelicidin HDPs, which can be helical or Gly/Ser-rich peptides, some of which may contain disulfide bridges.

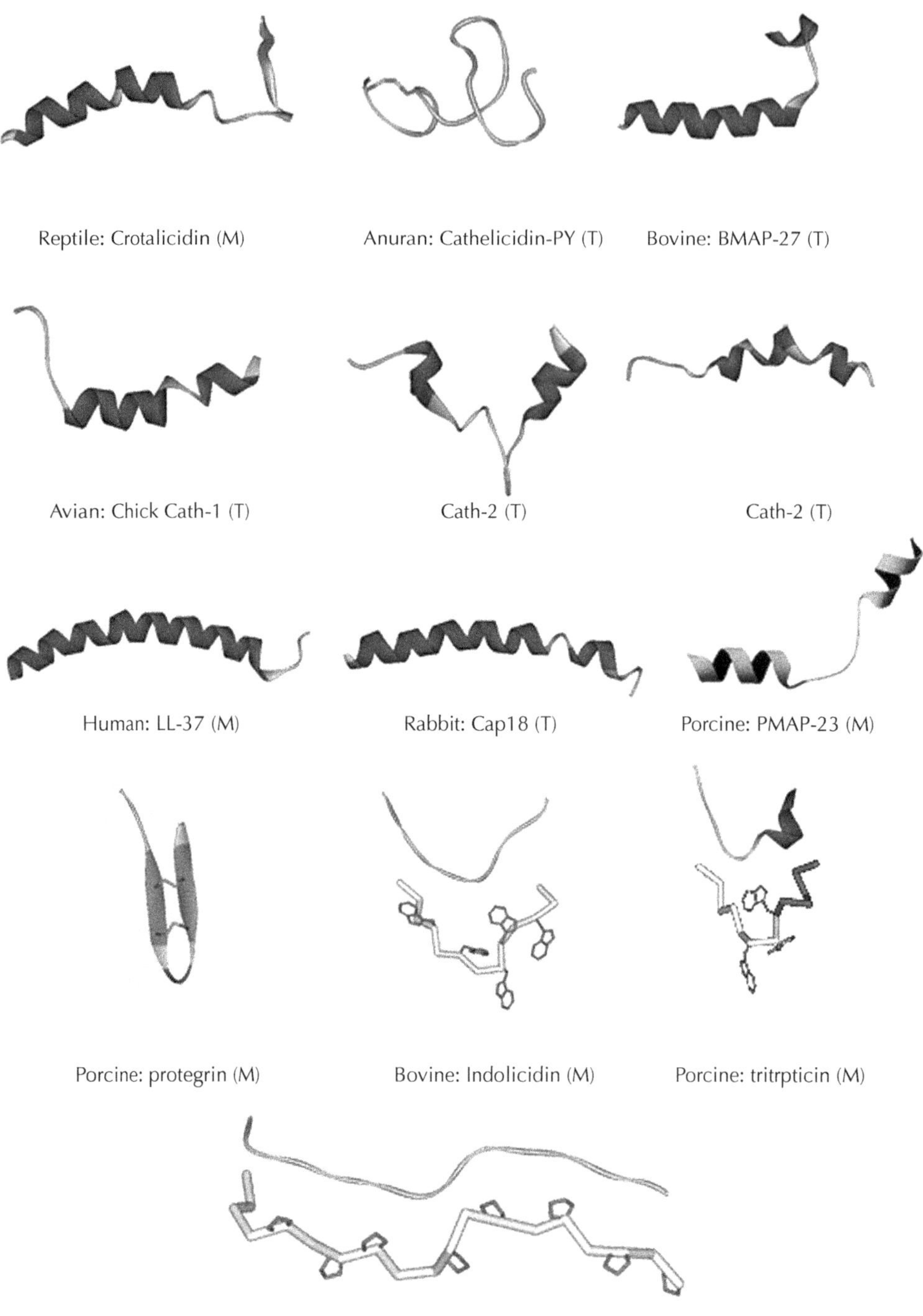

Fig. 2.2.   Solution structures of cathelicidin HDPs. Structures were obtained from the PDB database and prepared as ribbon models using DS Visualizer 2.0 (Accelrys). For indolicidin, tritrpticin and bactenecin, the Cα stick model with key side-chains is also shown. Peptides are indicated by their common name, followed by the conditions used in parentheses (M=phospholipid micelles, T=TFE). Bovine bactenecin was extracted

Continued

mechanism (Tossi *et al.*, 2000), suggesting convergent evolution of cathelicidin HDPs to this common function. These peptides are indicated as Type-α in Table 2.1.

Fish cathelicidins bear long, linear peptides that are particularly rich in Gly and Ser residues (Type-GS in Table 2.1). In salmonids they can be divided into two subgroups, due to the presence of two cysteine residues in the N-terminal part of the HDP region in *Cath1* type peptides, which is absent in *Cath2* type peptides (Maier *et al.*, 2008). The GS-rich stretch usually remains relatively unstructured even in membrane-like environments, suggesting they are low complexity, intrinsically disordered sequences (D'Este *et al.*, 2016). GS-rich cathelicidin peptides are also found in some amphibian species (see Table 2.1).

Cetartiodactyl cathelicidin HDPs show the most diversity of structural forms (see Figs. 2.1 and 2.2). Apart from different Type-α peptides, there are long, Pro- and Arg-rich peptides with extended structures (Type-PR in Table 2.1) (Scocchi *et al.*, 2011), and small, wedge-shaped, Trp- and Arg-rich peptides (Type-WR in Table 2.1 and Fig. 2.2) (Schibli *et al.*, 1999; Rozek *et al.*, 2000; Tomasinsig and Zanetti, 2005). Another type of cathelicidin HDPs peculiar to this mammalian order are small, β-hairpin peptides stapled by one or two disulfide bonds (Type-β in Table 2.1). These include the bovid dodecapeptides (Raj *et al.*, 2000), and the porcine protegrins (Fahrner *et al.*, 1996). Some fish and amphibian cathelicidins also show paired cysteine motifs, but these tend to be inserted in longer extended sequences (see Table 2.1).

2.3.3 Features of the proregion

Similar 3D structures have been determined for the CLD of porcine and human cathelicidins (PDB IDs: 2K6O) (see Fig. 2.1), consistent with a high level of sequence conservation (Sanchez *et al.*, 2002a,b; Pazgier *et al.*, 2013). The solution structures of the respective HDPs have been determined independently (see Fig. 2.2), but how these relate to the CLD when still attached to it in the pro-form has only been inferred by modelling (Sanchez *et al.*, 2002a). In the CLD structure, a concave β-sheet platform, stabilized by two conserved disulfide bridges, nestles a long helical segment at the N-terminus. This structure displays a cystatin-like fold, but lacks key sequence elements, present in cystatins, required for cysteine protease inhibition (Pazgier *et al.*, 2013).

Surprisingly little is known about the function/s of the proregion (Pazgier *et al.*, 2013). It was initially suggested that it kept the peptides inactive in the pro-peptide storage form, until release into the phagosome or into the extracellular medium (Scocchi *et al.*, 1992; Sørensen *et al.*, 1997; Zanetti *et al.*, 2002). However, it is questionable whether this function on its own could justify the high level of CLD conservation. Alternatively, the CLD might also have antimicrobial activity, complementing that of the HDP (Zaiou *et al.*, 2003), or act as a cathepsin inhibitor, given its homology with cathelin. Initial studies with bovine cathelicidins suggested it might have such activities (Ritonja *et al.*, 1989; Verbanac *et al.*, 1993), but this was later cast into doubt (Lenarčič *et al.*, 1993; Storici *et al.*, 1996). Furthermore, as already mentioned, the CLD in mammalian cathelicidins lacks key structural features necessary for cathepsin inhibition. Studies on its antibacterial and inhibitory activities came to conflicting conclusions making both these roles uncertain (Zaiou *et al.*, 2003; Zhu *et al.*, 2008; Pazgier *et al.*, 2013). Whether the CLD of non-mammalian

Fig. 2.2. (Continued) from the crystal structure when bound to a ribosome subunit. Coordinate files: crotalicidin (2MWT), (Falcao *et al.*, 2015); cathelicidin-PY (2LR7), (Wei *et al.*, 2013); BMAP-27 (2KET), (Yang *et al.*, 2009); chicken cathelicidins Cath-1,-2 and -3 (2AMN, 2GDL and 2HFR), (Bommineni *et al.*, 2007; Xiao *et al.*, 2006b, 2009); LL-37 (2K6O),(Wang, 2008);) Cap18 (1LYP), (Chen *et al.*, 1995); PMAP-23 (Park *et al.*, 2002); protegrin (2MZ6), (Usachev *et al.*, 2015); indolicidin (1G89), (Rozek *et al.*, 2000); tritrpticin (1D6X), (Schibli *et al.*, 1999); bactenecin (5HAU), (Gagnon *et al.*, 2016)

cathelicidins, which diverge significantly from mammalian ones (van Hoek, 2016), have these capacities remains an open question.

This brings us back to the hypothesis that the CLD could be a platform from which the HDP can be released in a controlled manner, by an appropriate protease, at the right time and in the right place. The protegrin pro-peptide is reported to change its conformation in a pH-dependent manner, leading to a model for activation/release (Sanchez *et al.*, 2002). Disengagement involves breaking electrostatic interactions, which may be consistent with the observation that relatively well conserved anionic residues form a strip on the surface of the CLD that might allow relevant interactions with the cationic HDP domain (Xhindoli *et al.*, 2016). The presentation platform hypothesis fits with the observation that a substantial fraction of the human cathelicidin remains as the intact pro-form on release from granulocytes, and is bound to the outside of the plasma membrane (Stie *et al.*, 2007). It accompanies granulocytes to the sites of infection, conferring a spatial specificity to activation by extracellular proteases and concentrating antimicrobial action where it is needed, minimizing damage to surrounding tissues. Furthermore, this prevents the active peptide from being sequestered by plasma lipoproteins, which could occur if it is released too early (Bals *et al.*, 1998; Sørensen *et al.*, 1999; Wang *et al.*, 2004). This hypothesis, if demonstrated, could present a potentially interesting strategy for the production of HDPs as prodrugs, improving their bioavailability and selectivity.

Whatever the role/roles of the proregion turns out to be, it has resulted in sufficient conservation of the CLD that recognizable features are present in widely divergent vertebrate species (Xhindoli *et al.*, 2016). This is a very useful characteristic when hunting for novel cathelicidins either *in vivo*, in tissue extracts (Tossi *et al.*, 1997), or *in silico*, as more and more vertebrate genomes come online.

2.4 Expression and Processing

Cathelicidins are expressed in, and secreted from, epithelial cells and circulating cells involved in immunity (including neutrophils or heterophils, monocytes, macrophages, dendritic cells, NK cells, lymphocytes and mast cells) (Zaiou and Gallo, 2002; Zanetti, 2005; Xhindoli *et al.*, 2016). Expression in tissues or cells that have an active role in host defence or constitute barriers to infection underlines their importance as host defence effectors. It is differentially regulated in different tissues, and this extends to single members from species with multiple cathelicidin genes.

In humans, the pattern of expression is varied, complex and regulated differently in different cell types (Lai and Gallo, 2009; Méndez-Samperio, 2010; van der Does *et al.*, 2012; Vandamme *et al.*, 2012). It can be stimulated by exogenous microbial components (bacterial products such as lipopolysaccharide/lipoteichoic acid (LPS/LTA), DNA or butyrate up-regulate its expression) (Nell *et al.*, 2004; Schauber *et al.*, 2004, 2006; Méndez-Samperio, 2010), but this appears to be less important than induction by endogenous factors (Lai and Gallo, 2009). Vitamin D_3 is a potent endogenous inducer because the *CAMP* gene promoter sequence in humans and other primates contains vitamin D response elements (VDRE) (Gombart, 2009) and this vitamin seems to play a significant role in enhancing cathelicidin-mediated antimicrobial defence both in circulation and at epithelial surfaces (Schauber and Gallo, 2008; Dixon *et al.*, 2012).

In mice, expression of the orthologous *CAMP* gene shows many analogies to that of the human peptide (Popsueva *et al.*, 1996; Iimura *et al.*, 2005). As with the human orthologue, its secretion is induced by bacterial products (Kovach *et al.*, 2012; Brandenburg *et al.*, 2013), but the gene lacks a VDRE so is not strongly induced by vitamin D (Segaert, 2008). An interesting common feature of the human and mouse cathelicidins is that they are particularly abundant in neonatal skin and in milk. Here they may act together with other HDPs as a first line of defence against infection in the immature defence system of newborns (Dorschner *et al.*, 2003; Yoshio *et al.*, 2004; Ménard *et al.*, 2008).

A similar expression pattern in leukocyte and epithelial cells is also observed for bovid and pig cathelicidins (Wu *et al.*, 1999; Gennaro and Zanetti, 2000; Zanetti *et al.*, 2000; Tomasinsig *et al.*, 2002; Hennig-Pauka *et al.*, 2006), but in these cases the presence of several different genes allows for differential expression at different sites. For example, helical and PR-rich peptides, but not indolicidin, are induced by LPS-treatment of neutrophils (Tomasinsig *et al.*, 2010b), whereas they are all constitutively expressed in healthy mammary tissue (Kościuczuk *et al.*, 2014; Whelehan *et al.*, 2014). The concentration of various cathelicidins is increased in milk during mastitis, probably due to infiltration of stimulated neutrophils, thus providing both protection from infection and useful biomarkers to assist in detection of mastitis (Boehmer *et al.*, 2008; Tomasinsig *et al.*, 2010b; Smolenski *et al.*, 2011).

The expression patterns for cathelicidins in non-mammalian vertebrates are less studied, but there are indications that avian heterophils are a major source during infection. In reptiles, cathelicidins are stored in granulocytes present in the blood or in connective tissues, but epithelial cells can be stimulated to produce them after injury and contribute to keeping regenerating tissue free of infection (van Dijk *et al.*, 2009; Alibardi, 2014). Cathelicidins are widely expressed in amphibians and fish tissues, both constitutively and upregulated by bacterial components during infection (Hao *et al.*, 2012; Zhang *et al.*, 2015). Manipulating this expression could be a means to increase the endogenous defence of the fish and reduce the risk of infection in aquaculture settings, due to both their direct antimicrobial and immunostimulatory capacities (D'Este *et al.*, 2016).

Regarding their processing, cathelicidin gene products are directed either to storage granules or secreted as the pro-forms.

Release of the active HDP occurs extracellularly, and requires serine proteases acting at the suitable conserved cleavage sites at the C-terminus of the CLD. Elastase has been identified as the operative protease in several mammals (Scocchi *et al.*, 1992; Shinnar *et al.*, 2003), but proteinase-3 acts in humans (Sørensen *et al.*, 2001; Zaiou and Gallo, 2002) (see Fig. 2.1), and an as yet unidentified protease in mice (Pestonjamasp *et al.*, 2001). The putative cleavage sites of avian, reptile, amphibian and fish cathelicidins suggests that elastase-like proteases are involved in release of their HDPs (Xiao *et al.*, 2006a; Sun *et al.*, 2015; Maier *et al.*, 2008; Wang *et al.*, 2008). However, cleavage sites present just upstream of the mature HDP in different species can be quite varied, and the operative proteases are unknown (Sun *et al.*, 2015), so that the actual sequence of several putative cathelicidin HDPs remains uncertain. Processing can be quite complex, and varies in different tissues. The human cathelicidin hCAP18 when secreted from eccrine glands or keratinocytes is processed by kallikrein serine proteases rather than proteinase-3, and the HDP further processed to shorter fragments (Murakami *et al.*, 2004; Yamasaki *et al.*, 2006). hCAP18 secreted in seminal plasma is processed by gastricsin, resulting in a longer peptide, ALL-38 (Andersson *et al.*, 2002). Cathelicidin HDPs sometimes end with a Gly residue at the stop-codon, which is a signal for amidation.

2.5 Structure-dependent Mode of Action

Cathelicidin HDPs essentially conform to the five structural types mentioned above: Type-α, -β, -PR, -WR and -GS, although some may contain features of more than one type (see Fig. 2.1). A common feature of all these peptides, in any case, is a marked cationicity that favours interaction with bacterial membranes. However, while most HDPs are assumed by default to be membrane active, the mode of action of cathelicidin HDPs does not necessarily involve bacterial membrane disruption as a primary mechanism.

Type-α helical peptides are considered to be primarily membranolytic, their cationic and amphipathic structure allowing efficient interaction with, and insertion into, the microbial membrane, followed by either a detergent-like disruption when a critical concentration is reached (carpet model), or cooperative formation of discrete cavities by a toroidal pore mechanism (see also Chapter 7 in Part IV). The active conformation of helical AMPs generally forms only on contact with the membrane, where the peptides undergo a transition from an unstructured globule present in bulk solution to a helical, rod-like conformation partly inserted into the lipid bilayer (see Fig. 2.3 steps ①+② and/or ③) (Xhindoli *et al.*, 2016). This behaviour is shown by several Type-α cathelicidins from both non-mammalian and mammalian vertebrates, but not by all of them.

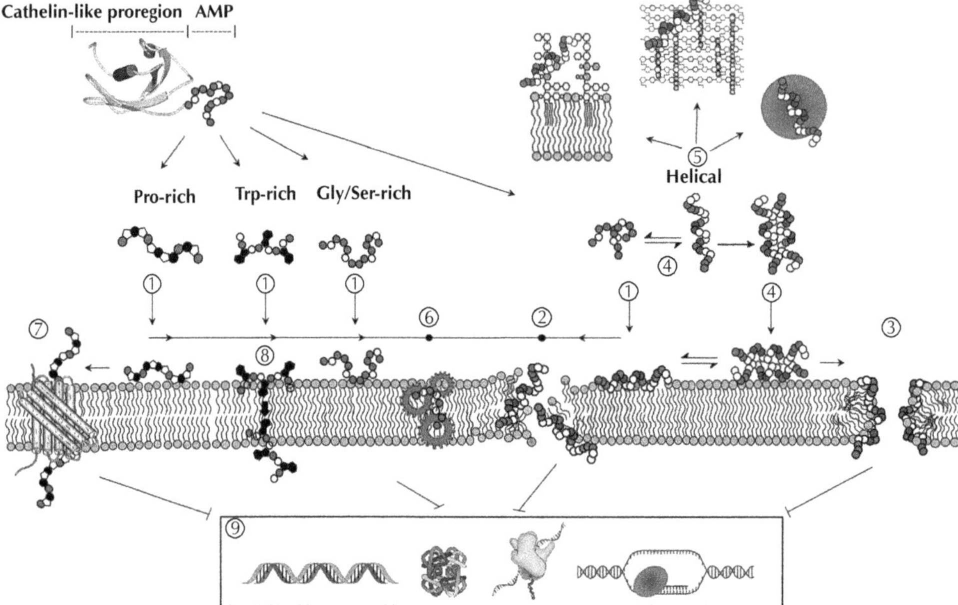

Fig. 2.3. Antibacterial modes of action of different cathelicidin HDPs. On release from the proregion, some cathelicidins have disordered structures in physiological bulk solution and approach bacterial membranes as such (1), and being cationic are electrostatically attracted to the anionic bacterial surface. Helical peptides undergo a transition from an unstructured globule to an extended, amphipathic, helical conformation that inserts into the membrane and when a critical concentration is reached, breach the membrane bilayer in a detergent-like manner (2), rather than forming discrete toroidal pores (3). Some helical peptides however adopt a helical structure already in bulk solution (4), and this drives aggregation. These peptides approach the membrane as oligomeric bundles and this favours the formation of toroidal pores. This type of helical peptide is more prone to interact with serum or medium components or outer components of the bacterial cell wall (5), so that their antimicrobial activity is more salt- and medium-sensitive. All structural types interact initially with the bacterial membrane surface, and at their active concentrations are likely to saturate it, so that interference with membrane-bound protein machinery is likely to contribute significantly to their activity (6). Pro/Arg-rich peptides such as bactenecins are then internalized by specific bacterial transport proteins (7) so that they can reach cytoplasmic targets (9) (ribosome sub-units and bacterial chaperones). Trp/Arg-rich peptides such as indolicidin have wedge-shaped structures that bind at the membrane surface interface and may then translocate into the bacterial cytoplasm in the manner of CPPs (cell penetrating peptides) (8). They also act on internal targets (9) selectively interfering with DNA transcription. Gly/Ser-rich peptides probably have intrinsically disordered structures and remain on the bacterial surface. Their precise mechanism of action is unknown, but the antimicrobial activity is quite salt-sensitive and not principally membranolytic.

Long helical peptides are present in all placental mammals (these are sometimes the only cathelicidin present, such as the human LL-37, and are indicated as Type-α° in Table 2.1) and can behave quite differently. They have evolved in different species to show a remarkable sequence diversity (which however mostly affects the balance of neutral polar, cationic and anionic residues) while the overall size, hydrophobicity and amphipathicity is well conserved (Xhindoli *et al.*, 2016). This results in a remarkable variation in the overall charge. Moreover, as all the charged residues (both cationic and anionic) cluster on one side when the helix forms, it also results in a diversified pattern of charged residues separated by 3 or 4 positions on the helix, which can engage in electrostatic attraction or repulsion. A preponderance of attractions (well balanced anionic and cationic residues, like in LL-37 at neutral pH) strongly increases the propensity for helix formation, even in the absence of membranes. This in turn drives a pH- and salt-dependent oligomerization so that the hydrophobic sector that forms on the other side of the helix can be removed from the aqueous environment (Johansson *et al.*, 1998; Zelezetsky and Tossi, 2006). As a consequence, these peptides tend to approach the membrane surface as oligomers, and this subsequently favours a toroidal mechanism for membrane permeabilization (Fig. 2.3 steps ④ + ③) (Morgera *et al.*, 2009; Xhindoli *et al.*, 2014, 2015), probably affecting the extent and kinetics of membrane permeabilization.

As another consequence, the preformed helices tend to be rather sticky and more prone to sequestering interactions with outer membrane or medium components (Fig. 2.3 steps ④ + ⑤) than peptides that remain as unstructured globules in bulk solution. This significantly affects their antimicrobial activity, making it more medium and salt sensitive (Tomasinsig *et al.*, 2009). In particular, it has been shown that the helical cathelicidin LL-37 interacts with phosphorylated *E. coli* lipopolysaccharide core sugars and *S. aureus* wall teichoic acid (Xhindoli *et al.*, 2014; Bociek

et al., 2015) in a manner that affects its antimicrobial activity differently to other helical cathelicidins. This observation cannot be explained only by differences in electrostatic interactions with these anionic cell wall components, as reported for other AMPs (Peschel *et al.*, 1999; Saar-Dover *et al.*, 2012).

Extending these considerations to known Type-α° orthologues in placental mammals, several show an excess of attractions over repulsions, and therefore likely have an augmented propensity for helix formation that favours toroidal pore formation. Several others instead show an excess of repulsions, and are therefore likely to act as unstructured monomers in bulk solution favouring a carpet-like mechanism (Xhindoli *et al.*, 2016).

With respect to the other types of linear peptides, Type-PR have a distinctive mode of action that does not involve membrane disruption, but an active transport mechanism, so that they can then interact with internal targets (Fig. 2.3 steps ① + ⑦ + ⑨). They have an extended structure in solution that does not greatly alter on contact with bacterial membranes, suggesting they remain surface bound (Cabiaux *et al.*, 1994; Tani *et al.*, 1995). They then accumulate on the surface and internalize into the cytoplasm of susceptible bacteria, at low micromolar concentrations, using specific membrane transporters. In *E. coli*, one transporter has been identified as the membrane protein SbmA (Mattiuzzo *et al.*, 2007; Runti *et al.*, 2013). This mechanism has been shown to hold also for unrelated PR-rich peptides from invertebrates, another example of convergent evolution of common structural and functional features. This mechanism is (i) highly selective, as only Gram-negative bacteria expressing this type of transport system are strongly affected (e.g. *E. coli*, *S. typhimurium* and *A. baumannii*, but not *P. aeruginosa* or Gram-positive bacteria), and (ii) highly stereoselective. Unlike membranolytic helical peptides that act equally well as left-handed helices formed by D-aminoacids, the all-D PR-rich peptides completely lose their activity (Scocchi *et al.*, 2011). This is probably due to the stereoselective interaction requirements for transport and/or cytoplasmic target inactivation (Guida *et al.*, 2015). The first internal target to be identified for PR-rich peptides in general (also confirmed for cathelicidins) was the chaperone DnaK (Cudic and Otvos Jr, 2002; Scocchi *et al.*, 2009), but a more important, recently identified target is the bacterial ribosome (Mardirossian *et al.*, 2014; Krizsan *et al.*, 2015; Gagnon *et al.*, 2016a; Seefeldt *et al.*, 2016). It appears that PR-rich bactenecins block the ribosomal peptide exit tunnel by occupying known antibiotic-binding sites, thus interfering with the initiation step and preventing entry into the elongation phase.

Type-WR peptides, such as bovine indolicidin and porcine tritrpticin (see Table 2.1 and Fig. 2.2), act by yet another apparently distinct mechanism. Given the abundance of both cationic Arg and aromatic Trp residues, they have a strong tendency to interact with bacterial membrane surfaces and then traverse the membrane to hit internal targets (Fig. 2.3 steps ⑧ + ⑨). These peptides adopt a wedge-shaped conformation (Schibli *et al.*, 1999; Rozek *et al.*, 2000) (see Fig. 2.2) and partition near the membrane–water interface (Chan *et al.*, 2006; Shagaghi *et al.*, 2016). Indolicidin then has the capacity, at its active concentration, to penetrate into the bacterial cell without causing massive membrane lysis (Hsu *et al.*, 2005), possibly aided by the abundance of Arg residues that confer the characteristics of cell penetrating peptides (Shagaghi *et al.*, 2016). Once in the bacterial cytoplasm it selectively inhibits DNA synthesis (Subbalakshmi and Sitaram, 1998; Hsu *et al.*, 2005; Ghosh *et al.*, 2014), by interacting with the DNA duplex. The mechanism for tritrpticin is not well defined but, given the similar structures, may be analogous.

Type-GS peptides have the least well defined mechanism of action, but again it appears to be distinctive, underlining how cathelicidins have sampled a very broad structural and functional space. These peptides tend to be quite long, and are sometimes heterogeneous in sequence with cysteine-bridged or other types of flanking domains (see Table 2.1). As a consequence, the mode of action has frequently been studied for rationally selected fragments rather than the whole peptide. In any case, the GS-rich domain is likely to have an intrinsically unstructured extended conformation that is not greatly affected by membrane interaction (Broekman *et al.*, 2011; D'Este *et al.*, 2016). They are also relatively poor in hydrophobic residues, so are likely to interact only with the surface of membranes, and their microbicidal mode of action, which is still uncertain, is quite salt sensitive. It is not as yet clear what steps follow membrane interaction (step ① in Fig. 2.3), and they seem to permeabilize the bacterial membrane relatively inefficiently and only under low salt conditions (Broekman *et al.*, 2011; D'Este *et al.*, 2016). Even less is known about how anuran GS-rich peptides function, but they are likely to have a similar characteristic to the fish peptides (Hao *et al.*, 2012).

Of the last group, the Type-β peptides, the interaction of protegrins with membranes has been extensively studied, using both NMR techniques and molecular modelling (Bolintineanu *et al.*, 2012; Lazaridis *et al.*, 2013; Usachev *et al.*, 2016). Their mode of action has not been inserted into Fig. 2.3 for space reasons, but these peptides are considered to act via a membranolytic mechanism with some analogies to that of the helical HDPs, including the fact that the mechanism of action is not sensitive to the stereochemistry (Chen *et al.*, 2000). Protegrins are monomeric but well structured in solution, due to the presence of disulfide bridges (Fahrner *et al.*, 1996), and initially interact electrostatically with the membrane, partly inserting hydrophobic residues on one face or tip of the hairpin into the lipid bilayer (Raj *et al.*, 2000; Lazaridis *et al.*, 2013). They then dimerize and further oligomerize and insert into the membrane to form an octameric pore. There is some debate as to how the dimerization and oligomerization steps proceed, and at what stage the peptide inserts into the membrane, but there is substantial agreement that these steps occur. Dodecapeptide also forms S-S-stabilized β-hairpins in solution and is thought to also dimerize at the bacterial surface (López-Oyama *et al.*, 2011; Madhongsa *et al.*, 2013), so they may act similarly. A twist to their mode of action may come from the possibility that they also form covalent dimers during biosynthesis, involving intermolecular disulfide bridge formation (P. Storici *et al.*, 1996). Curiously, an extended, parallel or antiparallel covalent dimeric arrangement does not have a dramatic effect on the antimicrobial activity with respect to that of the β-hairpin monomer (Lee *et al.*, 2008).

In summary, Type-α and Type-β peptides act via a membranolytic mechanism at low micromolar concentrations. Depending on the structure in bulk solution (disordered globule or preformed helix or β-hairpin conformation) they can then preferentially disrupt the membrane via a carpet-like detergent mechanism or pore formation. Type-WR, -PR and -GS peptides function by mechanisms other than membrane lysis in the same concentration range, and the first two types affect internal targets. All these peptides, however, first interact with and accumulate on the bacterial surface as a necessary part of their killing mechanism. If a sufficient concentration is reached, it can lead to membrane disruption in a detergent-like manner, irrespective of the structure (i.e. they all converge onto step ② of Fig. 2.3 at higher concentrations). Furthermore, one should always bear in mind that at their active concentrations HDPs completely saturate the bacterial surface, and so are likely to interfere with vital protein machinery residing in the bacterial membranes, thus affecting bioenergetics, transport and cell wall maintenance. This *sand-in-the-gearbox* effect could be a significant component of their killing mechanism (Fig. 2.3 step ⑥), irrespective of whether the peptides are membrane- or internally active (Pag *et al.*, 2008; Scocchi *et al.*, 2016). Furthermore, by the very nature of their mechanism, membrane-lytic peptides gain access to the bacterial cytoplasm, and there is mounting evidence that interaction with cytoplasmic targets (Fig. 2.3 step ⑨) contributes to their antimicrobial activity (see also Chapter 9 in

Part IV). For example, it has recently been shown that LL-37 can interfere with bacterial acyl-carrier protein (Chung *et al.*, 2015), and there are reports that lytic AMPs, being cationic, also interact with nucleic acids, which could affect replication or transcription.

2.6 Pleiotropic Roles of Cathelicidins in Host Defence and Potential Applications

On discovery, most cathelicidin HDPs are first evaluated for their direct antimicrobial activity *in vitro*, though this is not necessarily their principal role in host defence. They can affect other aspects of immunity and healing, by binding and sequestering bacterial components (e.g. LPS or LTA) (Nakamichi *et al.*, 2014) and thus reducing their pro-inflammatory effects, by helping to recruit or modulate the activities of host immune cells, or by stimulating cell growth in wound healing (Yang *et al.*, 2001; Ramanathan *et al.*, 2002; Lai and Gallo, 2009; Wu *et al.*, 2010; Chow *et al.*, 2013; Linde *et al.*, 2013). The literature on both direct antibiotic and host cell modulatory activities is burgeoning; more so considering the innumerable variants that have been designed through the years to obtain structure/function relationships or in the attempt to optimize the activity for potential therapeutic uses.

One could summarize the direct antibiotic activity of cathelicidin HDPs by indicating that those of Type-α and Type-β, acting via membranolytic mechanisms, tend to have the more potent and broad-spectrum antimicrobial activities *in vitro*. This also correlates with a discernible toxicity for eukaryotic cells at concentrations not appreciably higher than their active concentration. Much effort has been expended on sequence modifications that attempt to maintain the desirable antimicrobial activities while decreasing cytotoxicity, but it is objectively rather difficult to do this. For this reason, they are considered to have the best potential for topical uses. This includes use as inhalation agents to reduce airway infections, where efficacy, toxicity and susceptibility to degradation however still remain problematic (Kollef *et al.*, 2006; Vaara, 2009; Pompilio *et al.*, 2012; Mardirossian *et al.*, 2016).

The human helical cathelicidin LL-37 has received much attention as a potential therapeutic agent (Xhindoli *et al.*, 2016), with applications such as treatment of chronic, polymicrobially infected wounds (Duplantier and van Hoek, 2013). These exploit both its broad spectrum of activity, also against biofilm, and its capacity to stimulate re-epithelialization and angiogenesis. Results from a clinical study for the treatment of venous leg ulcers are encouraging (Grönberg *et al.*, 2014).

Type-β protegrins were developed for use in oral mucositis (Chen *et al.*, 2000), and a close analogue, iseganan, has been through clinical trials for use against oral mucositis, or for prevention of ventilator-associated pneumonia. In both cases, however, despite encouraging initial results, the trials failed due to insufficient efficacy. This lack of success has been ascribed to incorrect pharmacological usage (van Saene *et al.*, 2007), and recent clinical trials are more promising (Elad *et al.*, 2012).

The Type-WR cathelicidin indolicidin has been extensively tested for antimicrobial activity, which is quite broad spectrum (Chan *et al.*, 2006), but it has significant toxicity to host cells, probably due to the presence of numerous Trp residues (Ahmad *et al.*, 1995; Subbalakshmi *et al.*, 1996). For this reason it is also deemed most suitable for topical application and a close structural analogue of indolicidin, omiganan, is currently undergoing clinical testing for treatment of skin conditions and preventing catheter related infections (Sader *et al.*, 2004; Melo *et al.*, 2006).

Type-PR peptides are quite selective, acting principally by an intracellular mechanism on only a relatively narrow spectrum of Gram-negative bacteria, which includes enterobacteriaceae and Acinetobacter. *In vivo* tests have shown that bovine Bac7 has a good capacity to protect mice in a model of typhoid fever, with a very low toxicity, but unfortunately was rapidly cleared by renal excretion (Benincasa *et al.*, 2010). Polyethylene glycol/(PEG)ylated conjugates, linked either via a cleavable ester bond or non-hydrolysable amide bond, retained significant *in vitro* activity or significantly reduced clearance. The ester bond was cleaved in human serum or plasma, releasing the HDP and resulted in a higher activity, but it was interesting to note that the non-cleavable version still killed by internalizing into bacteria (Benincasa *et al.*, 2015). This suggests a capacity to internalize carrying quite sizeable cargos into bacterial cells, which could be a useful feature of this type of cathelicidins.

Type-GS peptides also tend to be broad-spectrum antimicrobials, but the antimicrobial activity is quite salt sensitive and the membrane permeabilization capacity is low (Broekman *et al.*, 2011; X.-J. Zhang *et al.*, 2015; D'Este *et al.*, 2016). Immunomodulatory activities were observed under isotonic conditions suggesting that they may have additional roles in defence beyond direct antimicrobial activity. In any case, they have not been as extensively studied as other cathelicidin AMPs, so that their potential is yet unclear.

Like other peptides involved in host defence, the effect of cathelicidin HDPs on host cells may be either beneficial (modulation of immune or inflammatory responses, stimulation of wound healing and angiogenesis), or detrimental (cytotoxic effects leading to necrosis or apoptosis). Concentrations leading to *in vitro* toxicity are generally higher than those required for *in vitro* antimicrobial activity or immunostimulatory effects, but this may not be sufficient for *in vivo* applications, thus requiring sequence optimization. As indicated above, Type-α, -β and -WR peptides have been investigated as therapeutic agents, but all show appreciable toxicity at active concentrations (Vaara, 2009). The human cathelicidin LL-37 has only a moderate and quite medium-sensitive selectivity for bacterial cells and has cytotoxic activities against erythrocytes, lymphocytes and fibroblasts (Oren *et al.*, 1999; Ciornei *et al.*, 2005). This is probably partly due to its helical, oligomeric nature in bulk solution (see Section

2.5). On the other hand this property may also underlie some of its immunomodulatory activities at non-toxic concentrations (Xhindoli *et al.*, 2016), as these are less evident in primate orthologues that do not oligomerize (Tomasinsig *et al.*, 2008).

It is interesting that some capacity to modulate host cell activities has been reported for all cathelicidin HDP types. Helical peptides, and in particular LL-37 and mouse CRAMP, have a plethora of reported activities (Kin *et al.*, 2011; Nakagawa and Gallo, 2015; Xhindoli *et al.*, 2016), but Type-WR indolicidin (Bowdish *et al.*, 2005; K. Yu *et al.*, 2015), Type-PR bactenecins (Djanani *et al.*, 2006; Tomasinsig *et al.*, 2006; Veldhuizen *et al.*, 2014) and Type-β protegrin analogues (Zughaier *et al.*, 2014; Gupta *et al.*, 2015) also show analogous activities, despite significant structural diversity. The capacity to neutralize bacterial endotoxin is another activity that is shared at comparable concentrations by all structural types of cathelicidins, as demonstrated using numerous *in vitro* and *in vivo* models (Ghiselli *et al.*, 2003; Zughaier *et al.*, 2005; Rosenfeld and Shai, 2006; Giuliani *et al.*, 2010; Xu-Jie Zhang *et al.*, 2015). Notably there are only a limited number of studies analysing in parallel the capacity of different cathelicidin types to affect host cell functions (e.g. chemotaxis, proliferation, cytokine gene expression (Verbanac *et al.*, 1993; Bowdish *et al.*, 2005; Tomasinsig *et al.*, 2010a, 2010b; Baumann *et al.*, 2014); autophagy (D'Este *et al.*, unpublished results) and angiogenesis (Tomasinsig *et al.*, unpublished results)). These studies highlight quantitative and qualitative differences among and within different structural types. Unfortunately, the lack of systematic comparative analyses does not yet allow us to assign precise biological functions to each of them.

It is generally supposed that cathelicidin peptides act on host cells via receptor activation, but how they exert their action is not well understood. For helical cathelicidins, it has been suggested that they interact with receptors in a non-canonical manner, by first interacting with and accumulating in the membrane surrounding different receptors, possibly preferring the cholesterol- and sphingomyelin-rich lipid rafts where they are located, and then interacting with their transmembrane domains rather than with specific ligand-binding sites (Tomasinsig *et al.*, 2008; Xhindoli *et al.*, 2016). It is possible that this also applies to the other structural types. This is consistent with the promiscuous and generally low-affinity type of activity that is generally observed, and is supported by the fact that for human LL-37, activation of different receptors by the all-*D* enantiomer is as effective as the native one (Braff *et al.*, 2005; Tomasinsig *et al.*, 2008). The enantiomer has a different stereochemistry but similar structuring, oligomerization and membrane interaction capacities.

It is interesting to note that different peptides may have evolved distinct mechanisms to accomplish the same tasks, as in the case of the angiogenic effect observed for LL-37 and PR-39. These appear to be mediated by interaction with quite different cellular targets (Li, J. *et al.*, 2000; Koczulla *et al.*, 2003). The former has a direct effect on endothelial cells specifically involving the receptor fPRL1, the latter by inhibiting the ubiquitin–proteasome-dependent degradation of hypoxia-inducible factor-1α protein. Another example of functional convergence may be represented by the capacity of these structurally distinct cathelicidins to promote healing (Gennaro *et al.*, 2002; Xhindoli *et al.*, 2016), further supporting the concept of convergent evolution towards protective roles in host defence.

2.7 Conclusions

Cathelicidins have a manifest role in vertebrate innate immunity, with a remarkably wide range of functions. These endogenous peptide antibiotics have accompanied vertebrate animals throughout their evolution, co-evolving with the host's immune system and the changing threats it has had to cope with. This has resulted in a comprehensive sampling of different active structures capable of inactivating bacteria with distinct mechanisms. Some cathelicidin HDPs have evolved the capacity to adopt stable helical or β-sheet conformations in physiological solutions, which determines how they approach biological membranes and then breach them by pore formation. Others adopt active structures only on contact with the membrane and disrupt it in a more detergent-like manner. Yet other types have extended, disordered or wedge-like structures in solution, interact more with the membrane surface and have evolved different ways to internalize into bacteria to inactivate cytoplasmic targets. This structural diversity also defines the toxicity of these endogenous antibiotics towards host cells and their capacity to modulate cellular activities in processes useful for host defence, at subtoxic concentrations. Our growing understanding of the interconnected factors that allow cathelicidins to carry out their important and wide-ranging immune functions may allow us to eventually exploit their considerable therapeutic potential, at a time when microbial resistance to conventional antibiotics has become a paramount global health problem.

References

Agerberth, B., Gunne, H., Odeberg, J., Kogner, P., Boman, H.G. and Gudmundsson, G.H. (1995) FALL-39, a putative human peptide antibiotic, is cysteine-free and expressed in bone marrow and testis. *Proceedings of the National Academy of Sciences of the United States of America* 92, 195–199.

Agerberth, B., Gunne, H., Odeberg, J., Kogner, P., Boman, H.G. and Gudmundsson, G.H. (1996) PR-39, a proline-rich peptide antibiotic from pig, and FALL-39, a tentative human counterpart. *Veterinary Immunology and Immunopathology* 54, 127–131.

Ahmad, I., Perkins, W.R., Lupan, D.M., Selsted, M.E. and Janoff, A.S. (1995) Liposomal entrapment of the neutrophil-derived peptide indolicidin endows it with in vivo antifungal activity. *Biochimica et Biophysica Acta (BBA) – Biomembranes* 1237, 109–114. DOI:10.1016/0005-2736(95)00087-J

Alibardi, L. (2014) Ultrastructural immunolocalization of chatelicidin-like peptides in granulocytes of normal and regenerating lizard tissues. *Acta Histochemica* 116, 363–371. DOI:10.1016/j.acthis.2013.08.014

Andersson, E., Sørensen, O.E., Frohm, B., Borregaard, N., Egesten, A. and Malm, J. (2002) Isolation of human cationic antimicrobial protein-18 from seminal plasma and its association with prostasomes. *Human Reproduction* 17, 2529–2534. DOI:10.1093/humrep/17.10.2529

Antcheva, N., Guida, F. and Tossi, A. (2013) Chapter 18, Defensins. In: Kastin, A.J. (ed.) *Handbook of Biologically Active Peptides* (2nd edn) Academic Press, Boston, MA, pp. 101–118.

Bals, R., Wang, X., Zasloff, M. and Wilson, J.M. (1998) The peptide antibiotic LL-37/hCAP-18 is expressed in epithelia of the human lung where it has broad antimicrobial activity at the airway surface. *Proceedings of the National Academy of Sciences of the United States of America* 95, 9541–9546.

Baumann, A., Démoulins, T., Python, S. and Summerfield, A. (2014) Porcine cathelicidins efficiently complex and deliver nucleic acids to plasmacytoid dendritic cells and can thereby mediate bacteria-induced IFN-α responses. *Journal of Immunology* 193, 364–371. DOI:10.4049/jimmunol.1303219

Benincasa, M., Pelillo, C., Zorzet, S., Garrovo, C., Biffi, S., Gennaro, R. and Scocchi, M. (2010) The proline-rich peptide Bac7(1-35) reduces mortality from *Salmonella typhimurium* in a mouse model of infection. *BMC Microbiology* 10, 178. DOI:10.1186/1471-2180-10-178

Benincasa, M., Zahariev, S., Pelillo, C., Milan, A., Gennaro, R. and Scocchi, M. (2015) PEGylation of the peptide Bac7(1-35) reduces renal clearance while retaining antibacterial activity and bacterial cell penetration capacity. *European Journal of Medicinal Chemistry* 95, 210–219. DOI:10.1016/j.ejmech.2015.03.028

Bociek, K., Ferluga, S., Mardirossian, M., Benincasa, M., Tossi, A., Gennaro, R. and Scocchi, M. (2015) Lipopolysaccharide phosphorylation by the WaaY Kinase affects the susceptibility of *Escherichia coli* to the human antimicrobial peptide LL-37. *Journal of Biological Chemistry* 290, 19933–19941. DOI:10.1074/jbc.M114.634758

Boehmer, J.L., Bannerman, D.D., Shefcheck, K. and Ward, J.L. (2008) Proteomic analysis of differentially expressed proteins in bovine milk during experimentally induced *Escherichia coli* mastitis. *Journal of Dairy Science* 91, 4206–4218. DOI:10.3168/jds.2008-1297

Bolintineanu, D.S., Vivcharuk, V. and Kaznessis, Y.N. (2012) Multiscale models of the antimicrobial peptide protegrin-1 on Gram-negative bacteria membranes. *International Journal of Molecular Sciences* 13, 11000–11011. DOI:10.3390/ijms130911000

Bommineni, Y.R., Dai, H., Gong, Y.-X., Soulages, J.L., Fernando, S.C., *et al.* (2007) Fowlicidin-3 is an alpha-helical cationic host defense peptide with potent antibacterial and lipopolysaccharide-neutralizing activities. *FEBS Journal* 274, 418–428. DOI:10.1111/j.1742-4658.2006.05589.x

Bowdish, D.M.E., Davidson, D.J., Scott, M.G. and Hancock, R.E.W. (2005) Immunomodulatory activities of small host defense peptides. *Antimicrobial Agents and Chemotherapy* 49, 1727–1732. DOI:10.1128/AAC.49.5.1727-1732.2005

Braff, M.H., Hawkins, M.A., Nardo, A.D., Lopez-Garcia, B. and Howell, M.D. (2005) Structure–function relationships among human cathelicidin peptides: dissociation of antimicrobial properties from host immunostimulatory activities. *Journal of Immunology* 174, 4271–4278. DOI:10.4049/jimmunol.174.7.4271

Brandenburg, L.-O., Jansen, S., Albrecht, L.-J., Merres, J., Gerber, J., Pufe, T. and Tauber, S.C. (2013) CpG oligodeoxynucleotides induce the expression of the antimicrobial peptide cathelicidin in glial cells. *Journal of Neuroimmunology* 255, 18–31. DOI:10.1016/j.jneuroim.2012.10.012

Broekman, D.C., Zenz, A., Gudmundsdottir, B.K., Lohner, K., Maier, V.H. and Gudmundsson, G.H. (2011) Functional characterization of codCath, the mature cathelicidin antimicrobial peptide from Atlantic cod (*Gadus morhua*) *Peptides* 32, 2044–2051. DOI:10.1016/j.peptides.2011.09.012

Cabiaux, V., Agerberth, B., Johansson, J., Homblé, F., Goormaghtigh, E. and Ruysschaert, J.-M. (1994) Secondary structure and membrane interaction of PR-39, a Pro+Arg-rich antibacterial peptide. *European Journal of Biochemistry* 224, 1019–1027. DOI:10.1111/j.1432-1033.1994.01019.x

Castiglioni, B., Scocchi, M., Zanetti, M. and Ferretti, L. (1996) Six antimicrobial peptide genes of the cathelicidin family map to bovine chromosome 22q24 by fluorescence in situ hybridization. *Cytogenetics and Cell Genetics* 75, 240–242.

Chan, D.I., Prenner, E.J. and Vogel, H.J. (2006) Tryptophan- and arginine-rich antimicrobial peptides: structures and mechanisms of action. *Biochimica et Biophysica Acta (BBA) – Biomembranes* 1758, 1184–1202. DOI:10.1016/j.bbamem.2006.04.006

Chen, C., Brock, R., Luh, F., Chou, P.-J., Larrick, J.W., Huang, R.-F. and Huang, T. (1995) The solution structure of the active domain of CAP18 – a lipopolysaccharide binding protein from rabbit leukocytes. *FEBS Letters* 370, 46–52. DOI:10.1016/0014-5793(95)00792-8

Chen, J., Falla, T.J., Liu, H., Hurst, M.A., Fujii, C.A., Mosca, D.A. and Embree, J.R., *et al.* (2000) Development of protegrins for the treatment and prevention of oral mucositis: structure–activity relationships of synthetic protegrin analogues. *Peptide Science* 55, 88–98. DOI:10.1002/1097-0282(2000)55:1<88::AID-BIP80>3.0.CO;2-K

Chow, J.Y.C., Li, Z.J., Wu, W.K.K. and Cho, C.H. (2013) Cathelicidin a potential therapeutic peptide for gastrointestinal inflammation and cancer. *World Journal of Gastroenterology* 19, 2731. DOI:10.3748/wjg.v19.i18.2731

Chung, M.-C., Dean, S.N. and Hoek, M.L. van, (2015) Acyl carrier protein is a bacterial cytoplasmic target of cationic antimicrobial peptide LL-37. *Biochemical Journal* 470, 243–253. DOI:10.1042/BJ20150432

Ciornei, C.D., Sigurdardottir, T., Schmidtchen, A. and Bodelsson, M. (2005) Antimicrobial and chemoattractant activity, lipopolysaccharide neutralization, cytotoxicity, and inhibition by serum of analogs of human cathelicidin LL-37. *Antimicrobial Agents and Chemotherapy* 49, 2845–2850. DOI:10.1128/AAC.49.7.2845-2850.2005

Cowland, J.B., Johnsen, A.H. and Borregaard, N. (1995) hCAP-18, a cathelin/pro-bactenecin-like protein of human neutrophil specific granules. *FEBS Letters* 368, 173–176. DOI:10.1016/0014-5793(95)00634-L

Cudic, M. and Otvos Jr, L. (2002) Intracellular targets of antibacterial peptides. *Current Drug Targets* 3, 101–106.

Del Sal, G., Storici, P., Schneider, C., Romeo, D. and Zanetti, M. (1992) CDNA cloning of the neutrophil bactericidal peptide indolicidin. *Biochemical and Biophysical Research Communications* 187, 467–472. DOI:10.1016/S0006-291X(05)81517-7

D'Este, F., Benincasa, M., Cannone, G., Furlan, M., Scarsini, M., *et al.* (2016) Antimicrobial and host cell-directed activities of Gly/Ser-rich peptides from salmonid cathelicidins. *Fish and Shellfish Immunology* 59, 456–468. DOI:10.1016/j.fsi.2016.11.004

Dixon, B.M., Barker, T., McKinnon, T., Cuomo, J., Frei, B., Borregaard, N. and Gombart, A.F. (2012) Positive correlation between circulating cathelicidin antimicrobial peptide (hCAP18/LL-37) and 25-hydroxyvitamin D levels in healthy adults. *BMC Research Notes* 5, 575.

Djanani, A., Mosheimer, B., Kaneider, N.C., Ross, C.R., Ricevuti, G., Patsch, J.R. and Wiedermann, C.J. (2006) Heparan sulfate proteoglycan-dependent neutrophil chemotaxis toward PR-39 cathelicidin. *Journal of Inflammation* 3, 14. DOI:10.1186/1476-9255-3-14

Dorschner, R.A., Lin, K.H., Murakami, M. and Gallo, R.L. (2003) Neonatal skin in mice and humans expresses increased levels of antimicrobial peptides: innate immunity during development of the adaptive response. *Pediatric Research* 53, 566–572. DOI:10.1203/01.PDR.0000057205.64451.B7

Doss, M., White, M.R., Tecle, T. and Hartshorn, K.L. (2010) Human defensins and LL-37 in mucosal immunity. *Journal of Leukocyte Biology* 87, 79–92. DOI:10.1189/jlb.0609382

Duplantier, A.J. and van Hoek, M.L. (2013) The human cathelicidin antimicrobial peptide LL-37 as a potential treatment for polymicrobial infected wounds. Front. *Immunology* 4. DOI:10.3389/fimmu.2013.00143

Elad, S., Epstein, J.B., Raber-Durlacher, J., Donnelly, P. and Strahilevitz, J. (2012) The antimicrobial effect of Iseganan HCl oral solution in patients receiving stomatotoxic chemotherapy: analysis from a multicenter, double-blind, placebo-controlled, randomized, phase III clinical trial. *Journal of Oral Pathology and Medicine* 41, 229–234. DOI:10.1111/j.1600-0714.2011.01094.x

Fahrner, R.L., Dieckmann, T., Harwig, S.S., Lehrer, R.I., Eisenberg, D. and Feigon, J. (1996) Solution structure of protegrin-1, a broad-spectrum antimicrobial peptide from porcine leukocytes. *Chemical Biology* 3, 543–550.

Falcao, C.B., Pérez-Peinado, C., de la Torre, B.G., Mayol, X., Zamora-Carreras, H., *et al.* (2015) Structural dissection of Crotalicidin, a rattlesnake venom cathelicidin, retrieves a fragment with antimicrobial and antitumor activity. *Journal of Medicinal Chemistry* 58, 8553–8563. DOI:10.1021/acs.jmedchem.5b01142

Frank, R.W., Gennaro, R., Schneider, K., Przybylski, M. and Romeo, D. (1990) Amino acid sequences of two proline-rich bactenecins: antimicrobial peptides of bovine neutrophils. *Journal of Biological Chemistry* 265, 18871–18874.

Gagnon, M.G., Roy, R.N., Lomakin, I.B., Florin, T., Mankin, A.S. and Steitz, T.A. (2016) Structures of proline-rich peptides bound to the ribosome reveal a common mechanism of protein synthesis inhibition. *Nucleic Acids Research* 44, 2439–2450. DOI:10.1093/nar/gkw018

Gennaro, R. and Zanetti, M. (2000) Structural features and biological activities of the cathelicidin-derived antimicrobial peptides. *Peptide Science* 55, 31–49. DOI:10.1002/1097-0282(2000)55:1<31::AID-BIP40>3.0.CO;2-9

Gennaro, R., Skerlavaj, B. and Romeo, D. (1989) Purification, composition, and activity of two bactenecins, antibacterial peptides of bovine neutrophils. *Infection and Immunity* 57, 3142–3146.

Gennaro, R., Zanetti, M., Benincasa, M., Podda, E. and Miani, M. (2002) Pro-rich antimicrobial peptides from animals: structure, biological functions and mechanism of action. *Current Pharmaceutical Design* 8, 763–778.

Ghiselli, R., Giacometti, A., Cirioni, O., Circo, R., Mocchegiani, F., *et al.* (2003) Neutralization of endotoxin *in vitro* and *in vivo* by Bac7(1-35), a proline-rich antibacterial peptide. *Shock (Augusta, Ga.)* 19, 577–581. DOI:10.1097/01.shk.0000055236.26446.c9

Ghosh, A., Kar, R.K., Jana, J., Saha, A., Jana, B., *et al.* (2014) Indolicidin targets duplex DNA: structural and mechanistic insight through a combination of spectroscopy and microscopy. *ChemMedChem* 9, 2052–2058. DOI:10.1002/cmdc.201402215

Giuliani, A., Pirri, G. and Rinaldi, A.C. (2010) Antimicrobial peptides: the LPS connection. *Methods Mol. Biol. Clifton NJ* 618, 137–154. DOI:10.1007/978-1-60761-594-1_10

Gombart, A.F. (2009) The vitamin D–antimicrobial peptide pathway and its role in protection against infection. *Future Microbiology* 4, 1151–1165. DOI:10.2217/fmb.09.87

Grönberg, A., Mahlapuu, M., Ståhle, M., Whately-Smith, C. and Rollman, O. (2014) Treatment with LL-37 is safe and effective in enhancing healing of hard-to-heal venous leg ulcers: a randomized, placebo-controlled clinical trial. *Wound Repair and Regeneration* 22, 613–621. DOI:10.1111/wrr.12211

Guida, F., Benincasa, M., Zahariev, S., Scocchi, M., Berti, F., Gennaro, R. and Tossi, A. (2015) Effect of size and N-terminal residue characteristics on bacterial cell penetration and antibacterial activity of the proline-rich peptide Bac7. *Journal of Medicinal Chemistry* 58, 1195–1204. DOI:10.1021/jm501367p

Gupta, K., Kotian, A., Subramanian, H., Daniell, H. and Ali, H. (2015) Activation of human mast cells by retrocyclin and protegrin highlight their immunomodulatory and antimicrobial properties. *Oncotarget* 6, 28573–28587.

Hao, X., Yang, H., Wei, L., Yang, S., Zhu, W., Ma, D., Yu, H. and Lai, R. (2012) Amphibian cathelicidin fills the evolutionary gap of cathelicidin in vertebrate. *Amino Acids* 43, 677–685. DOI:10.1007/s00726-011-1116-7

Hennig-Pauka, I., Jacobsen, I., Blecha, F., Waldmann, K.-H. and Gerlach, G.-F. (2006) Differential proteomic analysis reveals increased cathelicidin expression in porcine bronchoalveolar lavage fluid after an *Actinobacillus pleuropneumoniae* infection. *Veterinary Research* 37, 13. DOI:10.1051/vetres:2005043

Hsu, C.-H., Chen, C., Jou, M.-L., Lee, A.Y.-L., Lin, Y.-C., *et al.* (2005) Structural and DNA-binding studies on the bovine antimicrobial peptide, indolicidin: evidence for multiple conformations involved in binding to membranes and DNA. *Nucleic Acids Research* 33, 4053–4064. DOI:10.1093/nar/gki725

Huttner, K.M., Lambeth, M.R., Burkin, H.R., Burkin, D.J. and Broad, T.E. (1998) Localization and genomic organization of sheep antimicrobial peptide genes. *Gene* 206, 85–91.

Iimura, M., Gallo, R.L., Hase, K., Miyamoto, Y., Eckmann, L. and Kagnoff, M.F. (2005) Cathelicidin mediates innate intestinal defense against colonization with epithelial adherent bacterial pathogens. *Journal of Immunology* 174, 4901–4907. DOI:10.4049/jimmunol.174.8.4901

Jenssen, H., Hilpert, K. and Hancock, R.E. (2007) Antibacterial host defence peptides of bovine origin. *Chimica Oggi* 25, 17–19.

Johansson, J., Gudmundsson, G.H., Rottenberg, M.E., Berndt, K.D. and Agerberth, B. (1998) Conformation-dependent antibacterial activity of the naturally occurring human peptide LL-37. *Journal of Biological Chemistry* 273, 3718–3724. DOI:10.1074/jbc.273.6.3718

Kin, N.W., Chen, Y., Stefanov, E.K., Gallo, R.L. and Kearney, J.F. (2011) Cathelin-related antimicrobial peptide differentially regulates T- and B-cell function. *European Journal of Immunology* 41, 3006–3016. DOI:10.1002/eji.201141606

Koczulla, R., von Degenfeld, G., Kupatt, C., Krötz, F., Zahler, S., *et al.* (2003) An angiogenic role for the human peptide antibiotic LL-37/hCAP-18. *Journal of Clinical Investigation* 111, 1665–1672. DOI:10.1172/JCI200317545

Kollef, M., Pittet, D., Sánchez García, M., Chastre, J., Fagon, J.-Y., *et al.* (2006) A randomized double-blind trial of iseganan in prevention of ventilator-associated pneumonia. *American Journal of Respiratory and Critical Care Medicine* 173, 91–97. DOI:10.1164/rccm.200504-656OC

Kościuczuk, E.M., Lisowski, P., Jarczak, J., Krzyżewski, J., Zwierzchowski, L. and Bagnicka, E. (2014) Expression patterns of β-defensin and cathelicidin genes in parenchyma of bovine mammary gland infected with coagulase-positive or coagulase-negative Staphylococci. *Veterinary. Research* 10. DOI:10.1186/s12917-014-0246-z

Kovach, M.A., Ballinger, M.N., Newstead, M.W., Zeng, X., Bhan, U., *et al.* (2012) Cathelicidin related antimicrobial peptide is required for effective lung mucosal immunity in Gram-negative bacterial pneumonia. *Journal of Immunology* 189, 304–311. DOI:10.4049/jimmunol.1103196

Krizsan, A., Knappe, D. and Hoffmann, R. (2015) Influence of the *yjiL-mdtM* gene cluster on the antibacterial activity of proline-rich antimicrobial peptides overcoming *Escherichia coli* resistance induced by the missing SbmA transporter system. *Antimicrobial Agents and Chemotherapy* 59, 5992–5998. DOI:10.1128/AAC.01307-15

Lai, Y. and Gallo, R.L. (2009) AMPed up immunity: how antimicrobial peptides have multiple roles in immune defense. *Trends in Immunology* 30, 131–141. DOI:10.1016/j.it.2008.12.003

Larrick, J.W., Morgan, J.G., Palings, I., Hirata, M. and Yen, M.H. (1991) Complementary DNA sequence of rabbit CAP18 – a unique lipopolysaccharide binding protein. *Biochemical and Biophysical Research Communications* 179, 170–175. DOI:10.1016/0006-291X(91)91350-L

Larrick, J.W., Hirata, M., Balint, R.F., Lee, J., Zhong, J. and Wright, S.C. (1995) Human CAP18: a novel antimicrobial lipopolysaccharide-binding protein. *Infection and Immunity* 63, 1291–1297.

Larrick, J.W., Lee, J., Ma, S., Li, X., Francke, U., Wright, S.C. and Balint, R.F. (1996) Structural, functional analysis and localization of the human CAP18 gene. *FEBS Letters* 398, 74–80. DOI:10.1016/S0014-5793(96)01199-4

Lazaridis, T., He, Y., Prieto, L. (2013) Membrane interactions and pore formation by the antimicrobial peptide protegrin. *Biophysical Journal* 104, 633–642. DOI:10.1016/j.bpj.2012.12.038

Lee, J.Y., Yang, S.-T., Lee, S.K., Jung, H.H., Shin, S.Y., Hahm, K.-S. and Kim, J.I. (2008) Salt-resistant homodimeric bactenecin, a cathelicidin-derived antimicrobial peptide. *FEBS Journal* 275, 3911–3920. DOI:10.1111/j.1742-4658.2008.06536.x

Lenarčič, B., Ritonja, A., Dolenc, I., Stoka, V., Berbič, S., *et al.* (1993) Pig leukocyte cysteine proteinase inhibitor (PLCPI), a new member of the stefin family. *FEBS Letters* 336, 289–292. DOI:10.1016/0014-5793(93)80822-C

Li, J., Post, M., Volk, R., Gao, Y., Li, M., *et al.* (2000) PR39, a peptide regulator of angiogenesis. *Nature Medicine* 6, 49–55.

Linde, A., Lushington, G.H., Abello, J. and Melgarejo, T., (2013) Clinical relevance of cathelicidin in infectious disease. *Journal of Clinical and Cellular Immunology.* DOI:10.4172/2155-9899. S13-003

López-Oyama, A.B., Taboada, P., Burboa, M.G., Rodríguez, E., Mosquera, V., Valdez, M.A. (2011) Interaction of the cationic peptide bactenecin with mixed phospholipid monolayers at the air–water interface. *Journal of Colloid and Interface Science* 359, 279–288. DOI:10.1016/j.jcis.2011.03.081

Lu, Z., Wang, Y., Zhai, L., Che, Q., Wang, H., *et al.* (2010) Novel cathelicidin-derived antimicrobial peptides from *Equus asinus. FEBS Journal* 277, 2329–2339. DOI:10.1111/j.1742-4658.2010.07648.x

Madhongsa, K., Pasan, S., Phophetleb, O., Nasompag, S., Thammasirirak, S., *et al.* (2013) Antimicrobial action of the cyclic peptide Bactenecin on *Burkholderia pseudomallei* correlates with efficient membrane permeabilization. *PLoS Neglected Tropical Diseases* 7. DOI:10.1371/journal.pntd.0002267

Maier, V.H., Dorn, K.V., Gudmundsdottir, B.K. and Gudmundsson, G.H. (2008) Characterisation of cathelicidin gene family members in divergent fish species. *Molecular Immunology* 45, 3723–3730. DOI:10.1016/j.molimm.2008.06.002

Mardirossian, M., Grzela, R., Giglione, C., Meinnel, T., Gennaro, R., Mergaert, P. and Scocchi, M. (2014) The host antimicrobial peptide Bac71-35 binds to bacterial ribosomal proteins and inhibits protein synthesis. *Chemical Biology* 21, 1639–1647. DOI:10.1016/j.chembiol.2014.10.009

Mardirossian, M., Pompilio, A., Crocetta, V., Nicola, S.D., Guida, F., *et al.* (2016) In vitro and in vivo evaluation of BMAP-derived peptides for the treatment of cystic fibrosis-related pulmonary infections. *Amino Acids* 48, 2253–2260. DOI:10.1007/s00726-016-2266-4

Marzari, R., Scaggiante, B., Skerlavaj, B., Bittolo, M., Gennaro, R. and Romeo, D. (1988) Small, antibacterial and large, inactive peptides of neutrophil granules share immunoreactivity to a monoclonal antibody. *Infection and Immunity* 56, 2193–2197.

Mattiuzzo, M., Bandiera, A., Gennaro, R., Benincasa, M., Pacor, S., Antcheva, N. and Scocchi, M. (2007) Role of the *Escherichia coli* SbmA in the antimicrobial activity of proline-rich peptides. *Molecular Microbiology* 66, 151–163. DOI:10.1111/j.1365-2958.2007.05903.x

Melo, M.N., Dugourd, D. and Castanho, M.A.R.B. (2006) Omiganan pentahydrochloride in the front line of clinical applications of antimicrobial peptides. *Recent Patents on Anti-Infective Drug Discovery* 1, 201–207.

Ménard, S., Förster, V., Lotz, M., Gütle, D., Duerr, C.U., *et al.* (2008) Developmental switch of intestinal antimicrobial peptide expression. *Journal of Experimental Medicine* 205, 183–193. DOI:10.1084/jem.20071022

Méndez-Samperio, P. (2010) The human cathelicidin hCAP18/LL-37: a multifunctional peptide involved in mycobacterial infections. *Peptides* 31, 1791–1798. DOI:10.1016/j.peptides.2010.06.016

Mookherjee, N., Brown, K.L. and Hancock, R.E.W. (2013) Cathelicidin. In: *Handbook of Biologically Active Peptides.* Academic Press, pp. 77–84.

Morgera, F., Vaccari, L., Antcheva, N., Scaini, D., Pacor, S. and Tossi, A. (2009) Primate cathelicidin orthologues display different structures and membrane interactions. *Biochemical Journal* 417, 727. DOI:10.1042/BJ20081726

Murakami, M., Lopez-Garcia, B., Braff, M., Dorschner, R.A. and Gallo, R.L. (2004) Postsecretory processing generates multiple cathelicidins for enhanced topical antimicrobial defense. *Journal of Immunology* 172, 3070–3077. DOI:10.4049/jimmunol.172.5.3070

Nagaoka, I., Hirota, S., Yomogida, S., Ohwada, A. and Hirata, M. (2000) Synergistic actions of antibacterial neutrophil defensins and cathelicidins. *Inflammation Research* 49, 73–79. DOI:10.1007/s000110050561

Nakagawa, Y. and Gallo, R.L. (2015) Endogenous intracellular cathelicidin enhances TLR9 activation in dendritic cells and macrophages. *Journal of Immunology* 194, 1274–1284. DOI:10.4049/jimmunol.1402388

Nakamichi, Y., Horibe, K., Takahashi, N. and Udagawa, N. (2014) Roles of cathelicidins in inflammation and bone loss. *Odontology* 102, 137–146. DOI:10.1007/s10266-014-0167-0

Nell, M.J., Sandra Tjabringa, G., Vonk, M.J., Hiemstra, P.S. and Grote, J.J. (2004) Bacterial products increase expression of the human cathelicidin hCAP-18/LL-37 in cultured human sinus epithelial cells. *FEMS Immunology and Medical. Microbiology* 42, 225–231. DOI:10.1016/j.femsim.2004.05.013

Oren, Z., Lerman, J.C., Gudmundsson, G.H., Agerberth, B. and Shai, Y. (1999) Structure and organization of the human antimicrobial peptide LL-37 in phospholipid membranes: relevance to the molecular basis for its non-cell-selective activity. *Biochemical Journal* 341, 501–513.

Pag, U., Oedenkoven, M., Sass, V., Shai, Y., Shamova, O., *et al.* (2008) Analysis of in vitro activities and modes of action of synthetic antimicrobial peptides derived from an alpha-helical 'sequence template'. *Journal of Antimicrobial Chemotherapy* 61, 341–352. DOI:10.1093/jac/dkm479

Park, K., Oh, D., Yub Shin, S., Hahm, K.-S. and Kim, Y. (2002) Structural studies of porcine myeloid antibacterial peptide PMAP-23 and its analogues in DPC Micelles by NMR spectroscopy. *Biochemical and Biophysical Research Communications* 290, 204–212. DOI:10.1006/bbrc.2001.6173

Pazgier, M., Ericksen, B., Ling, M., Toth, E., Shi, J., *et al.* (2013) Structural and functional analysis of the pro-domain of human cathelicidin, LL-37. *Biochemistry* 52, 1547–1558. DOI:10.1021/bi301008r

Peschel, A., Otto, M., Jack, R.W., Kalbacher, H., Jung, G. and Götz, F. (1999) Inactivation of the dlt Operon in *Staphylococcus aureus* confers sensitivity to defensins, protegrins, and other antimicrobial peptides. *Journal of Biological Chemistry* 274, 8405–8410. DOI:10.1074/jbc.274.13.8405

Pestonjamasp, V.K., Huttner, K.H. and Gallo, R.L. (2001) Processing site and gene structure for the murine antimicrobial peptide CRAMP. *Peptides* 22, 1643–1650.

Pompilio, A., Crocetta, V., Scocchi, M., Pomponio, S., Di Vincenzo, V., *et al.* (2012) Potential novel therapeutic strategies in cystic fibrosis: antimicrobial and anti-biofilm activity of natural and designed α-helical peptides against *Staphylococcus aureus, Pseudomonas aeruginosa,* and *Stenotrophomonas maltophilia. BMC Microbiology* 12, 145. DOI:10.1186/1471-2180-12-145

Popsueva, A.E., Zinovjeva, M.V., Visser, J.W., Zijlmans, J.M., Fibbe, W.E. and Belyavsky, A.V. (1996) A novel murine cathelin-like protein expressed in bone marrow. *FEBS Letters* 391, 5–8.

Raj, P.A., Karunakaran T. and Sukumaran, D.K. (2000) Synthesis, microbicidal activity, and solution structure of the dodecapeptide from bovine neutrophils. *Biopolymers* 53, 281–292. DOI:10.1002/(SICI)1097-0282(20000405)53:4<281::AID-BIP1>3.0.CO;2-2

Ramanathan, B., Davis, E.G., Ross, C.R. and Blecha, F. (2002) Cathelicidins: microbicidal activity, mechanisms of action, and roles in innate immunity. *Microbes and Infection* 4, 361–372. DOI:10.1016/S1286-4579(02)01549-6

Ritonja, A., Kopitar, M., Jerala, R. and Turk, V. (1989) Primary structure of a new cysteine proteinase inhibitor from pig leucocytes. *FEBS Letters* 255, 211–214.

Romeo, D., Skerlavaj, B., Bolognesi, M. and Gennaro, R. (1988) Structure and bactericidal activity of an antibiotic dodecapeptide purified from bovine neutrophils. *Journal of Biological Chemistry* 263, 9573–9575.

Rosenfeld, Y. and Shai, Y. (2006) Lipopolysaccharide (endotoxin)-host defense antibacterial peptides interactions: role in bacterial resistance and prevention of sepsis. *Biochimica et Biophysica Acta (BBA) – Biomembranes* 1758, 1513–1522. DOI:10.1016/j.bbamem.2006.05.017

Rozek, A., Friedrich, C.L. and Hancock, R.E.W. (2000) Structure of the bovine antimicrobial peptide indolicidin bound to dodecylphosphocholine and sodium dodecyl sulfate micelles. *Biochemistry* 39, 15765–15774. DOI:10.1021/bi000714m

Runti, G., Lopez Ruiz, M.D.C., Stoilova, T., Hussain, R., Jennions, M., *et al.* (2013) Functional characterization of SbmA, a bacterial inner membrane transporter required for importing the antimicrobial peptide Bac7(1-35) *Journal of Bacteriology* 195, 5343–5351. DOI:10.1128/JB.00818-13

Saar-Dover, R., Bitler, A., Nezer, R., Shmuel-Galia, L., Firon, A., *et al.* (2012) D-alanylation of lipoteichoic acids confers resistance to cationic peptides in Group B streptococcus by increasing the cell wall density. *PLoS Pathogens* 8, e1002891. DOI:10.1371/journal.ppat.1002891

Sader, H.S., Fedler, K.A., Rennie, R.P., Stevens, S. and Jones, R.N. (2004) Omiganan pentahydrochloride (MBI 226), a topical 12-amino-acid cationic peptide: spectrum of antimicrobial activity and measurements of bactericidal activity. *Antimicrobial Agents and Chemotherapy* 48, 3112–3118. DOI:10.1128/AAC.48.8.3112-3118.2004

Sanchez, J.-F., Hoh, F., Strub, M.-P., Aumelas, A. and Dumas, C. (2002a) Structure of the cathelicidin motif of protegrin-3 precursor: structural insights into the activation mechanism of an antimicrobial protein. *Structure* 10, 1363–1370. DOI:10.1016/S0969-2126(02)00859-6

Sanchez, J.F., Wojcik, F., Yang, Y.-S., Strub, M.-P., Strub, J.M., *et al.* (2002b) Overexpression and structural study of the cathelicidin motif of the protegrin-3 precursor. *Biochemistry* 41, 21–30. DOI:10.1021/bi010930a

Sang, Y., Teresa Ortega, M., Rune, K., Xiau, W., Zhang, G., *et al.* (2007) Canine cathelicidin (K9CATH): gene cloning, expression, and biochemical activity of a novel pro-myeloid antimicrobial peptide. *Developmental and Comparative Immunology* 31, 1278–1296. DOI:10.1016/j.dci.2007.03.007

Schauber, J., Iffland, K., Frisch, S., Kudlich, T., Schmausser, B., *et al.* (2004) Histone-deacetylase inhibitors induce the cathelicidin LL-37 in gastrointestinal cells. *Molecular Immunology* 41, 847–854. DOI:10.1016/j.molimm.2004.05.005

Schauber, J., Dorschner, R.A., Yamasaki, K., Brouha, B. and Gallo, R.L. (2006) Control of the innate epithelial antimicrobial response is cell-type specific and dependent on relevant microenvironmental stimuli. *Immunology* 118, 509–519. DOI:10.1111/j.1365-2567.2006.02399.x

Schauber, J. and Gallo, R.L. (2008) Antimicrobial peptides and the skin immune defense system. *Journal of Allergy and Clinical Immunology* 122, 261–266. DOI:10.1016/j.jaci.2008.03.027

Schibli, D.J., Hwang, P.M. and Vogel, H.J. (1999) Structure of the antimicrobial peptide tritrpticin bound to micelles: a distinct membrane-bound peptide fold. *Biochemistry* 38, 16749–16755. DOI:10.1021/bi990701c

Scocchi, M., Skerlavaj, B., Romeo, D. and Gennaro, R. (1992) Proteolytic cleavage by neutrophil elastase converts inactive storage proforms to antibacterial bactenecins. *European Journal of Biochemistry* 209, 589–595. DOI:10.1111/j.1432-1033.1992.tb17324.x

Scocchi, M., Wang, S. and Zanetti, M. (1997) Structural organization of the bovine cathelicidin gene family and identification of a novel member. *FEBS Letters* 417, 311–315.

Scocchi, M., Lüthy, C., Decarli, P., Mignogna, G., Christen, P. and Gennaro, R. (2009) The proline-rich antibacterial peptide Bac7 binds to and inhibits in vitro the molecular chaperone DnaK. *International Journal of Peptide Research and Therapeutics* 15, 147–155. DOI:10.1007/s10989-009-9182-3

Scocchi, M., Tossi, A. and Gennaro, R. (2011) Proline-rich antimicrobial peptides: converging to a non-lytic mechanism of action. *Cellular and Molecular Life Sciences* 68, 2317–2330. DOI:10.1007/s00018-011-0721-7

Scocchi, M., Mardirossian, M., Runti, G. and Benincasa, M. (2016) Non-membrane permeabilizing modes of action of antimicrobial peptides on bacteria. *Current Topics in Medicinal Chemistry* 16, 76–88.

Seefeldt, A.C., Graf, M., Pérébaskine, N., Nguyen, F., Arenz, S., *et al.* (2016) Structure of the mammalian antimicrobial peptide Bac7(1-16) bound within the exit tunnel of a bacterial ribosome. *Nucleic Acids Research* 44, 2429–2438. DOI:10.1093/nar/gkv1545

Segaert, S. (2008) Vitamin D regulation of cathelicidin in the skin: toward a renaissance of vitamin D in dermatology? *Journal of Investigative Dermatology* 128, 773–775. DOI:10.1038/jid.2008.35

Selsted, M.E., Novotny, M.J., Morris, W.L., Tang, Y.Q., Smith, W. and Cullor, J.S. (1992) Indolicidin, a novel bactericidal tridecapeptide amide from neutrophils. *Journal of Biological Chemistry* 267, 4292–4295.

Shagaghi, N., Palombo, E.A., Clayton, A.H.A. and Bhave, M. (2016) Archetypal tryptophan-rich antimicrobial peptides: properties and applications. *World Journal of Microbiology and Biotechnology* 32, 31. DOI:10.1007/s11274-015-1986-z

Shinnar, A.E., Butler, K.L. and Park, H.J. (2003) Cathelicidin family of antimicrobial peptides: proteolytic processing and protease resistance. *Bioorganic Chemistry* 31, 425–436. DOI:10.1016/S0045-2068(03)00080-4

Smolenski, G.A., Wieliczko, R.J., Pryor, S.M., Broadhurst, M.K., Wheeler, T.T. and Haigh, B.J. (2011) The abundance of milk cathelicidin proteins during bovine mastitis. *Veterinary Immunology and Immunopathology* 143, 125–130. DOI:10.1016/j.vetimm.2011.06.034

Sørensen, O. and Borregaard, N. (2005) Cathelicidins – Nature's attempt at combinatorial chemistry. *Combinatorial Chemistry and High Throughput Screening* 8, 273–280.

Sørensen, O., Cowland, J.B., Askaa, J. and Borregaard, N. (1997) An ELISA for hCAP-18, the cathelicidin present in human neutrophils and plasma. *Journal of Immunological Methods* 206, 53–59. DOI:10.1016/S0022-1759(97)00084-7

Sørensen, O., Bratt, T., Johnsen, A.H., Madsen, M.T. and Borregaard, N. (1999) The human antibacterial cathelicidin, hCAP-18, is bound to lipoproteins in plasma. *Journal of Biological Chemistry* 274, 22445–22451.

Sørensen, O.E., Follin, P., Johnsen, A.H., Calafat, J., Tjabringa, G.S., Hiemstra, P.S. and Borregaard, N. (2001) Human cathelicidin, hCAP-18, is processed to the antimicrobial peptide LL-37 by extracellular cleavage with proteinase 3. *Blood* 97, 3951–3959.

Stie, J., Jesaitis, A.V., Lord, C.I., Gripentrog, J.M., Taylor, R.M., Burritt, J.B. and Jesaitis, A.J. (2007) Localization of hCAP-18 on the surface of chemoattractant-stimulated human granulocytes: analysis using two novel hCAP-18-specific monoclonal antibodies. *Journal of Leukocyte Biology* 82, 161–172. DOI:10.1189/jlb.0906586

Storici, P., Del Sal, G., Schneider, C. and Zanetti, M. (1992) cDNA sequence analysis of an antibiotic dodecapeptide from neutrophils. *FEBS Letters* 314, 187–190. DOI:10.1016/0014-5793(92)80971-I

Storici, P., Tossi, A., Lenarčič, B. and Romeo, D. (1996) Purification and structural characterization of bovine cathelicidins, precursors of antimicrobial peptides. *European Journal of Biochemistry* 238, 769–776. DOI:10.1111/j.1432-1033.1996.0769w.x

Subbalakshmi, C. and Sitaram, N. (1998) Mechanism of antimicrobial action of indolicidin. *FEMS Microbiology Letters* 160, 91–96.

Subbalakshmi, C., Krishnakumari, V., Nagaraj, R. and Sitaram, N. (1996) Requirements for antibacterial and hemolytic activities in the bovine neutrophil derived 13-residue peptide indolicidin. *FEBS Letters* 395, 48–52. DOI:10.1016/0014-5793(96)00996-9

Sun, T., Zhan, B., Gao, Y. (2015) A novel cathelicidin from *Bufo bufo gargarizans* Cantor showed specific activity to its habitat bacteria. *Gene* 571, 172–177. DOI:10.1016/j.gene.2015.06.034

Tani, A., Lee, S., Oishi, O., Aoyagi, H. and Ohno, M. (1995) Interaction of the fragments characteristic of bactenecin 7 with phospholipid bilayers and their antimicrobial activity. *Journal of Biochemistry* 117, 560–565.

Tomasinsig, L. and Zanetti, M. (2005) The cathelicidins--structure, function and evolution. *Current Protein and Peptide Science* 6, 23–34.

Tomasinsig, L., Scocchi, M., Di Loreto, C., Artico, D. and Zanetti, M. (2002) Inducible expression of an antimicrobial peptide of the innate immunity in polymorphonuclear leukocytes. *Journal of Leukocyte Biology* 72, 1003–1010.

Tomasinsig, L., Skerlavaj, B., Papo, N., Giabbai, B., Shai, Y. and Zanetti, M. (2006) Mechanistic and functional studies of the interaction of a proline-rich antimicrobial peptide with mammalian cells. *Journal of Biological Chemistry* 281, 383–391. DOI:10.1074/jbc.M510354200

Tomasinsig, L., Pizzirani, C., Skerlavaj, B., Pellegatti, P., Gulinelli, S., *et al.* (2008) The human cathelicidin LL-37 modulates the activities of the P2X7 receptor in a structure-dependent manner. *Journal of Biological Chemistry* 283, 30471–30481. DOI:10.1074/jbc.M802185200

Tomasinsig, L., Morgera, F., Antcheva, N., Pacor, S., Skerlavaj, B., Zanetti, M. and Tossi, A. (2009) Structure dependence of biological activities for primate cathelicidins. *Journal of Peptide Science* 15, 576–582. DOI:10.1002/psc.1143

Tomasinsig, L., Benincasa, M., Scocchi, M., Skerlavaj, B., Tossi, A., Zanetti, M. and Gennaro, R. (2010a) Role of cathelicidin peptides in bovine host defense and healing. *Probiotics and Antimicrobial Proteins* 2, 12–20. DOI:10.1007/s12602-010-9035-6

Tomasinsig, L., De Conti, G., Skerlavaj, B., Piccinini, R., Mazzilli, M., *et al.* (2010b) Broad-spectrum activity against bacterial mastitis pathogens and activation of mammary epithelial cells support a protective role of neutrophil cathelicidins in bovine mastitis. *Infection and Immunity* 78, 1781–1788. DOI:10.1128/IAI.01090-09

Tossi, A., Scocchi, M., Zanetti, M., Gennaro, R., Storici, P. and Romeo, D. (1997) An approach combining rapid cDNA amplification and chemical synthesis for the identification of novel, cathelicidin-derived, antimicrobial peptides. In: Shafer, W. (ed.) *Antibacterial Peptide Protocols: Methods in Molecular Biology*. Humana Press, pp. 133–150.

Tossi, A., Sandri, L. and Giangaspero, A. (2000) Amphipathic, α-helical antimicrobial peptides. *Peptide Science* 55, 4–30. DOI:10.1002/1097-0282(2000)55:1<4::AID-BIP30>3.0.CO;2-M

Usachev, K.S., Efimov, S.V., Kolosova, O.A., Klochkova, E.A., Aganov, A.V. and Klochkov, V.V. (2015) Antimicrobial peptide protegrin-3 adopt an antiparallel dimer in the presence of DPC micelles: a high-resolution NMR study. *Journal of Biomolecular NMR* 62, 71–79. DOI:10.1007/s10858-015-9920-0

Usachev, K.S., Kolosova, O.A., Klochkova, E.A., Yulmetov, A.R., Aganov, A.V. and Klochkov, V.V. (2016) Oligomerization of the antimicrobial peptide protegrin-5 in a membrane-mimicking environment: structural studies by high-resolution NMR spectroscopy. *European Biophysics Journal* 46, 293–300. DOI:10.1007/s00249-016-1167-5

Uzzell, T., Stolzenberg, E.D., Shinnar, A.E. and Zasloff, M. (2003) Hagfish intestinal antimicrobial peptides are ancient cathelicidins. *Peptides* 24, 1655–1667. DOI:10.1016/j.peptides.2003.08.024

Vaara, M. (2009) New approaches in peptide antibiotics. *Current Opinion in Pharmacology* 9, 571–576. DOI:10.1016/j.coph.2009.08.002

van der Does, A.M., Bergman, P., Agerberth, B. and Lindbom, L. (2012) Induction of the human cathelicidin LL-37 as a novel treatment against bacterial infections. *Journal of Leukocyte Biology* 92, 735–742. DOI:10.1189/jlb.0412178

van Dijk, A., Tersteeg-Zijderveld, M.H.G., Tjeerdsma-van Bokhoven, J.L.M., Jansman, A.J.M., Veldhuizen, E.J.A. and Haagsman, H.P. (2009) Chicken heterophils are recruited to the site of salmonella infection and release antibacterial mature cathelicidin-2 upon stimulation with LPS. *Molecular Immunology* 46, 1517–1526. DOI:10.1016/j.molimm.2008.12.015

van Hoek, M.L. (2014) Antimicrobial peptides in reptiles. *Pharmaceuticals* 7, 723–753. DOI:10.3390/ph7060723

van Hoek, M.L. (2016) Diversity in host defense antimicrobial peptides. In: Epand, R.M. (ed.) *Host Defense Peptides and Their Potential as Therapeutic Agents*. Springer, Heidelberg, pp. 3–26.

van Saene, H., van Saene, J., Silvestri, L., de la Cal, M., Sarginson, R. and Zandstra, D. (2007) ISeganan failure due to the wrong pharmaceutical technology. *Chest* 132, 1412–1412. DOI:10.1378/chest.07-0172

Vandamme, D., Landuyt, B., Luyten, W. and Schoofs, L. (2012) A comprehensive summary of LL-37, the factotum human cathelicidin peptide. *Cellular Immunology* 280, 22–35. DOI:10.1016/j.cellimm.2012.11.009

Veldhuizen, E.J.A., Schneider, V.A.F., Agustiandari, H., van Dijk, A., Tjeerdsma-van Bokhoven, J.L.M., Bikker, F.J. and Haagsman, H.P. (2014) Antimicrobial and immunomodulatory activities of PR-39 derived peptides. *PLoS ONE* 9, e95939. DOI:10.1371/journal.pone.0095939

Verbanac, D., Zanetti, M. and Romeo, D. (1993) Chemotactic and protease-inhibiting activities of antibiotic peptide precursors. *FEBS Letters* 317, 255–258. DOI:10.1016/0014-5793(93)81287-A

Wang, G. (2008) Structures of human host defense cathelicidin LL-37 and its smallest antimicrobial peptide KR-12 in lipid micelles. *Journal of Biological Chemistry* 283, 32637–32643. DOI:10.1074/jbc.M805533200

Wang, J., Wong, E.S.W., Whitley, J.C., Li, J., Stringer, J.M., Short, K.R., *et al.* (2011) Ancient antimicrobial peptides kill antibiotic-resistant pathogens: Australian mammals provide new options. *PLoS ONE* 6, e24030. DOI:10.1371/journal.pone.0024030

Wang, T.-T., Nestel, F.P., Bourdeau, V., Nagai, Y., Wang, Q., *et al.* (2004) Cutting edge: 1,25-Dihydroxyvitamin D3 is a direct inducer of antimicrobial peptide gene expression. *Journal of Immunology* 173, 2909–2912. DOI:10.4049/jimmunol.173.5.2909

Wang, Y., Hong, J., Liu, X., Yang, H., Liu, R., *et al.* (2008) Snake cathelicidin from *Bungarus fasciatus* is a potent peptide antibiotics. *PLoS ONE* 3, e3217. DOI:10.1371/journal.pone.0003217

Wei, L., Yang, J., He, X., Mo, G., Hong, J., *et al.* (2013) Structure and function of a potent lipopolysaccharide-binding antimicrobial and anti-inflammatory peptide. *Journal of Medicinal Chemistry* 56, 3546–3556. DOI:10.1021/jm4004158

Whelehan, C.J., Barry-Reidy, A., Meade, K.G., Eckersall, P.D., Chapwanya, A., *et al.* (2014) Characterisation and expression profile of the bovine cathelicidin gene repertoire in mammary tissue. *BMC Genomics* 15, 128. DOI:10.1186/1471-2164-15-128

Wu, H., Zhang, G., Ross, C.R. and Blecha, F. (1999) Cathelicidin gene expression in porcine tissues: roles in ontogeny and tissue specificity. *Infection and Immunity* 67, 439–442.

Wu, W.K.K., Wang, G., Coffelt, S.B., Betancourt, A.M., Lee, C.W., *et al.* (2010) Emerging roles of the host defense peptide LL-37 in human cancer and its potential therapeutic applications. *International Journal of Cancer* 127, 1741–1747. DOI:10.1002/ijc.25489

Xhindoli, D., Pacor, S., Guida, F., Antcheva, N. and Tossi, A. (2014) Native oligomerization determines the mode of action and biological activities of human cathelicidin LL-37. *Biochemical Journal* 457, 263–275. DOI:10.1042/BJ20131048

Xhindoli, D., Morgera, F., Zinth, U., Rizzo, R., Pacor, S. and Tossi, A. (2015) New aspects of the structure and mode of action of the human cathelicidin LL-37 revealed by the intrinsic probe p-cyanophenylalanine. *Biochemical Journal* 465, 443–457. DOI:10.1042/BJ20141016

Xhindoli, D., Pacor, S., Benincasa, M., Scocchi, M., Gennaro, R. and Tossi, A. (2016) The human cathelicidin LL-37 – a pore-forming antibacterial peptide and host-cell modulator. *Biochimica et Biophysica Acta (BBA) – Biomembranes* 1858, 546–566. DOI:10.1016/j.bbamem.2015.11.003

Xiao, Y., Cai, Y., Bommineni, Y.R., Fernando, S.C., Prakash, O., Gilliland, S.E. and Zhang, G. (2006a) Identification and functional characterization of three chicken cathelicidins with potent antimicrobial activity. *Journal of Biological Chemistry* 281, 2858–2867. DOI:10.1074/jbc.M507180200

Xiao, Y., Dai, H., Bommineni, Y.R., Soulages, J.L., Gong, Y.-X., Prakash, O. and Zhang, G. (2006b) Structure–activity relationships of fowlicidin-1, a cathelicidin antimicrobial peptide in chicken. *FEBS Journal* 273, 2581–2593. DOI:10.1111/j.1742-4658.2006.05261.x

Xiao, Y., Herrera, A.I., Bommineni, Y.R., Soulages, J.L., Prakash, O. and Zhang, G. (2009) The central kink region of fowlicidin-2, an alpha-helical host defense peptide, is critically involved in bacterial killing and endotoxin neutralization. *Journal of Innate Immunity* 1, 268–280. DOI:10.1159/000174822

Yamasaki, K., Schauber, J., Coda, A., Lin, H., Dorschner, R.A., *et al.* (2006) Kallikrein-mediated proteolysis regulates the antimicrobial effects of cathelicidins in skin. *FASEB Journal* 20, 2068–2080. DOI:10.1096/fj.06-6075com

Yang, D., Chertov, O. and Oppenheim, J.J. (2001) Participation of mammalian defensins and cathelicidins in anti-microbial immunity: receptors and activities of human defensins and cathelicidin (LL-37) *Journal of Leukocyte Biology* 69, 691–697.

Yang, S., Jung, H. and Kim, J. (2009) BMAP-27, p. online. Available at: http://www.rcsb.org/pdb/explore/explore.do?structureId=2KET (accessed 1 March 2017).

Yoshio, H., Lagercrantz, H., Gudmundsson, G.H. and Agerberth, B. (2004) First line of defense in early human life. *Seminars in Perinatology* 28, 304–311.

Yu, H., Lu, Y., Qiao, X., Wei, L., Fu, T., *et al.* (2015) Novel cathelicidins from pigeon highlights evolutionary convergence in avian cathelicidins and functions in modulation of innate immunity. *Scientific Reports* 5. DOI:10.1038/srep11082

Yu, K., Lai, B.F.L., Gani, J., Mikut, R., Hilpert, K. and Kizhakkedathu, J.N. (2015) Interaction of blood components with cathelicidins and their modified versions. *Biomaterials* 69, 201–211. DOI:10.1016/j.biomaterials.2015.08.003

Zaiou, M. and Gallo, R.L. (2002) Cathelicidins: essential gene-encoded mammalian antibiotics. *Journal of Molecular Medicine* 80, 549–561. DOI:10.1007/s00109-002-0350-6

Zaiou, M., Nizet, V. and Gallo, R.L. (2003) Antimicrobial and protease inhibitory functions of the human cathelicidin (hCAP18/LL-37) prosequence. *Journal of Investigative Dermatology* 120, 810–816.

Zanetti, M. (2004) Cathelicidins, multifunctional peptides of the innate immunity. *Journal of Leukocyte Biology* 75, 39–48. DOI:10.1189/jlb.0403147

Zanetti, M. (2005) The role of cathelicidins in the innate host defenses of mammals. *Current Issues in Molecular Biology* 7, 179–196.

Zanetti, M., Litteri, L., Gennaro, R., Horstmann, H. and Romeo, D. (1990) Bactenecins, defense polypeptides of bovine neutrophils, are generated from precursor molecules stored in the large granules. *Journal of Cell Biology* 111, 1363–1371. DOI:10.1083/jcb.111.4.1363

Zanetti, M., Litteri, L., Griffiths, G., Gennaro, R. and Romeo, D. (1991) Stimulus-induced maturation of probactenecins, precursors of neutrophil antimicrobial polypeptides. *Journal of Immunology* 146, 4295–4300.

Zanetti, M., Gennaro, R. and Romeo, D. (1995) Cathelicidins: a novel protein family with a common proregion and a variable C-terminal antimicrobial domain. *FEBS Letters* 374, 1–5. DOI:10.1016/0014-5793(95)01050-O

Zanetti, M., Gennaro, R., Scocchi, M. and Skerlavaj, B. (2000) Structure and biology of cathelicidins. *Advances in Experimental Medicine and Biology* 479, 203–218. DOI:10.1007/0-306-46831-X_17

Zanetti, M., Gennaro, R., Scocchi, M. and Skerlavaj, B. (2002) Structure and biology of cathelicidins. In: Keisari, Y. and Ofek, I. (eds) *The Biology and Pathology of Innate Immunity Mechanisms: Advances in Experimental Medicine and Biology.* Springer, pp. 203–218.

Zasloff, M. (2002) Antimicrobial peptides of multicellular organisms. *Nature* 415, 389–395. DOI:10.1038/415389a

Zelezetsky, I. and Tossi, A. (2006) Alpha-helical antimicrobial peptides – using a sequence template to guide structure–activity relationship studies. *Biochimica et Biophysica Acta (BBA) – Biomembranes* 1758, 1436–1449. DOI:10.1016/j.bbamem.2006.03.021

Zelezetsky, I., Pontillo, A., Puzzi, L., Antcheva, N., Segat, L., *et al.* (2006) Evolution of the primate cathelicidin: correlation between structural variations and antimicrobial activity. *Journal of Biological Chemistry* 281, 19861–19871. DOI:10.1074/jbc.M511108200

Zhang, X.-J., Zhang, X.-Y., Zhang, N., Guo, X., Peng, K.-S., *et al.* (2015) Distinctive structural hallmarks and biological activities of the multiple cathelicidin antimicrobial peptides in a primitive teleost fish. *Journal of Immunology* 194, 4974–4987. DOI:10.4049/jimmunol.1500182

Zhu, S. (2008) Did cathelicidins, a family of multifunctional host-defense peptides, arise from a cysteine protease inhibitor? *Trends in Microbiology* 16, 353–360. DOI:10.1016/j.tim.2008.05.007

Zhu, S. and Gao, B. (2009) A fossil antibacterial peptide gives clues to structural diversity of cathelicidin-derived host defense peptides. *FASEB Journal* 23, 13–20. DOI:10.1096/fj.08-114579

Zhu, S., Wei, L., Yamasaki, K. and Gallo, R.L. (2008) Activation of cathepsin L by the cathelin-like domain of protegrin-3. *Molecular Immunology* 45, 2531–2536. DOI:10.1016/j.molimm.2008.01.007

Zughaier, S.M., Shafer, W.M. and Stephens, D.S. (2005) Antimicrobial peptides and endotoxin inhibit cytokine and nitric oxide release but amplify respiratory burst response in human and murine macrophages. *Cellular Microbiology* 7, 1251–1262. DOI:10.1111/j.1462-5822.2005.00549.x

Zughaier, S.M., Svoboda, P. and Pohl, J. (2014) Structure-dependent immune modulatory activity of protegrin-1 analogs. *Antibiotics* 3, 694–713. DOI:10.3390/antibiotics3040694

3 Disulfide-linked Defensins

Monique L. van Hoek*

School of Systems Biology, George Mason University, Manassas, VA 20110, USA

Abstract

This chapter provides an overview of the literature on disulfide-linked defensin peptides. Key proteomic and genomic aspects of vertebrate defensins, including the characteristics of α-, β- and θ-defensins are described. The host-defence role of vertebrate defensins is reviewed, as well as possible implications for this activity of peptides in their development as potential therapeutics. Approaches for the synthesis or heterologous expression of the defensins are reviewed. The mechanism of action and *in vivo* role of each class of vertebrate defensins are discussed, as is the therapeutic potential of the defensin peptides. The similarities and differences of vertebrate, bivalve, arthropod and plant defensins are explored. Finally, a brief discussion is presented of other disulfide-linked antimicrobial peptides that may not meet the criteria for defensins.

3.1 Overview

3.1.1 Introduction to disulfide-linked defensins

Host-defence antimicrobial peptides are part of the innate immune system of organisms in multicellular eukaryotes. Defensins are a major class of typically small, disulfide-linked antimicrobial peptides (3–4 kDa) and have been found in reptiles, birds, mammals, arthropods including insects, and plants (Tu *et al.*, 2015). Defensin peptides demonstrate antimicrobial activity against a wide variety of microbes, including Gram-positive bacteria, Gram-negative bacteria, fungi and viruses. However, their dominant biological activity may be their host-directed, immunomodulatory activity (Hancock *et al.*, 2016). The number, activity and diversity of these antimicrobial peptides suggest that they could be a significant natural armamentarium to be drawn upon to design new compounds as bacterial resistance to standard antibiotics develops. Thus, defensins are a promising area of research for the potential development of new antimicrobials, possibly as host-directed therapeutics.

Defensin peptides characteristically have six cysteines arranged in three disulfide bonds, with the pairing pattern of the bonds being highly characteristic for each subclass of defensin (see below). Defensin peptides have a typical 'defensin fold', consisting of two or three anti-parallel β-sheets (Hoover *et al.*, 2001) and may have helical regions, especially at the N-terminus of β-defensins for example. Other molecules of the innate immune system also have disulfide bonds, but have very different numbers or patterns of disulfide bonding (discussed below). These defensin peptides share function,

* Corresponding author e-mail: mvanhoek@gmu.edu

structure and mechanism within their groups but often have very different sequences in between the highly conserved cysteines (Jenssen *et al.*, 2006). That is, they have significant structural conservation, often without significant sequence conservation.

Multiple defensin peptides are expressed in most tissues throughout the body, usually in response to infection, inflammation or injury (Ganz, 2003). Defensins are encoded in clusters in the genome (described later), and are cleaved to be processed from a pro-molecule by various proteases to the active form of the peptide (Wilson *et al.*, 2009).

Defensins are known to be critical components of innate immunity (Zhao and Lu, 2014). The expression of these defensin peptides is induced following bacterial or viral infection as part of the innate immune response, although some of the defensins are thought to be constitutively expressed (e.g. hBD-1 in humans).

3.1.2 Mechanisms of action

The dominant mode of action of defensin antimicrobial peptides appears to be in their immunomodulation of the host; thus, they are classified as host-defence peptides. These immunomodulatory activities include promoting macrophage phagocytosis, while also limiting their pro-inflammatory responses, being chemoattractants to other immune cells and promoting wound healing (Hancock *et al.*, 2016). The host-directed and immunomodulatory activities of human defensin peptides were recently reviewed in two excellent articles by Zhao and Lu (2014) and by Hancock *et al.* (2016).

The direct antibacterial activity of defensin peptides varies considerably, but is generally considered weak unless at high concentrations, due to impingement by salt, lipopolysaccharide (LPS) and proteins found *in vivo*. The interaction of cationic antimicrobial peptides with the anionic lipids within the bacterial outer membrane is the general mechanism proposed for cationic peptides to interact with bacterial membranes. This interaction can lead to thinning or pore-formation of the bacterial membrane and lysis of the bacterial cell (Wimley *et al.*, 1994; Wang, 2014).

Recent work has focused either on identifying additional molecular targets in bacteria of the antimicrobial peptides (including defensins) such as proteins in or on the pathogen, or on investigating nucleic acid binding properties. An interesting mechanism of action was found for some defensin peptides (Human defensins, HNP-1 and hBD-3; oyster defensins; and fungal defensin, Plectasin) in their ability to directly interfere with the bacterial lipid II enzyme, which is responsible for peptidoglycan synthesis, the dominant component of bacterial cell walls (Sass *et al.*, 2010; Schmitt *et al.*, 2010; Schneider *et al.*, 2010; Varney *et al.*, 2013; Witzke *et al.*, 2016). This bacterial target is mainly thought to be applicable to Gram-positive organisms, such as *Staphylococcus aureus*. By inhibiting lipid II, the defensin peptides inhibit cell wall synthesis, in much the same way as lantibiotics.

3.1.3 Structural features of defensins

The class of defensin peptides is structurally diverse. The main characteristic of this group is a disulfide-bond stabilized β-sheet ('defensin fold'), and significant conservation of the cysteines that form those bonds. Structurally, vertebrate defensins have predominantly β-sheet characteristics plus intra-molecular disulfide bonds while defensins from insects, plants and bivalves have more diverse structures, including prominent α-helical domains (Fig. 3.1). The disulfide bonding of the defensin peptides may significantly contribute to their physiological stability, as well as to their antimicrobial activity (Tu *et al.*, 2015). Specific cysteine-bonding patterns are characteristic for each class, such as α- and β-defensins, as described below.

As well as this structural diversity, defensins can vary in size and charge. Searching the Antimicrobial Peptide Database APD3 (Wang *et al.*, 2016) for 'defensin' antimicrobial peptides, 316 peptides were identified. On average, these 'defensin' peptides are 41.3 amino acids (aa) in length with an average net charge of +4.66 (Table 3.1). Wang (2014) reports an average of 32.4

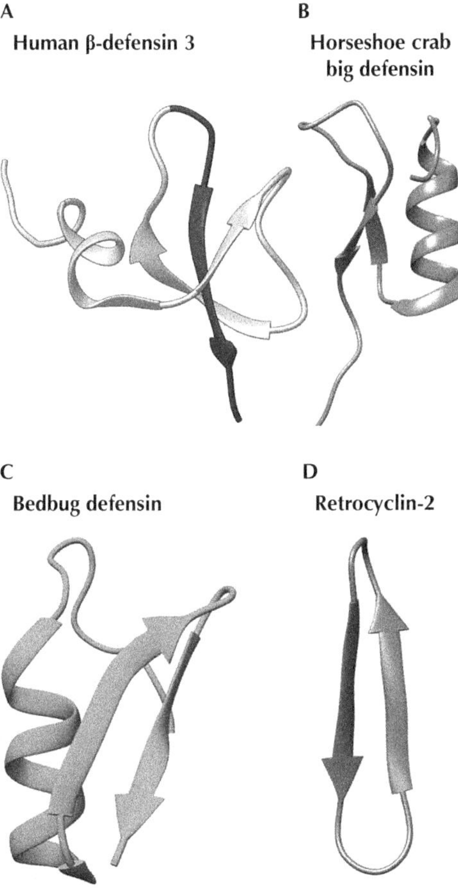

Fig. 3.1. Structure of various defensins as modelled by Chimera, molecular modelling system (disulfide bonds are not shown). (A) Human β-defensin 3: A three-dimensional view of the proposed structure of the human β-defensin with the linear fragment (peptide 4) region in darker tone (vertical) (PDB 1KJ6). (B) Horseshoe crab big defensin: The invertebrate defensin from *Tachypleus tridentatus* (Japanese horseshoe crab) (PDB 2RNG) (Kouno *et al*, 2008). (C) Bedbug (*Cimex lectularis*) defensin: A three-dimensional view of the NMR structure of the insect defensin. In the figure the N-terminal loop, α-helix and antiparallel β-sheets of sapecin A are shown (PDB 1L4V). (D) Retrocyclin-2: Structure of antiviral synthetic θ-defensin bound to membrane-mimetic SDS micelles (PDB 2ATG).

residues and an average net charge of +3.2) for all human AMPs in the APD. Thus defensin peptides as a group are slightly longer and more highly charged than the 'average' human AMP in the database. However, as described in each section below, each subclass of defensin has distinctive size and charge characteristics, from small θ-defensins to the large big defensins.

3.2 Vertebrate Defensins

3.2.1 β-defensins

β-defensin definition

The β-defensin peptides are the most conserved defensins among the vertebrates, with very characteristic cysteine patterns in their sequence. β-defensins are defined as peptides that contain a highly conserved pattern of six cysteines with a clearly defined pattern of intramolecular bonding: Cys1-Cys5, Cys2-Cys4, and Cys3-Cys6 (Wu *et al.*, 2003) (Fig. 3.1A). On average, β-defensin peptides have a net charge of +5.7 and are 43.2 amino acids (aa) long (Table 3.1). This length is greater than the average for α-defensins (~33 aa), much greater than θ-defensins (18 aa) and considerably smaller than the big defensins (~80 aa). β-defensin peptides typically have more α-helical structure than α-defensins, perhaps accounted for in the increased length of the peptides. Other than the highly conserved cysteines, however, there is significant diversity in the intervening sequences of β-defensin peptides (Cheng *et al.*, 2015b; Semple *et al.*, 2006) (Table 3.1).

β-defensins are widely expressed in the epithelial cells, gastrointestinal tract and in the reproductive tract as well as in the respiratory system (Garcia *et al.*, 2001a). Human β-defensin 2 (hBD-2) and human β-defensin 3 (hBD-3) are expressed by keratinocytes and healthy skin, as well as in the middle ear epithelial cells (Wang, 2014). β-defensin expression has been found to be high throughout the male reproductive tract and may play a role in sperm maturation and capacitation, perhaps unrelated to the

Table 3.1. Sequence, size and charge of selected defensin peptides listed in the Antimicrobial Peptide Database (APD) (Wang *et al.*, 2016). Averages are calculated as indicated.

Sequence, length and charge of selected defensin peptides from APD3 (from 316 total)

Name	Sequence	Length (aa)	Net charge
Human α-defensin peptides			
HNP-1	ACYCRIPACIAGERRYGTCIYQGRLWAFCC	30	3
HNP-2	CYCRIPACIAGERRYGTCIYQGRLWAFCC	29	3
HNP-3	DCYCRIPACIAGERRYGTCIYQGRLWAFCC	30	2
HNP-4	VCSCRLVFCRRTELRVGNCLIGGVSFTYCCTRV	33	4
HD-5	ATCYCRTGRCATRESLSGVCEISGRLYRLCCR	32	4
HD-6	AFTCHCRRSCYSTEYSYGTCTVMGINHRFCCL	32	2
Other α-defensin peptides (excluding eNAPs)			
Cryptdin-1 (Crp1), mouse	LRDLVCYCRTRGCKRRERMNGTCRKGHLMYTLCCR	35	8
Cryptdin-2 (Crp2), mouse	LRDLVCYCRARGCKGRERMNGTCRKGHLLYMLCCR	35	7
Cryptdin-5 (Crp5) mouse	LSKKLICYCRIRGCKRRERVFGTCRNLFLTFVFCCS	36	8
Rabbit neutrophil defensin 3a (NP-3a)	GICACRRRFCPNSERFSGYCRVNGARYVRCCSRR	34	8
Rabbit neutrophil peptide 3b (NP-3b)	GRCVCRKQLLCSYRERRIGDCKIRGVRFPFCCPR	34	8
Rabbit neutrophil peptide 4 (NP-4)	VSCTCRRFSCGFGERASGSCTVNGVRHTLCCRR	33	5
Rabbit neutrophil peptide 5 (NP-5)	VFCTCRGFLCGSGERASGSCTINGVRHTLCCRR	33	4
Average (from 13 α-defensin sequences)		32.77	5.08
Human β-defensin peptides			
hBD-1	DHYNCVSSGGQCLYSACPIFTKIQGTCYRGKAKCCK	36	4
hBD-2	GIGDPVTCLKSGAICHPVFCPRRYKQIGTCGLPGTKCCKKP	41	7
hBD-3	GIINTLQKYYCRVRGGRCAVLSCLPKEEQIGKCSTRGRKCCRRKK	45	11
hBD-4	FELDRICGYGTARCRKKCRSQEYRIGRCPNTYACCLRKWDESLLNRTKP	49	7
DEFB114	DRCTKRYGRCKRDCLESEKQIDICSLPRKICCTEKLYEEDDMF	43	0
hBD-26	WYVKKCLNDVGICKKKCKPEEMHVKNGWAMCGKGRDCCVPAD	42	4
hBD-27	QLKKCWNNYVQGHCRKICRVNEVPEALCENGRYCCLNIKELEAC	44	2
Other β-defensin peptides			
mBD-1, mouse	DQYKCLQHGGFCLRSSCPSNTKLQGTCKPDKPNCCKS	37	4
mBD-3, mouse	KINNPVSCLRKGGRCWNRCIGNTRQIGSCGVPFLKCCKRK	40	10
mBD-4 (Defb4), mouse	QIINNPITCMTNGAICWGPCPTAFRQIGNCGHFKVRCCKIR	41	5

mBD-7, mouse	NSKRACYREGGECLQRCIGLFHKIGTCNFRFKCCKFQ	37	6
mBD-8, mouse	NEPVSCIRNGGICQYRCIGLRHKIGTCGSPFKCCK	35	5
mBD-14, mouse	FLPKTLRKFFCRIRGGRCAVLNCLGKEEQIGRCSNSGRKCCRKKK	45	12
TAP, β-defensin, cattle	NPVSCVRNKGICVPIRCPGSMKQIGTCVGRAVKCCRKK	38	9
TAP 20N, cattle	NPVSCVRNKGICVPIRCPGNMKQIGTCVGRAVKCCRKK	38	9
bBD-1, cattle	DFASCHTNGGICLPNRCPGHMIQIGICFRPRVKCCRSW	38	4
bBD-2, cattle	VRNHVTCRINRGFCVPIRCPGRTRQIGTCFGPRIKCCRSW	40	9
bBD-3, cattle	QGVRNHVTCRINRGFCVPIRCPGRTRQIGTCFGPRIKCCRSW	42	9
bBD-4, cattle	QRVRNPQSCRWNMGVCIPFLCRVGMRQIGTCFGPRVPCCRR	41	8
bBD-5, cattle	QVVRNPQSCRWNMGVCIPISCPGNMRQIGTCFGPRVPCCRRW	42	6
bBD-6, cattle	QGVRNHVTCRIYGGFCVPIRCPGRTRQIGTCFGRPVKCCRRW	42	9
bBD-7, cattle,	QGVRNFVTCRINRGFCVPIRCPGHRRQIGTCLGPRIKCCR	40	9
bBD-8, cattle	VRNFVTCRINRGFCVPIRCPGHRRQIGTCLGPQIKCCR	38	8
bBD-9, cattle	QGVRNFVTCRINRGFCVPIRCPGHRRQIGTCLAPQIKCCR	40	8
bBD-10, cattle	QGVRSYLSCWGNRGICLLNRCPGRMRQIGTCLAPRVKCCR	40	8
bBD-11, cattle	GPLSCRRNGGVCIPIRCPGPMRQIGTCFGRPVKCCRSW	38	7
bBD-12, cattle	GPLSCCRNGGVCIPIRCPVPMRQIGTCFGRPVKCCRSW	38	6
bBD-13, cattle	SGISGPLSCGRNGGVCIPIRCPVPMRQIGTCFGRPVKCCRSW	42	6
sBD-1, sheep	NRLSCHRNKGVCVPSRCPRHMRQIGTCRGPPVKCCRKK	38	11
LAP, β-defensin, cattle	GFTQGVRNSQSCRRNKGICVPIRCPGSMRQIGTCLGAQVKCCRRK	45	10
saBD, seabream (fish)	ASFPWSCPSLSGVCRKVCLPTELFFGPLGCGKGFLCGVSHFL	42	3
cod beta defensin (fish)	WSCPTLSGVCRKVCLPTEMFFGPLGCGKEFQCCVSHFF	38	1
pdBD-2 (fish)	YDTGIQGWTCGSRGLCRKHCYAQEHTVGYHGCPRRYRCCALRF	43	5
CFBD-1 (salamander)	FAVWGCADYRGYCRAACFAFEYSLGPKGCTEGYVCCVPNTF	41	0
Panusin , β-defensin, crustacean	SYVGDCGSNGGSCVSSYCPYGNRLNYFCPLGRTCCRRSY	39	4
AvBD1, Ostrich, Ostricacin-2	APGNKAECEREKGYCGFLKCSFPFVVSGKCSRFFFCCKNIW	41	4
AvBD2, Ostrich, Ostricacin-1	LFCRKGTCHFGGCPAHLVKVGSCFGFRACCKWPWDV	36	4
AvBD4 (gallinacin 7), chicken	RYHMQCGYRGTFCTPGKCPYGNAYLGLCRPKYSCCRWL	38	6
AvBD5 (gallinacin 9), Chicken	GLPQDCERRGGFCSHKSCPPGIGRIGLCSKEDFCCRSRWYS	41	3
AvBD6 (gallinacin 4), Chicken	SPIHACRYQRGVCIPGPCRWPYYRVGSCGSGLKSCCVRNRWA	42	7
AvBD7 (Gallinacin-5), Chicken	QPFIPRPIDTCRLRNGICFPGICRRPYYWIGTCNNGIGSCCARGWRS	47	6
AvBD7, Ostrich, Ostricacin-3	IPRPLDPCIAQNGRCFTGICRYPYFWIGTCRNGKSCCRRR	40	7

Continued

Table 3.1. Continued.

Name	Sequence	Length (aa)	Net charge
AvBD8, Ostrich, Ostricacin-4	LPVNEAQCRQVGGYCGLRICNFPSRFLGLCTRNHPCCSRVWV	42	4
Duck AvBD9 (gallinacin-6)	ADTLACRQSHQSCSFVACRAPSVDIGTCRGGKLKCCKWAPSS	42	4
Duck AvBD10	VLLFLFQAAPGSADAPFADTAACRSQGNFCRAGACPPTFAASGSCHGGLLNCCAK	55	1
Chicken AvBD12 (Gallinacin-10)	GPDSCNHDRGLCRVGNCNPGEYLAKYCFEPVILCCKPLSPTPTKT	45	1
Apl-AvBD16, ducks	FFLLFLQGAAGNSVLCRIRGGRCHVGSCHFPERHIGRCSGFQACCIRTWG	50	5
TBD-1, Turtle β-defensin 1	YDLSKNCRLRGGICYIGKCPRRFFRSGSCSRGNVCCLRFG	40	8
TEWP, Turtle-reptilian defensin	QKKCPGRCTLKCGKHERPTLPYNCGKYICCVPVKVK	36	8
Pelovaterin, Turtle	DDTPSSRCGSGGWGPCLPIVDLLCIVHVTVGCSGGFGCCRIG	42	-1
β-defensin Average (77 peptides)		43.19	5.69
Big Defensin Peptides			
BjBD (B. japonicum)	AVPLAVPLVYMGASVSPAVWNWLLVTFGAAAVAAAAVTVSDNDSHSCANNRGWCRSRCFSHEYIDSWHSDVCGSYDCCRPRY	82	−1
VpBD (V. philippinarum)	LCLDQKPEMEPFRKDAQQALEPSRQRRWLHRRCLSGRGFCRAICSIFEEPVRGNIDCYFGYNCCRRMFSHYRTS	74	6
BDEF_TACTR, Horseshoe Crab	NPLIPAIYIGATVGPSVWAYLVALVGAAAVTAANIRRASSDNHSCAGNRGWCRSKCFRHEYVDTYYSAVCGRYFCCRSR	79	6
Average		78.33	3.67
Primate θ-Defensin Peptides			
RTD-1 (Rhesus θ-defensin-1)	GFCRCLCRRGVCRCICTR	18	5
RTD-2 (Rhesus θ-defensin 2)	GVCRCLCRRGVCRCLCRR	18	6
RTD-3 (Rhesus θ-defensin 3)	GFCRCICTRGFCRCICTR	18	4
RTD-4 (Rhesus macaque θ-defensin-4)	GICRCICTRGFCRCICVL	18	3
RTD-5 (rhesus macaque θ-defensin-5)	GICRCLCRRGVCRCICVL	18	4
BTD-1 (Baboon θ-defensin-1)	RCVCTRGFCRCVCRRGVC	18	5
BTD-2 (Baboon θ-defensin-2)	RCVCRRGVCRCVCRRGVC	18	6
BTD-3 (Baboon θ-defensin-3)	RCVCTRGFCRCVCTRGFC	18	4
BTD-4 (Baboon θ-defensin-4)	RCVCTRGFCRCICLLGIC	18	3
BTD-7 (Baboon θ-defensin-7)	RCVCTRGFCRCFCRRGVC	18	5
PhTD1 (P. hamadryas θ-defensin-1)	RCVCRRGVCRCVCTRGFC	18	5
PhTD3 (P. hamadryas θ-defensin-3)	RCVCTRGFCRCVCTRGFC	18	4
Average		18	4.5

host-defence activities of these peptides (Zhou *et al.*, 2004; Patil *et al.*, 2005).

Expression of β-defensin gene clusters

β-defensin genes are found to be clustered on chromosomal DNA in many species of animals. For example, in addition to the four well-studied human β-defensins, hBD-1 to hBD-4, 28 new defensin genes have been identified (Schutte *et al.*, 2002), including hBD-5, -6, -8, -9, and -18; many of them are clustered together on chromosome 8p23 (Sparkes *et al.*, 1989; Linzmeier *et al.*, 1999). In more than 50 avian genomes examined so far, there is a very large cluster of β-defensin genes (Xiao *et al.*, 2004; Cuperus *et al.*, 2013; Zhang and Sunkara, 2014; Cheng *et al.*, 2015b). In the mouse (C57BL/6J), the β-defensin genes are also found to be clustered on a few chromosomes (Amid *et al.*, 2009). The regulation of these gene clusters is the subject of current study. A recent study suggests that β-defensin gene copy number variation may play a role in the outcome of host innate immune response (Machado and Ottolini, 2015). The studies of the regulation of the clusters and of the effect of copy number variation will lead to important new understanding of the role of β-defensin peptides.

β-defensin expression – constitutive or inducible

Expression of many of the vertebrate defensins is known to be inducible (Cociancich *et al.*, 1993; Han *et al.*, 2008), and is induced mainly through TLR receptor binding to microbial components (PAMPs) and subsequent NF-κB activation, or via pro-inflammatory cytokines, such as TNF-α and IL1-β. β-defensin gene expression can also be induced by exposure of lung epithelial cells to cigarette smoke (Pierson *et al.*, 2013) and other environmental factors. Various β-defensins can also be induced by fungal infection in respiratory epithelial cells (Alekseeva *et al.*, 2009).

Human β-defensin 2 (hBD-2) gene expression is highly inducible by exposure to microbial products such as the presence of Gram-negative pathogens such as mucoid *Pseudomonas (P.) aeruginosa* (McCray and Bentley, 1997; Harder *et al.*, 2001), *Francisella* (Han *et al.*, 2008) or bacterial pneumonia (Hiratsuka *et al.*, 1998). The gene for hBD-2 was localized to the chromosome region 8p22, where many other human defensin genes cluster together (Garcia *et al.*, 2001b; Schutte *et al.*, 2002). hBD-2 expression is inducible in keratinocytes, the gingival mucosa and the tracheal epithelium (O'Neil *et al.*, 1999; Schutte and McCray, 2002). Among other tissues, altered hBD-2 gene expression has been found in many diseases, such as cystic fibrosis and lupus erythematosus (Niyonsaba and Ogawa, 2005; Yanagi *et al.*, 2005; Kreuter *et al.*, 2011).

hBD-3 is also highly inducible and is an effective *in vitro* antimicrobial peptide (Harder *et al.*, 2001; Han *et al.*, 2008). Importantly, hBD-3 exhibits salt tolerance in its antimicrobial activity, which is unlike many of the other defensin peptides (Harder *et al.*, 2001). hBD-3 expression is highly induced by microbial products, including LPS and *Aspergillus* (Han *et al.*, 2008; Alekseeva *et al.*, 2009).

hBD-8 is a human β-defensin gene recently predicted by HMMER, a computational search tool. It is a peptide with a 52 amino acid length (longer than the average, Table 3.1) and its gene chromosomal location is 8p23-p22, where it co-locates with hBD-1 to -9 (Schutte *et al.*, 2002). Studies have found hBD-8 is not constitutively expressed, but can be slightly induced by IL-1β in human gingival keratinocytes (Premratanachai *et al.*, 2004).

Some of the defensin genes are constitutively expressed. The most often cited example is hBD-1, which does not appear to be inducible by microbial PAMPs and is constitutively expressed in the tissues that have been examined (O'Neil *et al.*, 1999; Eckmann, 2005).

In vivo roles of β-defensin expression

Many studies have suggested *in vivo* roles for β-defensins, particularly in modulating the host response to infection (Hancock *et al.*, 2016). β-defensins may play roles in skin physiology and in response to wounding of the skin. One interesting report of an *in vivo* role for β-defensin peptide expression has been in the tail regeneration of the anole lizard, *Anolis carolinensis.* These small lizards can lose their tail to a predator and then regrow the tail from the wound-bed, which also remains remarkably uninfected. In addition to the cathelicidin-like peptides, β-defensin peptides were expressed in both the azurophilic granulocytes located in the wound-bed as well as in the surrounding epithelium (Alibardi, 2013; Alibardi, 2014). β-defensin peptides are also observed in phagosomes containing degraded bacteria, thus further protecting the wound-bed from reinfection. There is a distinct lack of inflammation in the wound (which is important for regeneration) (Alibardi *et al.*, 2012). In addition, there is a high level of expression of two of the most highly expressed β-defensins in that tissue, AcBD15 and AcBD27 (Alibardi, 2013). Thus, there is a potential role of β-defensins in infection prevention, wound healing and regeneration of the anole lizard tail.

Reptile eggs contain a large amount of readily available biological material and thus are a good potential resource for discovering antimicrobial peptides (Mine *et al.*, 2003). Recently, pelovaterin (Table 3.1), a β-defensin-like peptide first identified in the Chinese soft-shelled turtle eggshell, was shown to have antimicrobial activity. It was suggested that these peptides may also play an additional role through aggregation in the formation of the eggshell (Lakshminarayanan *et al.*, 2008). This is similar to the role of gallin, an ovo-defensin which is a β-defensin-like peptide in avian eggs (Mine *et al.*, 2003; Lakshminarayanan *et al.*, 2008; Herve-Grepinet *et al.*, 2010). Turtle genomes also encode at least one defensin-type peptide (gallinacin-like) that is similar to 'avian'-type β-defensin peptides (van Hoek, 2014) (Table 3.1).

Diverse requirements for folding of β-defensin antimicrobial activity

The β-defensin peptides demonstrate diverse requirements of folding for

antimicrobial activity. For example, human β-defensin 2 (hBD-2) must be folded correctly with the cystines in the correct bonded pattern to exhibit its full antimicrobial activity (Wu *et al.*, 2003). hBD-4 can demonstrate antimicrobial activity with non-native disulfide bridges (Sharma and Nagaraj, 2015).

For human β-defensin 3, hBD-3, it has been demonstrated that the disulfide bonds are dispensable for antimicrobial activity but required for chemotactic activity (Hoover *et al.*, 2001; Hoover *et al.*, 2003; Wu *et al.*, 2003). Furthermore, small C-terminal fragments of hBD-3 that are designed to be linear also have high antimicrobial activity (Hoover *et al.*, 2003; Taylor *et al.*, 2008; Papanastasiou *et al.*, 2009). This finding has important implications for the potential mechanism of hBD-3 action on the host and on pathogens. A separation of these two activities was demonstrated through testing different regions of the peptides. Thus, the host-directed activity of hBD-3 requires proper folding, while the antimicrobial activity does not. The host targets of hBD-3 by which immunomodulation is achieved are beginning to be elucidated (Hancock *et al.*, 2016).

Interestingly, almost the opposite is true for hBD-1, the constitutively expressed AMP. Schroeder *et al.* (2011) demonstrated that by reducing all the disulfide bonds within hBD-1, the antimicrobial activity is significantly increased (Schroeder *et al.*, 2011a; Schroeder *et al.*, 2011b) compared to the fully oxidized form, which is usually inactive for antimicrobial activity. This finding, combined with an evaluation of the redox potential in the lung and other epithelial surfaces, has led to a new appreciation for the potential role of hBD-1 in host defence, and suggests that this peptide should be further examined for potential therapeutic uses.

Biological expression systems for the expression of β-defensins

Due to the complex folding patterns of the β- and α-defensins, chemical synthesis with correct folding is onerous and costly. Thus, researchers have sought alternative and biological expression systems that may reduce the cost and increase the ease of production of correctly folded disulfide-linked defensin peptides (Corrales-Garcia *et al.*, 2011). Some successful examples include expression of β-defensin peptides in *Pichia pastoris* (Zhang *et al.*, 2011; Cao *et al.*, 2012; Peng *et al.*, 2014; Zhang *et al.*, 2014), generation of various fusion constructs (Huang *et al.*, 2009; Li *et al.*, 2010; Dong *et al.*, 2011; Xin *et al.*, 2014; Chang *et al.*, 2015), or other bacterial protein expression techniques (Luan *et al.*, 2014; Tomisawa *et al.*, 2015). Additional techniques for producing large quantities of properly folded defensin peptides include their heterologous expression in plants (Aerts *et al.*, 2005), as plants already can express defensin peptides of their own (Gazzaneo *et al.*, 2016). The production of fully glycosylated and properly folded disulfide-linked defensin proteins in these systems will be highly enabling to their further development as therapeutics.

The ability to generate active, antimicrobial linear fragments of β-defensin peptide has potential for generating a possible therapeutic molecule, although it will no longer be a defensin. Such a short peptide would be less expensive to chemically synthesize than the full-length defensin and would not require extensive synthetic folding processes. Indeed, in many cases easier-to-synthesize linearized versions have been shown to be as antibacterial or even more effective than natural, folded versions, even in high salt environments (Hoover *et al.*, 2003; Taylor *et al.*, 2008; Papanastasiou *et al.*, 2009). Of interest for their potential use as therapeutics, these small fragments do not appear to be inhibited by LPS (Gupta *et al.*, 2016), so while they are no longer defensin peptides, they may have the potential to be developed as antimicrobial compounds.

Therapeutic potential of β-defensins

Overall the therapeutic potential of β-defensins as antimicrobial agents might be challenging to implement, given the preponderance of evidence of their host-directed activities as their main biological function (Hancock *et al.*, 2016). Folding requirements for producing β-defensin peptides in chemical synthesis can be onerous, but progress has been made using various biological expression systems. The direct antimicrobial activity of defensin peptides is generally weak, except in locations where the local concentration may be quite high, such as when a neutrophil has dumped its granule contents or in an intestinal crypt near the Paneth cells (Hancock *et al.*, 2016).

The expression of β-defensins in wounded tissues of the anole lizard, and their expression pattern in human keratinocytes and epithelial cells suggests that these peptides may play an important role in wound healing, thus these peptides are excellent candidates for further study as topical salves to promote wound healing, reduce inflammation and, as a potential side benefit, perhaps exert some antibacterial activity as well. Some of the complexities of understanding the immunomodulation by these peptides in a therapeutic context are discussed by Hancock *et al.* (2016).

3.2.2 *α*-defensins

Definition of α-defensins

α-defensin peptides are a critical part of mammalian innate immunity (Wilson *et al.*, 2009; Zhao and Lu, 2014; Lehrer and Lu, 2012; Tongaonkar *et al.*, 2012). α-defensins are highly expressed in many, but not all, higher vertebrates (Das *et al.*, 2010). Similar to β-defensins, their direct antimicrobial activity *in vivo* is probably limited to physiological locations where high local concentrations can be achieved (e.g., a neutrophil granule) (Hancock *et al.*, 2016). They are small (3–4 kDa) peptides that contain a highly conserved pattern of six cysteines with a clearly defined pattern of intramolecular bonding: Cys1–Cys6, Cys2–Cys4, and Cys3–Cys5 (Wu *et al.*, 2003). α-defensins are differentiated from β-defensins in their bonding pattern of the six characteristic cysteines, and their more limited tissue expression pattern. The bonding pattern in β-defensins versus α-defensins differs in the first and third disulfide bond connection, while the Cys2–Cys4 disulfide bond is conserved between the two classes. α-defensins have an average length of 32.8 amino acids and an average net charge of +5 (Table 3.1), which is smaller than the average size of β-defensin peptides and larger than θ-defensin peptides.

Human neutrophil peptide HNP-1, also called α-defensin 1, is highly expressed in neutrophils and other leukocytes in humans. HNP-1 is important in the ability of white blood cells to deal with bacterial pathogens (Lehrer and Lu, 2012). It has recently been demonstrated that in addition to their first identified key role as antimicrobial peptides in neutrophil granules (Selsted *et al.*, 1985; Wilde *et al.*, 1989), HNPs also play an important role in neutrophil extracellular traps (NETs) (Saitoh *et al.*, 2012; Van Avondt *et al.*, 2013; Hu *et al.*, 2016).

α-defensins are classified as antimicrobial peptides, but their direct antimicrobial activity is not very robust at low concentrations (Hancock *et al.*, 2016). Although α-defensins (HNPs) can be antibacterial against many bacterial pathogens (de Leeuw *et al.*, 2010), they are ineffective against bacterial pathogens with generally high resistance to cationic peptides, such as *Burkholderia* (Blower *et al.*, 2015). The requirement for the disulfide bonds for antimicrobial activity was shown not to be absolute for HNP-1 (Varkey and Nagaraj, 2005), suggesting that the antimicrobial activity could be present in truncated or smaller fragments, providing an opportunity for synthetic approaches to develop an antimicrobial peptide fragment of the parental molecule.

Phylogenetic diversity of α-defensin expression

Although α-defensin expression is found in the neutrophils of many mammals, it has been reported that α-defensins are not found in the neutrophils of pigs or mice (Ganz, 2001). In addition, neither avians nor reptilians encode α-defensin antimicrobial peptides (Xiao *et al.*, 2004). Reptile neutrophil-like cells have granules that contain both cathelicidin-like and β-defensin peptides but not α-defensin peptides, unlike most mammals. By doing an in-depth analysis of multiple α- and β-defensin genes, Xiao *et al.* concluded that mammalian α-defensin genes may have arisen from early β-defensin genes through a process of gene duplication and evolution (Xiao *et al.*, 2004).

In vivo role of α-defensins

α-defensins play a very important antibacterial role *in vivo* in locations where their local concentration can be quite high. Firstly the function of HNPs as neutrophil-associated peptides reveals their critical role in fighting infection throughout the body (Rice *et al.*, 1987). HNPs have also been recently demonstrated to be associated with neutrophil extracellular traps (NETs, as described above), which may play a critical role in the ability to attack pathogens. Dysregulation of this process may be involved in systemic diseases such as lupus.

The α-defensins HD-5 and HD-6 (Table 3.1) have been shown to be expressed in Paneth cells in the intestine, suggesting an important role in interacting with the gut microbiome (Porter *et al.*, 1997a; Porter *et al.*, 1997b; Linzmeier *et al.*, 1999; Ghosh *et al.*, 2002; Furci *et al.*, 2015; Schroeder *et al.*, 2015).

Therapeutic potential of α-defensins

Similarly to β-defensins, if the main *in vivo* role of α-defensins is the modulation of the host innate immune response, then therapeutic interventions that are host-directed would represent a complex but emerging opportunity, yet unexplored. As antibacterial peptides, α-defensin (HNP-derived) peptides have been shown to be antibacterial even in high salt concentrations without requiring disulfide bonding (i.e. in linear form). This suggests that they may have potential use as antimicrobial agents in physiological salt conditions (Varkey and Nagaraj, 2005). The host-directed effects of α-defensins are likely to be complicated.

Mechanism of action of α-defensins

Recently, the ability of HNP-1 to modulate inflammation by affecting bystander macrophage mRNA translation was reported (Brook *et al.*, 2016), suggesting a direct mechanism by which the α-defensin peptide can modulate the host response, control inflammation and promote pathogen clearance. This important result suggests that host-targets for other defensin peptides will also be identified.

A bacterial target of the α-defensin HNP-1 has been identified as the bacterial cell wall precursor molecule (de Leeuw *et al.*, 2010). A fungal defensin, plectasin (Schneider *et al.*, 2010; Witzke *et al.*, 2016), as well as the oyster big defensins (Schmitt *et al.*, 2010), also target lipid II suggesting this target may be useful for the development of new antibacterial compounds. These findings have led to the development of a synthetic small molecule that targets lipid II and is being studied as a potential new antimicrobial agent (Varney *et al.*, 2013), underlining the importance of identifying such molecular targets.

3.2.3 θ-defensins

Definition of θ-defensins

The third class of defensins is the θ-defensins, which are expressed only in non-human 'old-world' primates (e.g. rhesus macaques and baboons) (Tran *et al.*, 2002; Trabi *et al.*, 2001), due to the presence of a premature stop codon in the corresponding human gene. θ-defensins have a fully cyclized peptide structure (Lehrer *et al.*, 2012; Selsted, 2004; Tran *et al.*, 2002; Trabi *et al.*, 2001). This cyclic cystine-ladder structure makes these peptides very resistant to protease attack, and thus they are likely to be stable *in vivo* (Conibear *et al.*, 2014; Conibear *et al.*, 2013). θ-defensins are formed through the cyclization of two 9-aa peptides. θ-defensin peptides are 18 amino acids long, making them the shortest of the defensin peptides, and have an average net charge of +4.5 (ranging between 3 and 6) (Table 3.1).

Host-directed activity of θ-defensin

θ-defensins have been shown to have an immunomodulatory effect to increase macrophage performance against *B. anthracis* (Welkos *et al.*, 2011) and thus also illustrate the property of a 'host-directed' antimicrobial action common to defensins. Indeed, retrocyclin (see below) has been demonstrated to activate human mast cells, suggesting that this synthetic peptide may have more than direct antiviral activities (Gupta *et al.*, 2015).

Therapeutic potential of θ-defensin derivatives

The primate θ-defensins are highly active antiviral peptides (Zhao and Lu, 2014; Tran *et al.*, 2008; Yasin *et al.*, 2004). Due to an early stop-codon, θ-defensins are not naturally expressed in humans, although a vestige of the gene can be found in the human genome. However, 'corrected' or 'normalized' synthetic versions of the human θ-defensin have been made; these are called retrocyclins (Yasin *et al.*, 2004), and they are being developed as a potential therapeutic microbicide (Gupta *et al.*, 2013; Lehrer *et al.*, 2012) (Table 3.2). The structure of retrocyclin-2 (Daly *et al.*, 2007) is shown in Fig. 3.1D. Thus, θ-defensins have demonstrated significant therapeutic potential (Lehrer *et al.*, 2012) already as antiviral peptides and are among the first antimicrobial peptide therapeutics to be used clinically.

3.3 Arthropod Defensins

3.3.1 Insect defensins

Insect defensins are small positively charged peptides of 34–51 residues (~3–5 kDa) that have six conserved cysteine residues and three overall disulfide bonds (Yi *et al.*, 2014). Their structure consists of N-terminal loop, an α-helix and antiparallel β-sheets (Fig. 3.1C). The α-helix and the antiparallel β-sheets are linked by two disulfide bonds and the third disulfide bridge which is the S-S bridge between N-terminal loop and β-sheet (Cornet *et al.*,

Table 3.2. Potential applications of disulfide-linked defensins.

Peptide	Potential application	References
All defensins	Modulation of host directed activities: immune cell recruitment, dampening of inflammation, improved wound healing.	(Brook *et al.*, 2016; Hancock *et al.*, 2016)
Retrocyclin synthetic peptides: Retrocyclin-1 (RC1), GICRCICGRGICRCICGR (+4), Retrocyclin-2 (RC2), GICRCICGRRICRCICGR (+5), Retrocyclin-3 (RC3), RICRCICGRRICRCICGR (+6)	Antiviral compound, retrocyclin inhibits host cell entry of HSV, HIV, IAV. Also protects against *Bacillus anthracis* spore infection through host-directed effects.	(Lehrer *et al.*, 2012)
hBD-1	Higher, salt-resistant activity when unfolded.	(Schroeder *et al.*, 2011a; Schroeder *et al.*, 2011b)
hBD-2	Over-expressed in psoriasis.	(Li *et al.*, 2004; Jansen *et al.*, 2009; Stuart *et al.*, 2012; Hu *et al.*, 2016; Kolbinger *et al.*; 2016)
hBD-3	Expressed in keratinocytes and epithelial cells.	
Linear fragment of hBD-3 (Peptide 4)	Antibacterial properties in a much smaller fragment (no longer a defensin)	(Hoover *et al.*, 2003; Taylor *et al.*, 2008; Papanastasiou *et al.*, 2009).
Big defensin from horseshoe crabs and oysters.	Both domains have antimicrobial activity.	(Saito *et al.*, 1995; Kouno *et al.*, 2008; Rosa *et al.*, 2015; van Hoek, 2016)
A defensins HNP1, HNP2, HNP3	Components of neutrophil extracellular traps, NETs, possible role in lupus.	(Van Avondt *et al.*, 2013; Cheng *et al.*, 2015a)
HD-5	Active against *Clostridium difficile* strains.	(Furci *et al.*, 2015)
HD-6	Selective activity against gut commensal bacteria.	(Schroeder *et al.*, 2015)
Potential Antibiotic Synergy with hNP1.	Combination of antibiotics acting in synergy with AMPs may increase their antibacterial activity, especially in high salt conditions.	(Sakoulas *et al.*, 2012)
Insect defensins	Strong activity against Gram-positive bacteria.	(Bulet and Stocklin, 2005; Yi *et al.*, 2014; Kaushal *et al.*, 2016b)

1995; Maget-Dana *et al.*, 1995). Their structural components include three domains: an amino-terminal loop, an amphipathic α-helix, and a carboxy-terminal antiparallel β-sheet (Bonmatin *et al.*, 1992). The insect defensins differ from vertebrate defensins mainly by the significant α-helix structural element (Compare Fig. 3.1A to Fig. 3.1C). These insect defensins are inducible and may form voltage-dependent channels in bacteria (Cociancich *et al.*, 1993).

Insect defensins are strongly active against Gram-positive bacteria (Otvos, 2000; Yi *et al.*, 2014; Bulet and Stocklin, 2005) and generally inactive against Gram-negative bacteria (Kaushal *et al.*, 2016b). Their primary mode of action is thought to be pore or channel formation in cytoplasmic membrane of the Gram-positive bacteria (Yi *et al.*, 2014). Defensins have been isolated from mosquitos and other insects (Gao *et al.*, 1999; Bulet and Stocklin, 2005) including their recent identification in the bedbug (Kaushal *et al.*, 2016b) (Fig. 3.1C). Common vectors of diseases such as the mosquito can also express various antimicrobial peptides, including forms of insect defensin as well as cecropin peptides (Kaushal *et al.*, 2016a).

3.3.2 Therapeutic potential of insect defensins

One interesting feature of insect defensins is that the sizeable N-terminal helical region (Fig. 3.1C) is not required for antimicrobial activity of the peptide, and thus could be removed to generate shorter peptides that may retain antimicrobial activity (Varkey *et al.*, 2006). In addition, for some insect defensins, the disulfide bonding is not required for antimicrobial activity of the linear peptide (Varkey *et al.*, 2006). This is a very useful characteristic, as linear peptides are more easily synthesized for therapeutic development than those requiring proper folding for activity (Yi *et al.*, 2014), as previously discussed.

It has been suggested that some of the beneficial effect of the ancient practice of 'maggot therapy' for infected-wound treatment may be attributable to the expression of lucifensin, an insect defensin produced by those insects (Cerovsky and Bem, 2014).

3.3.3 Antiparasitic activity of arthropod defensin peptides

Recent work has identified antiparasitic activity of some insect antimicrobial peptides, including insect defensins (Lacerda *et al.*, 2016), especially the defensin peptides of the hard tick, *Ixodes ricinus* (Tonk *et al.*, 2015). Additional defensins from other arthropods, in this case scorpions, have also demonstrated antiparasitic activity (Conde *et al.*, 2000). This is a promising area of research against the somewhat neglected parasitic diseases, which are re-emerging.

3.3.4 Horseshoe crab and oyster big-defensins

Big defensins (Schulenburg *et al.*, 2007; Schmitt *et al.*, 2012), first identified in horseshoe crabs in 1995 (Saito *et al.*, 1995), are peptides involved in innate immunity in organisms such as horseshoe crabs, oysters and mussels. Big defensins are an unusual antimicrobial peptide when compared to mammalian or vertebrate defensins and further reflect the diversity of antimicrobial peptides found in nature (Schmitt *et al.*, 2012). These peptides, approximately 80 amino acids in length, have two distinct domains: a highly hydrophobic, cationic (often +6 charge), probably helical, N-terminal domain, and a cationic C-terminal domain with six cysteines that closely resembles vertebrate β-defensins (Saito *et al.*, 1995; Kouno *et al.*, 2008) (Fig. 3.1B; Table 3.1). Each of these domains can exert separate antimicrobial activity. The N-terminal region was shown to be antimicrobial against Gram-positive bacteria, while the C-terminal region was shown to be antimicrobial against Gram-negative bacteria, and there appears to be some combined synergy of the two domains together with regards to LPS binding (Saito *et al.*, 1995; Rosa *et al.*, 2011; Kouno *et al.*, 2009). Many of the big defensin genes are inducible by bacterial products; for example, their expression is not observed in uninfected oysters (Rosa *et al.*, 2011).

These 'big-defensins' are evolutionarily related to vertebrate defensins in their C-terminal domain in terms of structure, but still surprisingly distant from human β-defensins by sequence (Schmitt *et al.*, 2012; Rosa *et al.*, 2015). The N-terminal domain of the big defensin is a hydrophobic, globular domain that may participate in binding LPS, while the C-terminal domain adopts a more typical β-defensin fold with the signature β-defensin bonding pattern (Cys1–5, 2–4, 3–6) (Kouno *et al.*, 2008).

There are at least 17 different big defensins known or predicted in different invertebrates (Schmitt *et al.*, 2012). Oysters, such as *Crassostrea gigas* (Gueguen *et al.*, 2006; Gonzalez *et al.*, 2007; Rosa *et al.*,

2015), have big defensins that are active only against Gram-positive bacteria. Oyster big defensins were shown to exert their antibacterial activity by interfering with *Staphylococcus aureus* lipid II and thus interfering with the bacteria's peptidoglycan synthesis (Schmitt *et al.*, 2010), revealing the diversity of bacterial targets for antimicrobial peptides. Horseshoe crabs express a big defensin, tachyplesin (Table 3.1), which can bind LPS and has activity against both Gram-positive and Gram-negative organisms under MIC conditions (Saito *et al.*, 1995; Kouno *et al.*, 2008; Kushibiki *et al.*, 2014).

3.4 Plant Defensins

Plants express a wide range of antibacterial, antiviral and antifungal compounds (Oard and Enright, 2006; Maroti *et al.*, 2011; Salas *et al.*, 2015). Plant defensins have a structure similar to insect defensins, with a significant α-helix domain attached to the β-pleated sheets by disulfide bonds (Tam *et al.*, 2015). Plant defensins generally do not have antibacterial activity but appear to be involved in defence against a broad range of fungi, demonstrating antifungal activity against many phyto-pathogenic fungi and yeast. Several recent reviews discuss these peptides in greater detail (Stotz *et al.*, 2009; Salas *et al.*, 2015; Tam *et al.*, 2015; Bolouri Moghaddam *et al.*, 2016). The mechanism of action of these peptides is a subject of active research, and may reveal new therapeutic approaches to the development of antifungal therapeutics.

In addition, plants express many other kinds of antimicrobial peptides, including cyclic peptides, which are very stable to protease degradation (Silverstein *et al.*, 2007; Tam *et al.*, 2015). There are hundreds of antimicrobial peptide-like genes identified in plants, such as in *Arabidopsis* (Silverstein *et al.*, 2005; Silverstein *et al.*, 2007). The very significant number of antifungal compounds found in plants represents a sizeable resource for development of novel antifungal therapeutics, which are a critical clinical need.

3.5 When Is a Disulfide-linked Antimicrobial Peptide not a Defensin?

Defensins are an example of a cystine-stabilized polypeptide with antimicrobial function, defined by a strict set of sequence criteria described in the sections above. Another family of cystine-stabilized peptides is the crotamine toxin family, first isolated from rattlesnakes with a similar 'gamma-core' motif to defensins (Kerkis *et al.*, 2010; Radis-Baptista and Kerkis, 2011). Crotamine is considered to be a cell-penetrating peptide. Many reptiles are known to express crotamine-like peptides. The sequence of crotamine is YKQCHKKG-GHCFPKEKICLPPSSDFGKMD-CRWRWKCCKKGSG (+8) (Wang *et al.*, 2009). This cationic peptide is highly charged with nine lysines (K), three disulfide bonds between six cysteines (C) and has a defensin-like fold. It is a matter of debate whether crotamine peptides are actually defensin peptides or if they just contain a similar cystine-stabilized core structure. Crotamine toxin displays limited-to-poor antimicrobial activity against *Bacillus subtilis*, and with permeabilized *Staphylococcus aureus* cells (Yount *et al.*, 2009). In addition, crotamine has been shown to have some antifungal activity (Yamane *et al.*, 2013). Despite arguments about whether they are antimicrobial or not (van Hoek, 2014), crotamines are not strictly considered to be defensin peptides.

Hepcidins are interesting disulfide-stabilized peptides with four disulfide bonds (eight cysteines). These small antimicrobial peptides are highly expressed in liver tissue and have a hairpin-like structure, rather than a β-defensin fold (Nemeth *et al.*, 2004). These peptides are widely expressed in the animal kingdom (van Hoek, 2014), but their poor *in vitro* antibacterial activity has dampened enthusiasm for their development as a new antimicrobial agent. Researchers now refer to hepcidin as a hormone rather than consider it an antibacterial peptide (Hunter *et al.* 2002; Ganz, 2006), highlighting its role as a host-defence peptide. However, the hepcidin peptides do play a critical role in the regulation of bacterial infection *in vivo* through their activity in iron homeostasis (Nemeth *et al.*, 2004; Ganz, 2009; Nairz *et al.*, 2014) and thus may still have significant therapeutic potential (Rochette *et al.*, 2015).

3.6 Therapeutic Potential of Synthetic Disulfide-linked Defensin Peptides

The main *in vivo* effect of disulfide-linked defensin peptides may be through their host-directed immunomodulatory effect. However, this has not yet been well explored for therapeutic potential. Significant complexities exist regarding the interaction of peptides with the host immune system (Hancock *et al.*, 2016).

Considerable work has been done to develop the antimicrobial activity of these peptides. Some of the therapeutic options for disulfide-linked peptides are summarized in Table 3.2. While synthesis and correct folding of the full-length defensin peptides can be highly challenging, new systems are being developed to address these technical issues. The production of fully glycosylated and properly folded disulfide-linked defensin proteins in these systems will be highly enabling to their further development as therapeutics.

Recent research in antimicrobial peptide development has focused on modifications to generate synthetic peptides that improve the therapeutic properties while minimizing the undesireable features of the natural peptides (Brogden and Brogden, 2011). Modifications made to the θ-defensin peptides have resulted in at least three synthetic retrocyclin peptides and further derivatives, with charges ranging from +3 to +6 (Table 3.2).

Other approaches include the development of fragments of peptides that retain antimicrobial function. Synthetic peptides based on desirable features of natural peptides have been made by combining fragments of diverse natural peptides. Recently, a combination of a fragment of hBD-1 was made with the retrocyclin peptide, then cyclized, and this hybrid peptide was found to have significant, salt-resistant antimicrobial and antifungal activity (Olli *et al.*, 2015). The antimicrobial activity of hBD-3 can be isolated to a small linear fragment not dependent on disulfide-bonded configurations. The antimicrobial activity can be separated from the chemo-attractant activity, suggesting that this small, linear fragment could be developed into a topical antimicrobial agent, for example. Alternatively the chemotactic fragment could be developed as a host-directed therapeutic.

3.7 Summary

3.7.1 Phylogenetic diversity of defensin gene expression

Genes encoding defensin peptides are widely expressed throughout the Animalia and Plantae kingdoms. β-defensin genes are highly conserved between bivalves, insects, plants and humans, but mostly due to the conserved sequence constraints of the six-cysteine pattern. The intervening sequences and N-terminal sequences can vary significantly, and these differences appear to have significant functional consequences. Many examples of α- and β-defensin gene clusters have been identified, suggesting additional levels of regulation of their expression. α-defensins are also highly conserved within the animal kingdom, but interestingly are not expressed in the avian or non-avian reptiles, nor are they found in lower eukaryotes such as bivalves, insects or plants. θ-defensins are only expressed in Old-world primates. Plants and arthropods also express defensin peptides with six cysteines, but have varied other domains and sequences.

3.7.2 Defensin activity

The main *in vivo* role of disulfide-linked defensin peptides is probably not their antimicrobial activity, but their host-directed, immunomodulatory activities. Defensins have shown antimicrobial or antiviral activity against a very wide range of bacterial, fungal and viral pathogens, reflecting their central contribution to innate immunity. While this broad range of activity may be beneficial *in vivo*, focusing development and research on the specific properties of each individual defensin peptide will allow its development for particular applications, such as antifungal therapeutics, perhaps through its host-directed effects.

Some bacteria that are inherently resistant to cationic peptides overall – such as *Burkholderia* species – are also resistant to these small peptides (Blower *et al.*, 2015). Overall, there is good potential to develop antimicrobial peptides into peptide-mimetic fragments for use against multi-drug resistant bacteria, either alone or in combination with antibiotics.

Defensin therapeutic potential

The most advanced therapeutic use of defensin peptides is retrocyclin, which shows significant promise against several viral pathogens. Several versions of retrocyclin are currently in clinical trials (Gupta *et al.*, 2013). The host-directed effects of retrocylins are currently being explored.

Although the structures of the α- and β-defensin peptides can be complex, with disulfide-linkages and mixed helical structures, many of these peptides show strong activity against various bacteria (Table 3.2). The most promising human defensin peptide candidates include hBD-1, which has increased activity when unfolded, and hBD-3, which is generally more salt resistant in its activity. In addition, small, linear peptides that have been derived from full-length defensins (although no longer themselves defensins) have been shown to have good antimicrobial activity and thus have significant potential for development as antimicrobial agents. Combinations of defensin antimicrobial peptides with antibiotics may demonstrate *in vitro* and *in vivo* synergy against various bacteria and may provide a new opportunity to develop novel therapeutic approaches for the treatment of multi-drug resistant bacteria.

Future work is needed to develop these host-defence peptides into potential therapeutics to exploit their host-directed activities in immune recruitment, wound healing or dampening inflammation. Production of large quantities of properly folded peptide, perhaps in a heterologous plant expression system may facilitate such studies.

Acknowledgements

Ryan J. Blower provided technical assistance in the preparation of figures. MVH is partially supported by HDTRA1-12-C-0039 from the Defense Threat Reduction Agency.

References

Aerts, A., Thevissen, K., Bresseleers, S., Wouters, P., Cammue, B. and Francois, I. (2005) Heterologous production of human beta-defensin-2 in *Arabidopsis thaliana*. *Communications in Agricultural and Applied Biological Sciences* 70, 51–55.

Alekseeva, L., Huet, D., Femenia, F., Mouyna, I., Abdelouahab, M., *et al.* (2009) Inducible expression of beta defensins by human respiratory epithelial cells exposed to *Aspergillus fumigatus* organisms. *BMC Microbiology* 9, 33.

Alibardi, L. (2013) Granulocytes of reptilian sauropsids contain beta-defensin-like peptides: a comparative ultrastructural survey. *Journal of Morphology* 274, 877–886.

Alibardi, L. (2014) Histochemical, biochemical and cell biological aspects of tail regeneration in lizards: an amniote model for studies on tissue regeneration. *Progress in Histochemistry and Cytochemistry* 48, 143–244.

Alibardi, L., Celeghin, A. and Dalla Valle, L. (2012) Wounding in lizards results in the release of beta-defensins at the wound site and formation of an antimicrobial barrier. *Developmental and Comparative Immunology* 36, 557–565.

Amid, C., Rehaume, L.M., Brown, K.L., Gilbert, J.G., Dougan, G., Hancock, R.E. and Harrow, J.L. (2009) Manual annotation and analysis of the defensin gene cluster in the C57bl/6j mouse reference genome. *BMC Genomics* 10, 606.

Blower, R.J., Barksdale, S.M. and Van Hoek, M.L. (2015) Snake cathelicidin Na-Cath and smaller helical antimicrobial peptides are effective against *Burkholderia thailandensis*. *PLOS Neglected Tropical Diseases* 9, E0003862.

Bolouri Moghaddam, M.R., Vilcinskas, A. and Rahnamaeian, M. (2016) Cooperative interaction of antimicrobial peptides with the interrelated immune pathways in plants. *Molecular Plant Pathology* 17, 464–471.

Bonmatin, J.M., Bonnat, J.L., Gallet, X., Vovelle, F., Ptak, M., *et al.* (1992) Two-dimensional H NMR study of recombinant insect defensin A in water: resonance assignments, secondary structure and global folding. *Journal of Biomolecular NMR* 2, 235–256.

Brogden, N.K. and Brogden, K.A. (2011) Will new generations of modified antimicrobial peptides improve their potential as pharmaceuticals? *International Journal of Antimicrobial Agents* 38, 217–225.

Brook, M., Tomlinson, G.H., Miles, K., Smith, R.W., Rossi, A.G., *et al.* (2016) Neutrophil-derived alpha defensins control inflammation by inhibiting macrophage Mrna translation. *Proceedings of the National Academy of Sciences of the United States of America* 113, 4350–4355.

Bulet, P. and Stocklin, R. (2005) Insect antimicrobial peptides: structures, properties and gene regulation. *Protein Peptide Letters* 12, 3–11.

Cao, Y., Ma, Q., Shan, A. and Dong, N. (2012) Expression in *Pichia pastoris* and biological activity of avian beta-defensin 6 and its mutant peptide without cysteines. *Protein Peptide Letters* 19, 1064–1070.

Cerovsky, V. and Bem, R. (2014). Lucifensins, the insect defensins of biomedical importance: the story behind maggot therapy. *Pharmaceuticals* 7, 251–264.

Chang, Z., Lu, M., Ma, Y., Kwag, D.G., Kim, S.H., Park, J.M., Nam, B.H., Kim, Y.O., An, C.M., Li, H., Jung, J.H. and Park, J.S. (2015) Production of disulfide bond-rich peptides by fusion expression using small transmembrane proteins of *Escherichia coli*. *Amino Acids* 47, 579–587.

Cheng, F.J., Zhou, X.J., Zhao, Y.F., Zhao, M.H. and Zhang, H. (2015a) Human neutrophil peptide 1-3, a component of the neutrophil extracellular trap, as a potential biomarker of lupus nephritis. *International Journal of Rheumatic Diseases* 18, 533–540.

Cheng, Y., Prickett, M.D., Gutowska, W., Kuo, R., Belov, K. and Burt, D.W. (2015b) Evolution of the avian beta-defensin and cathelicidin genes. *BMC Evolutionary Biology* 15, 188.

Cociancich, S., Ghazi, A., Hetru, C., Hoffmann, J.A. and Letellier, L. (1993) Insect defensin, an inducible antibacterial peptide, forms voltage-dependent channels in *Micrococcus luteus*. *Journal of Biological Chemistry*, 268, 19239–19245.

Conde, R., Zamudio, F.Z., Rodriguez, M.H. and Possani, L.D. (2000) Scorpine, an anti-malaria and anti-bacterial agent purified from scorpion venom. *FEBS Letters* 471, 165–168.

Conibear, A.C., Rosengren, K.J., Daly, N.L., Henriques, S.T. and Craik, D.J. (2013) The cyclic cystine ladder in theta-defensins is important for structure and stability, but not antibacterial activity. *Journal of Biological Chemistry* 288, 10830–10840.

Conibear, A.C., Bochen, A., Rosengren, K.J., Stupar, P., Wang, C., Kessler, H. and Craik, D.J. (2014) The cyclic cystine ladder of theta-defensins as a stable, bifunctional scaffold: a proof-of-concept study using the integrin-binding RGD motif. *ChemBioChem* 15, 451–459.

Cornet, B., Bonmatin, J.M., Hetru, C., Hoffmann, J.A., Ptak, M. and Vovelle, F. (1995) Refined three-dimensional solution structure of insect defensin A. *Structure*, 3, 435–448.

Corrales-Garcia, L.L., Possani, L.D. and Corzo, G. (2011) Expression systems of human beta-defensins: vectors, purification and biological activities. *Amino Acids* 40, 5–13.

Cuperus, T., Coorens, M., Van Dijk, A. and Haagsman, H.P. (2013) Avian host defense peptides. *Developmental and Comparative Immunology* 41, 352–369.

Daly, N.L., Chen, Y.K., Rosengren, K.J., Marx, U.C., Phillips, M.L., *et al.* (2007) Retrocyclin-2: structural analysis of a potent anti-HIV theta-defensin. *Biochemistry* 46, 9920–9928.

Das, S., Nikolaidis, N., Goto, H., McCallister, C., Li, J., Hirano, M. and Cooper, M.D. (2010) Comparative genomics and evolution of the alpha-defensin multigene family in primates. *Molecular Biology and Evolution* 27, 2333–2343.

De Leeuw, E., Li, C., Zeng, P., Li, C., Diepeveen-De Buin, M., Lu, W.Y., Breukink, E. and Lu, W. (2010) Functional interaction of human neutrophil peptide-1 with the cell wall precursor lipid II. *FEBS Letters* 584, 1543–1548.

Dong, J., Yu, H., Zhang, Y., Diao, H. and Lin, D. (2011) Soluble fusion expression and characterization of human beta-defensin 3 using a novel approach. *Protein Peptide Letters* 18, 1126–1132.

Eckmann, L. (2005) Defence molecules in intestinal innate immunity against bacterial infections. *Current Opinion in Gastroenterology* 21, 147–151.

Furci, L., Baldan, R., Bianchini, V., Trovato, A., Ossi, C., Cichero, P. and Cirillo, D.M. (2015) New role for human alpha-defensin 5 in the fight against hypervirulent *Clostridium difficile* strains. *Infection and Immunity* 83, 986–995.

Ganz, T. (2001) Defensins in the urinary tract and other tissues. *Journal of Infectious Diseases* 183 Suppl 1, S41–42.

Ganz, T. (2003) Defensins: antimicrobial peptides of innate immunity. *Nature Reviews Immunology* 3, 710–720.

Ganz, T. (2006) Hepcidin – peptide hormone at the interface of innate immunity and iron metabolism. *Current Topics in Microbiology and Immunology* 306, 183–198.

Ganz, T. (2009) Iron in innate immunity: starve the invaders. *Current Opinion in Immunology* 21, 63–67.

Gao, Y., Hernandez, V.P. and Fallon, A.M. (1999) Immunity proteins from mosquito cell lines include three defensin A isoforms from *Aedes aegypti* and A Defensin D From *Aedes albopictus*. *Insect Molecular Biology* 8, 311–331.

Garcia, J.R., Jaumann, F., Schulz, S., Krause, A., Rodriguez-Jimenez, J., *et al.* (2001a) Identification of a novel, multifunctional beta-defensin (human beta-defensin 3) with specific antimicrobial activity: its interaction with plasma membranes of Xenopus oocytes and the induction of macrophage chemoattraction. *Cell Tissue Research* 306, 257–264.

Garcia, J.R., Krause, A., Schulz, S., Rodriguez-Jimenez, F.J., Kluver, E., *et al.* (2001b) Human beta-defensin 4: a novel inducible peptide with a specific salt-sensitive spectrum of antimicrobial activity. *FASEB Journal* 15, 1819–1821.

Gazzaneo, L.R., Pandolfi, V., Jesus, A.L., Crovella, S., Benko-Iseppon, A.M. and Freitas, A.C. (2017) Heterologous expression systems for plant defensin expression: examples of success and pitfalls. *Current Protein and Peptide Science* 18, 391–399.

Ghosh, D., Porter, E., Shen, B., Lee, S.K., Wilk, D., *et al.* (2002) Paneth cell trypsin is the processing enzyme for human defensin-5. *Nature Immunology* 3, 583–590.

Gonzalez, M., Gueguen, Y., Desserre, G., De Lorgeril, J., Romestand, B. and Bachere, E. (2007) Molecular characterization of two isoforms of defensin from hemocytes of the oyster *Crassostrea gigas*. *Developmental and Comparative Immunology* 31, 332–339.

Gueguen, Y., Herpin, A., Aumelas, A., Garnier, J., Fievet, J., *et al.* (2006) Characterization of a defensin from the oyster *Crassostrea gigas*: recombinant production, folding, solution structure, antimicrobial activities, and gene expression. *Journal of Biological Chemistry* 281, 313–323.

Gupta, K., Kotian, A., Subramanian, H., Daniell, H. and Ali, H. (2015) Activation of human mast cells by retrocyclin and protegrin highlight their immunomodulatory and antimicrobial properties. *Oncotarget* 6, 28573–28587.

Gupta, K., Subramanian, H. and Ali, H. (2016) Modulation of host defense peptide-mediated human mast cell activation by LPS. *Innate Immunity* 22, 21–30.

Gupta, P., Lackman-Smith, C., Snyder, B., Ratner, D., Rohan, L.C., *et al.* (2013) Antiviral activity of retrocyclin rc-101, a candidate microbicide against cell-associated HIV-1. *Aids Research and Human Retroviruses* 29, 391–396.

Han, S., Bishop, B.M. and Van Hoek, M.L. (2008) Antimicrobial activity of human beta-defensins and induction by *Francisella*. *Biochemical and Biophysical Research Communications* 371, 670–674.

Hancock, R.E., Haney, E.F. and Gill, E.E. (2016) The immunology of host defence peptides: beyond antimicrobial activity. *Nature Reviews Immunology* 16, 321–334.

Harder, J., Bartels, J., Christophers, E. and Schroder, J.M. (2001) Isolation and characterization of human beta-defensin-3, a novel human inducible peptide antibiotic. *Journal of Biological Chemistry* 276, 5707–5713.

Herve-Grepinet, V., Rehault-Godbert, S., Labas, V., Magallon, T., Derache, C., *et al.* (2010). Purification and characterization of avian beta-defensin 11, an antimicrobial peptide of the hen egg. *Antimicrobial Agents and Chemotherapy* 54, 4401–4409.

Hiratsuka, T., Nakazato, M., Date, Y., Ashitani, J., Minematsu, T., Chino, N. and Matsukura, S. (1998) Identification of human beta-defensin-2 in respiratory tract and plasma and its increase in bacterial pneumonia. *Biochemical and Biophysical Research Communications* 249, 943–947.

Hoover, D.M., Chertov, O. and Lubkowski, J. (2001) The structure of human beta-defensin-1: new insights into structural properties of beta-defensins. *Journal of Biological Chemistry* 276, 39021–39026.

Hoover, D.M., Wu, Z., Tucker, K., Lu, W. and Lubkowski, J. (2003) Antimicrobial characterization of human beta-defensin 3 derivatives. *Antimicrobial Agents and Chemotherapy* 47, 2804–2809.

Hu, S.C., Yu, H.S., Yen, F.L., Lin, C.L., Chen, G.S. and Lan, C.C. (2016) Neutrophil extracellular trap formation is increased in psoriasis and induces human beta-defensin-2 production in epidermal keratinocytes. *Science Reports* 6, 311–319.

Huang, L., Leong, S.S. and Jiang, R. (2009) Soluble fusion expression and characterization of bioactive human beta-defensin 26 and 27. *Applied Microbiology and Biotechnology* 84, 301–308.

Hunter, H.N., Fulton, D.B., Ganz, T. and Vogel, H.J. (2002) The solution structure of human hepcidin: a peptide hormone with antimicrobial activity that is involved in iron uptake and hereditary hemochromatosis. *Journal of Biological Chemistry* 277, 37597–37603.

Jansen, P.A., Rodijk-Olthuis, D., Hollox, E.J., Kamsteeg, M., Tjabringa, G.S., *et al.* (2009) Beta-defensin-2 protein is a serum biomarker for disease activity in psoriasis and reaches biologically relevant concentrations in lesional skin. *PLOS One*, 4, E4725.

Jenssen, H., Hamill, P. and Hancock, R.E. (2006) Peptide antimicrobial agents. *Clinical Microbiology Reviews* 19, 491–511.

Kaushal, A., Gupta, K., Shah, R. and Van Hoek, M.L. (2016a) Antimicrobial activity of mosquito cecropin peptides against *Francisella*. *Developmental and Comparative Immunology* 63, 171–180.

Kaushal, A., Gupta, K. and Van Hoek, M.L. (2016b) Characterization of *Cimex lectularius* (bedbug) defensin peptide and its antimicrobial activity against human skin microflora. *Biochemical and Biophysical Research Communications* 470, 955–960.

Kerkis, I., Silva Fde, S., Pereira, A., Kerkis, A. and Radis-Baptista, G. (2010) Biological versatility of crotamine – a cationic peptide from the venom of a South American rattlesnake. *Expert Opinion on Investigational Drugs* 19, 1515–1525.

Kolbinger, F., Loesche, C., Valentin, M.A., Jiang, X., Cheng, Y., *et al.* (2016) Beta-defensin-2 is a responsive biomarker of Il-17a-driven skin pathology in psoriasis. *Journal of Allergy and Clinical Immunology* 139, 923–932.

Kouno, T., Fujitani, N., Mizuguchi, M., Osaki, T., Nishimura, S., *et al.* (2008) A novel beta-defensin structure: a potential strategy of big defensin for overcoming resistance by Gram-positive bacteria. *Biochemistry* 47, 10611–10619.

Kouno, T., Mizuguchi, M., Aizawa, T., Shinoda, H., Demura, M., Kawabata, S. and Kawano, K. (2009) A novel beta-defensin structure: big defensin changes its N-terminal structure to associate with the target membrane. *Biochemistry* 48, 7629–7635.

Kreuter, A., Jaouhar, M., Skrygan, M., Tigges, C., Stucker, M., *et al.* (2011) Expression of antimicrobial peptides in different subtypes of cutaneous Lupus erythematosus. *Journal of the American Academy of Dermatology* 65, 125–133.

Kushibiki, T., Kamiya, M., Aizawa, T., Kumaki, Y., Kikukawa, T., *et al.* (2014) Interaction between tachyplesin I, an antimicrobial peptide derived from horseshoe crab, and lipopolysaccharide. *Biochimica et Biophysica Acta* 1844, 527–534.

Lacerda, A.F., Pelegrini, P.B., De Oliveira, D.M., Vasconcelos, E.A. and Grossi-De-Sa, M.F. (2016) Antiparasitic peptides from arthropods and their application in drug therapy. *Frontiers in Microbiology* 7, 91.

Lakshminarayanan, R., Vivekanandan, S., Samy, R.P., Banerjee, Y., Chi-Jin, E.O., *et al.* (2008) Structure, self-assembly, and dual role of a beta-defensin-like peptide from the Chinese soft-shelled turtle eggshell matrix. *Journal of the American Chemical Society* 130, 4660–4668.

Lehrer, R.I. and Lu, W. (2012) Alpha-defensins in human innate immunity. *Immunology Reviews* 245, 84–112.

Lehrer, R.I., Cole, A.M. and Selsted, M.E. (2012) Theta-defensins: cyclic peptides with endless potential. *Journal of Biological Chemistry* 287, 27014–27019.

Li, D., Li, J., Duan, Y. and Zhou, X. (2004) Expression of LL-37, human beta defensin-2, and Ccr6 mRNA in patients with psoriasis vulgaris. *Journal of Huazhong University of Science and Technology (Medical Sciences)* 24, 404–406.

Li, J.F., Zhang, J., Zhang, Z., Ma, H.W., Zhang, J.X. and Zhang, S.Q. (2010) Production of bioactive human beta-defensin-4 in *Escherichia coli* using sumo fusion partner. *Protein Journal* 29, 314–319.

Linzmeier, R., Ho, C.H., Hoang, B.V. and Ganz, T. (1999) A 450-Kb contig of defensin genes on human chromosome 8p23. *Gene* 233, 205–211.

Luan, C., Xie, Y.G., Pu, Y.T., Zhang, H.W., Han, F.F., Feng, J. and Wang, Y.Z. (2014) Recombinant expression of antimicrobial peptides using a novel self-cleaving aggregation tag in *Escherichia coli*. *Canadian Journal of Microbiology* 60, 113–120.

Machado, L.R. and Ottolini, B. (2015) An evolutionary history of defensins: a role for copy number variation in maximizing host innate and adaptive immune responses. *Frontiers in Immunology* 6, 115.

Maget-Dana, R., Bonmatin, J.M., Hetru, C., Ptak, M. and Maurizot, J.C. (1995) The secondary structure of the insect defensin a depends on its environment: a circular dichroism study. *Biochimie* 77, 240–244.

Maroti, G., Kereszt, A., Kondorosi, E. and Mergaert, P. (2011) Natural roles of antimicrobial peptides in microbes, plants and animals. *Research in Microbiology* 162, 363–374.

McCray, P.B., Jr and Bentley, L. (1997) Human airway epithelia express a beta-defensin. *American Journal of Respiratory Cell and Molecular Biology* 16, 343–349.

Mine, Y., Oberle, C. and Kassaify, Z. (2003) Eggshell matrix proteins as defense mechanism of avian eggs. *Journal of Agricultural and Food Chemistry* 51, 249–253.

Nairz, M., Haschka, D., Demetz, E. and Weiss, G. (2014) Iron at the interface of immunity and infection. *Frontiers in Pharmacology* 5, 152.

Nemeth, E., Tuttle, M.S., Powelson, J., Vaughn, M.B., Donovan, A., *et al.* (2004) Hepcidin regulates cellular iron efflux by binding to ferroportin and inducing its internalization. *Science* 306, 2090–2093.

Niyonsaba, F. and Ogawa, H. (2005) Protective roles of the skin against infection: implication of naturally occurring human antimicrobial agents beta-defensins, cathelicidin Ll-37 and lysozyme. *Journal of Dermatological Science* 40, 157–168.

Oard, S.V. and Enright, F.M. (2006) Expression of the antimicrobial peptides in plants to control phytopathogenic bacteria and fungi. *Plant Cell Reports* 25, 561–572.

Olli, S., Nagaraj, R. and Motukupally, S.R. (2015) A hybrid cationic peptide composed of human beta-defensin-1 and humanized theta-defensin sequences exhibits salt-resistant antimicrobial activity. *Antimicrobial Agents and Chemotherapy* 59, 217–225.

O'Neil, D.A., Porter, E.M., Elewaut, D., Anderson, G.M., Eckmann, L., Ganz, T. and Kagnoff, M.F. (1999) Expression and regulation of the human beta-defensins hBD-1 And hBD-2 in intestinal epithelium. *Journal of Immunology* 163, 6718–6724.

Otvos, L., Jr (2000) Antibacterial peptides isolated from insects. *Journal of Peptide Science* 6, 497–511.

Papanastasiou, E.A., Hua, Q., Sandouk, A., Son, U.H., Christenson, A.J., Van Hoek, M.L. and Bishop, B.M. (2009) Role of acetylation and charge in antimicrobial peptides based on human beta-defensin-3. *APMIS* 117, 492–499.

Patil, A.A., Cai, Y., Sang, Y., Blecha, F. and Zhang, G. (2005) Cross-species analysis of the mammalian beta-defensin gene family: presence of syntenic gene clusters and preferential expression in the male reproductive tract. *Physiological Genomics* 23, 5–17.

Peng, Z., Wang, A., Feng, Q., Wang, Z., Ivanova, I.V., *et al.* (2014) High-level expression, purification and characterisation of porcine beta-defensin 2 in *Pichia pastoris* and its potential as a cost-efficient growth promoter in porcine feed. *Applied Microbiology and Biotechnology* 98, 5487–5497.

Pierson, T., Learmonth-Pierson, S., Pinto, D. and Van Hoek, M.L. (2013) Cigarette smoke extract induces differential expression levels of beta-defensin peptides in human alveolar epithelial cells. *Tobacco Induced Diseases* 11, 10.

Porter, E.M., Liu, L., Oren, A., Anton, P.A. and Ganz, T. (1997a) Localization of human intestinal defensin 5 in paneth cell granules. *Infection and Immunity* 65, 2389–2395.

Porter, E.M., Van Dam, E., Valore, E.V. and Ganz, T. (1997b) Broad-spectrum antimicrobial activity of human intestinal defensin 5. *Infection and Immunity* 65, 2396–2401.

Premratanachai, P., Joly, S., Johnson, G.K., Mccray, P.B., Jr, Jia, H.P. and Guthmiller, J.M. (2004) Expression and regulation of novel human beta-defensins in gingival keratinocytes. *Oral Microbiology and Immunology* 19, 111–117.

Radis-Baptista, G. and Kerkis, I. (2011) Crotamine, a small basic polypeptide myotoxin from rattlesnake venom with cell-penetrating properties. *Current Pharmaceutical Design* 17, 4351–4361.

Rice, W.G., Ganz, T., Kinkade, J.M., Jr, Selsted, M.E., Lehrer, R.I. and Parmley, R.T. (1987) Defensin-rich dense granules of human neutrophils. *Blood* 70, 757–65.

Rochette, L., Gudjoncik, A., Guenancia, C., Zeller, M., Cottin, Y. and Vergely, C. (2015) The iron-regulatory hormone hepcidin: a possible therapeutic target? *Pharmacology and Therapeutics* 146, 35–52.

Rosa, R.D., Santini, A., Fievet, J., Bulet, P., Destoumieux-Garzon, D. and Bachere, E. (2011) Big defensins, a diverse family of antimicrobial peptides that follows different patterns of expression in hemocytes of the oyster *Crassostrea gigas*. *PLOS One*, 6, E25594.

Rosa, R.D., Alonso, P., Santini, A., Vergnes, A. and Bachere, E. (2015) High polymorphism in big defensin gene expression reveals presence-absence gene variability (PAV) in the oyster *Crassostrea gigas*. *Developmental and Comparative Immunology* 49, 231–238.

Saito, T., Kawabata, S., Shigenaga, T., Takayenoki, Y., Cho, J., *et al.* (1995) A novel big defensin identified in horseshoe crab hemocytes: isolation, amino acid sequence, and antibacterial activity. *Journal of Biochemistry* 117, 1131–1137.

Saitoh, T., Komano, J., Saitoh, Y., Misawa, T., Takahama, M., *et al.* (2012) Neutrophil extracellular traps mediate a host defense response to Human Immunodeficiency Virus-1. *Cell Host & Microbe* 12, 109–116.

Sakoulas, G., Bayer, A.S., Pogliano, J., Tsuji, B.T., Yang, S.J., *et al.* (2012) Ampicillin enhances daptomycin- and cationic host defense peptide-mediated killing of ampicillin- and vancomycin-resistant *Enterococcus faecium*. *Antimicrobial Agents and Chemotherapy* 56, 838–844.

Salas, C.E., Badillo-Corona, J.A., Ramirez-Sotelo, G. and Oliver-Salvador, C. (2015) Biologically active and antimicrobial peptides from plants. *Biomedical Research Intearnational* 2015, 1021–1029.

Sass, V., Schneider, T., Wilmes, M., Korner, C., Tossi, A., *et al.* (2010) Human beta-defensin 3 inhibits cell wall biosynthesis in Staphylococci. *Infection and Immunity* 78, 2793–2800.

Schmitt, P., Wilmes, M., Pugniere, M., Aumelas, A., Bachere, E., *et al.* (2010) Insight into invertebrate defensin mechanism of action: oyster defensins inhibit peptidoglycan biosynthesis by binding to lipid II. *Journal of Biological Chemistry* 285, 29208–29216.

Schmitt, P., Rosa, R.D., Duperthuy, M., De Lorgeril, J., Bachere, E. and Destoumieux-Garzon, D. (2012) The antimicrobial defense of the pacific oyster, *Crassostrea gigas*: how diversity may compensate for scarcity in the regulation of resident/pathogenic microflora. *Frontiers in Microbiology* 3, 160.

Schneider, T., Kruse, T., Wimmer, R., Wiedemann, I., Sass, V., *et al.* (2010) Plectasin, a fungal defensin, targets the bacterial cell wall precursor lipid II. *Science* 328, 1168–1172.

Schroeder, B.O., Stange, E.F. and Wehkamp, J. (2011a) Waking the wimp: redox-modulation activates human beta-defensin 1. *Gut Microbes* 2, 262–266.

Schroeder, B.O., Wu, Z., Nuding, S., Groscurth, S., Marcinowski, M., *et al.* (2011b) Reduction of disulphide bonds unmasks potent antimicrobial activity of human beta-defensin 1. *Nature* 469, 419–423.

Schroeder, B.O., Ehmann, D., Precht, J.C., Castillo, P.A., Kuchler, R., *et al.* (2015) Paneth cell alpha-defensin 6 (Hd-6) is an antimicrobial peptide. *Mucosal Immunology* 8, 661–671.

Schulenburg, H., Boehnisch, C. and Michiels, N.K. (2007) How do invertebrates generate a highly specific innate immune response? *Molecular Immunology* 44, 3338–3344.

Schutte, B.C. and McCray, P.B., Jr (2002) [Beta]-defensins in lung host defense. *Annual Reviews of Physiology* 64, 709–748.

Schutte, B.C., Mitros, J.P., Bartlett, J.A., Walters, J.D., Jia, H.P., *et al.* (2002) Discovery of five conserved beta:defensin gene clusters using a computational search strategy. *Proceedings of the National Academy of Sciences of the United States of America* 99, 2129–2133.

Selsted, M.E. (2004) Theta-defensins: cyclic antimicrobial peptides produced by binary ligation of truncated alpha-defensins. *Current Protein & Peptide Science* 5, 365–371.

Selsted, M.E., Harwig, S.S., Ganz, T., Schilling, J.W. and Lehrer, R.I. (1985) Primary structures of three human neutrophil defensins. *Journal of Clinical Investigation* 76, 1436–1439.

Semple, C.A., Gautier, P., Taylor, K. and Dorin, J.R. (2006) The changing of the guard: molecular diversity and rapid evolution of beta-defensins. *Molecular Diversity* 10, 575–584.

Sharma, H. and Nagaraj, R. (2015) Human beta-defensin 4 with non-native disulfide bridges exhibit antimicrobial activity. *PLOS One* 10, E0119525.

Silverstein, K.A., Graham, M.A., Paape, T.D. and Vandenbosch, K.A. (2005) Genome organization of more than 300 defensin-like genes in *Arabidopsis*. *Plant Physiology* 138, 600–610.

Silverstein, K.A., Moskal, W.A., Jr, Wu, H.C., Underwood, B.A., Graham, M.A., *et al.* (2007) Small cysteine-rich peptides resembling antimicrobial peptides have been under-predicted in plants. *Plant Journal* 51, 262–280.

Sparkes, R.S., Kronenberg, M., Heinzmann, C., Daher, K.A., Klisak, I., Ganz, T. and Mohandas, T. (1989) Assignment of defensin gene(s) to human chromosome 8p23. *Genomics* 5, 240–244.

Stotz, H.U., Thomson, J.G. and Wang, Y. (2009) Plant defensins: defense, development and application. *Plant Signal Behaviour* 4, 1010–1012.

Stuart, P.E., Huffmeier, U., Nair, R.P., Palla, R., Tejasvi, T., *et al.* (2012) Association of beta-defensin copy number and psoriasis in three cohorts of European origin. *Journal of Investigative Dermatology* 132, 2407–2413.

Tam, J.P., Wang, S., Wong, K.H. and Tan, W.L. (2015) Antimicrobial peptides from plants. *Pharmaceuticals* 8, 711–757.

Taylor, K., Clarke, D.J., McCullough, B., Chin, W., Seo, E., *et al.* (2008) Analysis and separation of residues important for the chemoattractant and antimicrobial activities of beta-defensin 3. *Journal of Biological Chemistry* 283, 6631–6639.

Tomisawa, S., Sato, Y., Kamiya, M., Kumaki, Y., Kikukawa, T., *et al.* (2015) Efficient production of a correctly folded mouse alpha-defensin, cryptdin-4, by refolding during inclusion body solubilization. *Protein Expression and Purification* 112, 21–28.

Tongaonkar, P., Golji, A.E., Tran, P., Ouellette, A.J. and Selsted, M.E. (2012) High fidelity processing and activation of the human alpha-defensin hnp1 precursor by neutrophil elastase and proteinase 3. *PLOS One* 7, E32469.

Tonk, M., Cabezas-Cruz, A., Valdes, J.J., Rego, R.O., Grubhoffer, L., *et al.* (2015) Ixodes ricinus defensins attack distantly-related pathogens. *Developmental and Comparative Immunology* 53, 358–365.

Trabi, M., Schirra, H.J. and Craik, D.J. (2001) Three-dimensional structure of RTD-1, a cyclic antimicrobial defensin from rhesus macaque leukocytes. *Biochemistry* 40, 4211–4221.

Tran, D., Tran, P.A., Tang, Y.Q., Yuan, J., Cole, T. and Selsted, M.E. (2002) Homodimeric theta-defensins from rhesus macaque leukocytes: isolation, synthesis, antimicrobial activities, and bacterial binding properties of the cyclic peptides. *Journal of Biological Chemistry* 277, 3079–3084.

Tran, D., Tran, P.A., Roberts, K., Osapay, G., Schaal, J., Ouellette, A. and Selsted, M.E. (2008) Microbicidal properties and cytocidal selectivity of rhesus macaque theta defensins. *Antimicrobial Agents and Chemotherapy* 52, 944–953.

Tu, J., Li, D., Li, Q., Zhang, L., Zhu, Q., *et al.* (2015) Molecular evolutionary analysis of beta-defensin peptides in vertebrates. *Evolutionary Bioinformatics Online* 11, 105–114.

Van Avondt, K., Fritsch-Stork, R., Derksen, R.H. and Meyaard, L. (2013) Ligation of signal inhibitory receptor on leukocytes-1 suppresses the release of neutrophil extracellular traps in systemic Lupus erythematosus. *PLOS One* 8, E78459.

Van Hoek, M.L. (2014) Antimicrobial peptides in reptiles. *Pharmaceuticals* 7, 723–753.

Van Hoek, M.L. (2016) Diversity in host defense antimicrobial peptides. In: Epand, R.M. (ed.) *Host Defense Peptides and Their Potential as Therapeutic Agents.* Springer, New York.

Varkey, J. and Nagaraj, R. (2005) Antibacterial activity of human neutrophil defensin HNP-1 analogs without cysteines. *Antimicrobial Agents and Chemotherapy* 49, 4561–4566.

Varkey, J., Singh, S. and Nagaraj, R. (2006) Antibacterial activity of linear peptides spanning the carboxy-terminal beta-sheet domain of arthropod defensins. *Peptides* 27, 2614–2623.

Varney, K.M., Bonvin, A.M., Pazgier, M., Malin, J., Yu, W., *et al.* (2013) Turning defense into offense: defensin mimetics as novel antibiotics targeting lipid II. *PLOS Pathogens* 9, E1003732.

Wang, G. (2014) Human antimicrobial peptides and proteins. *Pharmaceuticals* 7, 545–594.

Wang, G., Li, X. and Wang, Z. (2009) APD2: the updated antimicrobial peptide database and its application in peptide design. *Nucleic Acids Research* 37, D933–937.

Wang, G., Li, X. and Wang, Z. (2016) APD3: the antimicrobial peptide database as a tool for research and education. *Nucleic Acids Research* 44, D1087–1093.

Welkos, S., Cote, C.K., Hahn, U., Shastak, O., Jedermann, J., *et al.* (2011) Humanized theta-defensins (retrocyclins) enhance macrophage performance and protect mice from experimental anthrax infections. *Antimicrobial Agents and Chemotherapy* 55, 4238–4250.

Wilde, C.G., Griffith, J.E., Marra, M.N., Snable, J.L. and Scott, R.W. (1989) Purification and characterization of human neutrophil peptide 4, a novel member of the defensin family. *Journal of Biological Chemistry* 264, 11200–11203.

Wilson, C.L., Schmidt, A.P., Pirila, E., Valore, E.V., Ferri, N., Sorsa, T., Ganz, T. and Parks, W.C. (2009) Differential processing of {alpha}- and {beta}-defensin precursors by matrix metalloproteinase-7 (MMP-7). *Journal of Biological Chemistry* 284, 8301–8311.

Wimley, W.C., Selsted, M.E. and White, S.H. (1994) Interactions between human defensins and lipid bilayers: evidence for formation of multimeric pores. *Protein Science* 3, 1362–1373.

Witzke, S., Petersen, M., Carpenter, T.S. and Khalid, S. (2016) Molecular dynamics simulations reveal the conformational flexibility of lipid II and its loose association with the defensin plectasin in the *Staphylococcus aureus* membrane. *Biochemistry* 55, 3303–3314.

Wu, Z., Hoover, D.M., Yang, D., Boulegue, C., Santamaria, F., *et al.* (2003) Engineering disulfide bridges to dissect antimicrobial and chemotactic activities of human beta-defensin 3. *Proceedings of the National Academies of Science of the United States of America* 100, 8880–8885.

Xiao, Y., Hughes, A.L., Ando, J., Matsuda, Y., Cheng, J.F., Skinner-Noble, D. and Zhang, G. (2004) A genome-wide screen identifies a single beta-defensin gene cluster in the chicken: implications for the origin and evolution of mammalian defensins. *BMC Genomics* 5, 56.

Xin, A., Zhao, Y., Yu, H., Shi, H., Liu, H., Diao, H. and Zhang, Y. (2014) Soluble fusion expression, characterization and localization of human beta-defensin 6. *Molecular Medicine Reports* 9, 149–155.

Yamane, E.S., Bizerra, F.C., Oliveira, E.B., Moreira, J.T., Rajabi, M., *et al.* (2013) Unraveling the anti-fungal activity of a South American rattlesnake toxin crotamine. *Biochimie* 95, 231–240.

Yanagi, S., Ashitani, J., Ishimoto, H., Date, Y., Mukae, H., Chino, N. and Nakazato, M. (2005) Isolation of human beta-defensin-4 in lung tissue and its increase in lower respiratory tract infection. *Respiratory Research* 6, 130.

Yasin, B., Wang, W., Pang, M., Cheshenko, N., Hong, T., *et al.* (2004) Theta defensins protect cells from infection by herpes simplex virus by inhibiting viral adhesion and entry. *Journal of Virology* 78, 5147–5156.

Yi, H.Y., Chowdhury, M., Huang, Y.D. and Yu, X.Q. (2014) Insect antimicrobial peptides and their applications. *Applied Microbiology and Biotechnology* 98, 5807–5822.

Yount, N.Y., Kupferwasser, D., Spisni, A., Dutz, S.M., Ramjan, Z.H., *et al.* (2009). Selective reciprocity in antimicrobial activity versus cytotoxicity of HBD-2 and crotamine. *Proceedings of the National Academies of Science of the United States of America* 106, 14972–14977.

Zhang, G. and Sunkara, L.T. (2014) Avian antimicrobial host defense peptides: from biology to thera-peutic applications. *Pharmaceuticals* 7, 220–247.

Zhang, J., Yang, Y., Teng, D., Tian, Z., Wang, S. and Wang, J. (2011) Expression of plectasin in *Pichia pastoris* and its characterization as a new antimicrobial peptide against *Staphyloccocus* and *Streptococcus*. *Protein Expression and Purification* 78, 189–196.

Zhang, Y., Teng, D., Mao, R., Wang, X., Xi, D., Hu, X. and Wang, J. (2014) High expression of a plectasin-derived peptide NZ2114 in *Pichia pastoris* and its pharmacodynamics, postantibiotic and syn-ergy against *Staphylococcus aureus*. *Applied Microbiology and Biotechnology* 98, 681–694.

Zhao, L. and Lu, W. (2014) Defensins in innate immunity. *Current Opinion in Hematology* 21, 37–42.

Zhou, C.X., Zhang, Y.L., Xiao, L., Zheng, M., Leung, K.M., *et al.* (2004) An epididymis-specific beta-defensin is important for the initiation of sperm maturation. *Nature Cell Biology* 6, 458–564.

4 Lantibiotics: Bioengineering and Applications

Brian Healy[1,2] and Paul D. Cotter[1,2,*]

[1]*Teagasc Food Research Centre, Moorepark, Fermoy, Co. Cork, Ireland;*
[2]*APC Microbiome Institute, Cork, Ireland*

Abstract

Bacteriocins from Gram-positive bacteria are a large and heterogeneous group of gene-encoded antimicrobial peptides that display antagonism against other bacteria. Although they have been employed for decades as food preservatives, bacteriocins have more recently also been regarded as viable successors to classical antibiotics due to their potentially wide array of applications in the pharmaceutical and veterinary fields. These peptides are also of considerable fundamental interest due to the associated unique structures, modifications and modes of action. In this review, recent developments relating to the Class I (modified) group of bacteriocins known as the lantibiotics are discussed with an emphasis on the various engineering strategies that have been employed to further enhance their potency and physicochemical properties.

4.1 Lantibiotics: Background, Structure, Mode of Action and Classification

As a post-antibiotic era would seem to be drawing ever closer, the discovery and application of new classes of antimicrobial peptides has become increasingly important. Coupled with this, modern consumers are seeking more natural methods of food bio-preservation to replace the chemical preservatives currently in use. One class of antimicrobial peptides, the lantibiotics, has the potential to address one, or both, of these needs.

Bacteriocins are a large heterogeneous group of ribosomally synthesized peptides that are active against other bacteria and against which the producer has a specific immunity mechanism. Bacteriocins that undergo post-translational modifications are classified as Class I bacteriocins and, within this class, the most extensively studied group are the lantibiotics (*Lant*-hionine-containing ant-*ibiotics*). The lantibiotics are lanthionine-containing peptides which display antimicrobial activity and comprise close to 100 members (Field *et al.*, 2015a). These are a somewhat unique class of antimicrobials due to the incorporation of post-translationally modified amino acids, such as dehydroalanines, dehydrobutyrines, lanthionines and methyl lanthionines, S-[(Z)-2-aminovinyl]-(*3S*)-3-methyl-D-cysteines and labionins into their mature structure (Allgaier *et al.*, 1986; Sahl and Bierbaum, 1998; Cotter *et al.*, 2005b; Meindl *et al.*, 2010). It is these 'rare', non-genetically

---

* Corresponding author e-mail: paul.cotter@teagasc.ie

encoded amino acids, and associated structures such as lanthionine bridges, that confer desirable characteristics. For example, in many cases, they provide potent activity against multiple Gram-positive clinical pathogens (Cotter *et al.*, 2005a; Dischinger *et al.*, 2014) and food spoilage microorganisms (Deegan *et al.*, 2006); they have notably high levels of physicochemical stability (van Heel *et al.*, 2011) and, very often, have a low frequency (relative to conventional antibiotics) of resistance – probably because lantibiotics are not extensively used in a clinical setting, and because of their target sites/modes of action (van Heel *et al.*, 2011; Draper *et al.*, 2015).

The most studied Class I bacteriocin is nisin, whose activity was first noted by Rogers in 1928 (Rogers, 1928). This 34 amino acid peptide, produced by many *Lactococcus lactis* strains, is currently the only class I bacteriocin to be commercialized in its application as a food preservative (additive E234) (Delves-Broughton *et al.*, 1996). It is also used for the prevention of bovine mastitis, in the form of a teat wipe (Wipe Out) and has also been investigated as a potential anti-mastitis treatment (Mast Out), due to its antagonist activity against the aetiological agents of the condition (Cao *et al.*, 2007).

In general, the genetic components required for the biosynthesis of bacteriocins are clustered and can be found on the chromosome, plasmids or transposons (Klaenhammer, 1993). Here we refer to the nisin gene cluster as an example. Briefly, the genes involved are organized into four distinct operons: *nisABTCIPRK*, *nisI*, *nisRK* and *nisFEG* (Lubelski *et al.*, 2008) (Fig. 4.1).

Specific serines and threonines are dehydrated and converted to dehydroalanines and dehydrobutyrines, respectively,

in the prepropeptide by the dehydratase enzyme, encoded by *nisB* (Karakas Sen *et al.*, 1999). This is followed by the formation of the (methyl) lanthionine bridges, giving the peptide its signature polycyclic form, through coupling of these dehydroamino acids with neighbouring cysteines, crosslinked via a thioether bond through Michael addition catalysed by the *nisC*-encoded enzyme (Meyer *et al.*, 1995). The ABC transporter, NisT, transports the inactive peptide precursor out of the cell where the serine protease, NisP, cleaves the leader sequence and renders the peptide active (Siezen *et al.*, 1996; Qiao and Saris, 1996) (Fig. 4.2).

In order for the producer to maintain immunity (i.e. self-protection), a single immunity protein is produced, NisI, along with a dedicated transport system, NisFEG (Draper *et al.*, 2008; AlKhatib *et al.*, 2014). While nisin remains a good example of lantibiotic post-translational modifications (PTMs), it should be noted that these modifications are not limited to dehydration and thioether bridge formation. For example, amino acid residues in NAI-107 (microbisporicin) and a variant of such, NAI-108, undergo halogenation and hydroxylation modifications (Cruz *et al.*, 2015).

Many antimicrobial peptides inhibit the biosynthesis of peptidoglycan by sequestering lipid II, a lipid intermediate responsible for the translocation of essential precursors across the plasma membrane to the periplasmic exterior of the cell where they are incorporated into the cell wall (Breukink and de Kruijff, 2006). These antimicrobial peptides include, but are not limited to, glycopeptides (including vancomycin and teicoplanin which bind to the last two D-amino acid residues of the lipid II

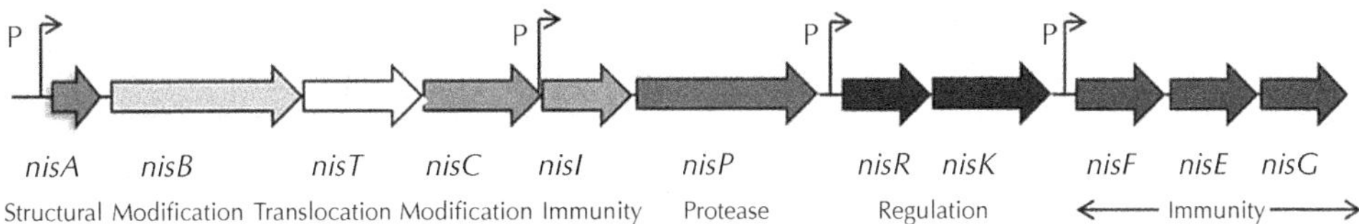

Fig. 4.1. Graphical representation of the nisin A gene cluster including all structural, modification, biosynthesis, immunity and regulation genes required. P denotes the promoter position for each of the distinct operons.

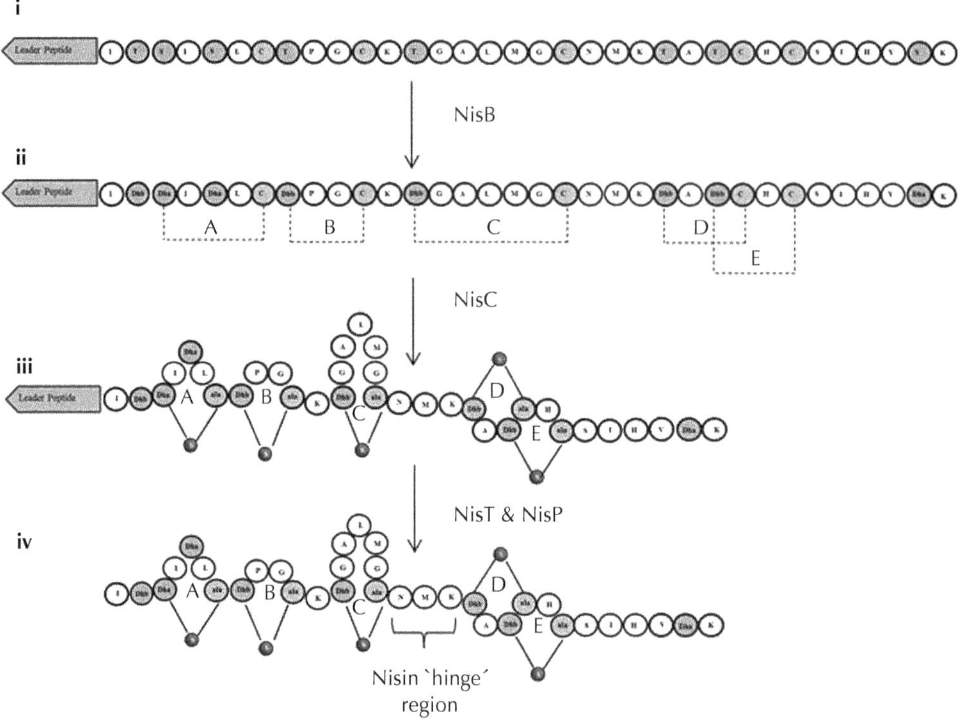

Fig. 4.2. (i) Before the commencement of the post-translational modification (PTM), nisin is transcribed as a 34 amino acid prepeptide with a leader attached at the N-terminal region. Residues involved in PTMs are shaded; (ii) NisB acts on a select number of serine and threonine residues converting them to dehydroalanines (Dha) and dehydrobutyrines (Dhb); (iii) The polycyclic form of the peptide arises from the coupling of these dehydrated amino acids with proximal cysteines catalysed by NisC; (iv). Finally, the peptide is transported from the cell and the leader sequence cleaved leading to the formation of active mature nisin. A–E denote the lanthionine ring structures.

pentapeptide side chain), defensins, non-ribosomally synthesized peptides, depsipeptides such as teixobactin, and the lantibiotics (Dischinger *et al.*, 2014; Scheffers and Tol, 2015).

Using nisin A to model lantibiotic-lipid II interactions, it has been established that sequestering begins when the N-terminus region forms a complex with lipid II, thereby terminating peptidoglycan synthesis through the formation of a 'pyrophosphate cage' structure (Breukink and de Kruijff, 2006). This method of cell inhibition is maintained even in truncated nisin analogues cleaved after position 22, albeit at levels 10-fold lower than the wild-type parent (Plat *et al.*, 2011). A conformational flexibility afforded to the peptide by the central 'hinge' region of the peptide (asparagine 20, methionine 21 and lysine 22) (Fig. 4.2, iv) allows for the permeabilization of the cell membrane of sensitive cells by the nisin C-terminus, leading to a rapid efflux of intercellular components and cell death (Wiedemann *et al.*, 2001). It should be noted however that certain lantibiotics such as mersacidin and actagardine lack this pore-forming mode of action and rely on lipid II interactions alone for activity (Brötz *et al.*, 1995; Boakes *et al.*, 2012). Furthermore, cinnamycin and related lantibiotics differ here in that they bind to phosphatidylethanolamine, leading to the inhibition of phospholipase A2 (Märki *et al.*, 1991).

In general, lantibiotics are most active against Gram-positive cells, but do exhibit some activity against Gram-negative strains which can be increased when used in conjunction with outer membrane destabilizing reagents or antibiotics. For example, the use of lacticin 3147 with polymyxin B or E, polypeptide antibiotics which exclusively target Gram-negative cells, results in a synergistic effect against a range of Gram-negative species such as *Cronobacter sakazakii* and *E. coli* (Draper *et al.*, 2013). A synergistic effect was also noted when nisin and colistin were used in combination against Gram-negative clinical pathogens (Naghmouchi *et al.*, 2013). Pre-treatment of Gram-negative cell wall with an outer membrane permeabilizing agent such as EDTA also increases their sensitivity to lantibiotics (Martin-Visscher *et al.*, 2011).

The classification of lantibiotics, and of bacteriocins in general, continues to evolve due to the ongoing discovery of new compounds with unique structural features and modification enzymes. Lantibiotics were originally classified as either Class A (elongated, positively charged and cell wall permeabilizing) or B (globular, net negative charge and inhibition of essential cell wall components) (Jung, 1991), but these groupings lacked the flexibility to accurately classify the ever-expanding spectrum. This system has since been refined to reflect the biosynthetic machinery employed in the formation of the (methyl)lanthionines and, as a result, now contains four classes. Class I lantibiotics are those modified by two modification enzymes, LanB and LanC, and include nisin. The Class II lantibiotics are those which are modified by a single bifunctional enzyme, generically termed LanM, the N-terminal domain of which houses the dehydration machinery while the C-terminal region contains the cyclization domain. Lacticin 3147 and lacticin 481 are two of the most studied members of this class. The next two classes, III and IV, relate to lanthipeptides, i.e. lanthionine-containing peptides that lack antimicrobial activity, only. Dehydration in both cases is achieved through the actions of a central kinase domain and an N-terminal phosphoSer/ phosphoThr lyase domain but with differing cyclization domains. Class III lantibiotics

are modified by LanKC proteins and include the labyrinthopeptins. This class is unique in that its structures contain, in addition to (methyl)lanthionines rings, labionin rings. Finally, Class IV lanthipeptides are those modified by LanL and include venezuelin and streptocollin (Goto *et al.*, 2010; Arnison *et al.*, 2013; Iftime *et al.*, 2015).

4.2 Lantibiotics as Clinical and Chemotherapeutic Agents

Lantibiotics are regarded as viable candidates to combat the threat posed by the emergence of multi-drug resistance (MDR) bacteria from both nosocomial and community environments. This class of antimicrobial offers a number of desirable traits such as (i) *in vitro* and *in vivo* activity against clinical and MDR pathogens; (ii) employment of bioengineering strategies for biological improvement; and (iii) implementation of large-scale *in silico* screens due to their gene encoded nature (Cotter *et al.*, 2005a; Piper *et al.*, 2009a; van Heel *et al.*, 2011). There are, however, bottlenecks which impede the employment of lantibiotics as biomedical and pharmaceutical agents, i.e. (i) although not as sensitive as unmodified bacteriocins, lantibiotics are somewhat susceptible to proteases such as the intestinal proteases trypsin and α-chymotrypsin; (ii) the challenge of large-scale production and, as noted above; (iii) a generally poor activity against Gram-negative pathogens.

The impressive *in vitro* activity of a number of lantibiotics against clinical and MDR pathogens has been reported on multiple occasions. For example, strains of methicillin resistant *Staphylococcus aureus* (MRSA) are inhibited by a large number of lantibiotics including NAI-107, nisin, lacticin 3147, mersacidin, planosporicin and mutacin B-Ny266 (Mota-Meira *et al.*, 2000; Castiglione *et al.*, 2008; Appleyard *et al.*, 2009; Piper *et al.*, 2009b; Thomsen *et al.*, 2016). *In vitro* assays have also highlighted the potential for the use of lacticin 3147 as a chemotherapeutic agent against a range of clinically relevant strains of *Mycobacterium* including *Mycobacterium tuberculosis* H37Ra, *Mycobacterium avium* subsp. *paratuberculosis* (MAP) ATCC 19698 and *Mycobacterium kansasii* CIT11/06 (Carroll *et al.*, 2010). Similarly, the causative agent of *Clostridium difficile* associated disease, *C. difficile*, is sensitive to lacticin 3147 and NVB302, a semi-synthetic analogue of deoxyactagardine B (Rea *et al.*, 2007; Crowther *et al.*, 2013;). Gallidermin has been shown to be effective in controlling biofilm formation from some species of *Staphylococcus* (Saising *et al.*, 2012) .

The *in vivo* activity of a number of these lantibiotics also supports their consideration as alternatives to antibiotics. More specifically, lantibiotics have been shown to effectively eradicate *S. aureus* infection in mouse models, with NAI-107 and lacticin 3147 emerging as potential chemotherapeutic agent against this pathogen, including MDR strains (Jabés *et al.*, 2011; Piper *et al.*, 2012). Similarly, Campion *et al.* (2013) demonstrated the ability of nisin A and a bioengineered derivative, nisin V, to efficiently control levels of *Listeria monocytogenes* in a murine model when the peptide was injected intraperitoneally. Promisingly, a number of lantibiotics are currently being assessed in pre-clinical trials. MU1140-S (mutacin 1140) is in late pre-clinical trials against MRSA, VRE (vancomycin-resistant enterococci) and interestingly, the Gram-negative causative agent of peptic ulcers, *Helicobacter pylori* (Oragenics Inc.). Other examples include NAI-107, which is currently undergoing pre-clinical trials (Thomsen *et al.*, 2016), NVB302, which has successfully completed Phase I clinical trials (Novacta Biosciences Limited), and duramycin (Moli1901), which has recently completed Class II clinical trials, and has been shown to be effective against cystic fibrosis through the stimulation of calcium-activated chloride channels (Donaldson and Galietta, 2013).

Interestingly, research into the application of nisin as an anticancer therapeutic has yielded positive results. It has been shown to give favourable results when used as an adjunct to doxorubicin to combat skin carcinogenesis (Preet *et al.*, 2015). Nisin has also displayed very positive outcomes in the treatment of head and neck squamous cell carcinoma (HNSCC) with follow on *in vivo* trials showing reduced tumorigenesis without any long-term negative effects on the mice (Kamarajan *et al.*, 2015).

Other potential applications for lantibiotics lay in oral health applications (Van Staden *et al.*, 2012), topical creams for the prevention of acne (Bowe *et al.*, 2006), treatment of mastitis (Cao *et al.*, 2007), or as potential microbiocides in the prevention of sexually transmitted diseases (Férir *et al.*, 2013).

4.3 Lantibiotics as Biopreservatives

In recent times, consumers have become more conscious of the importance of food safety while at the same time less satisified with the use of chemical preservatives due to the long-term health effects assiociated with consumption, e.g. nitrates and sulfur dioxide. This provides a challenge to the food industry as it must now provide foods which do not contain synthetic chemicals, are low in salt and sugar, but yet continue to be nutritious and safe (Egan *et al.*, 2016). Bacteriocins provide a tangible solution, in particular those produced from lactic acid bacteria (LAB) (Cotter *et al.*, 2005b), as they have a long history of safe use in food and many display a lack of cytotoxity. Furthermore, a number of the aforementioned LAB and their by-products are deemed Generally Regarded as Safe (GRAS) by the US FDA and have a Qualified Presumption of Safety (QPS) classification by the EU (Cotter *et al.*, 2005b). It should also be noted that bacteriocins are broken down by proteases within the digestive tract and therefore do not impact negatively on the gut microbiome and display antagonism against an array of food pathogens and spoilage microorganisms (Cotter *et al.*, 2005b; Deegan *et al.*, 2006).

Despite the aforementioned benefits of LAB-associated lantibiotics, nisin is the only lantibiotic to have been commerically marketed as a food biopreservative, having been approved for use by the FDA and the EU (E234). An under-appreciation of the potential benefits of bacteriocins coupled with a reluctance to move away from current preservation techniques may account for the underuse of these peptides (Cotter *et al.*, 2005b).

In situ lantibiotic production in dairy systems has often been reported as a possible route of application. Recently a study into the use of a nisin in Minas, a Brazilain goats milk cheese into which a nisin producer was added, showed that the levels of coagulase-positive cocci and biogenic amines decreased and a higher number of species was evident compared to a cheese without the addition of nisin (Perin *et al.*, 2015). Dal Bello *et al.* (2013) have shown that the addition of a starter culture producing nisin Z, a natural variant of nisin A, reduced the levels of *S. aureus* by 3.54 log cfu/ml in a ripened cheese compared to a control cheese. Positive results have also been reported for controlling the growth of *L. monocytogenes* through the *in situ* production of nisin A, nisin Z and lacticin 481 in a cottage cheese food model (Dal Bello *et al.*, 2012). Another possible application for nisin involves its use as a replacement for nitrate in the prevention of late blowing in hard cheeses from butyric acid fermentation. This phenomenon is caused by the outgrowth of *C. tyrobutyricum* in cheese, which results in flavour defects and economic losses (*Ávila et al.*, 2014). Indeed many bacteriocins, including a number of lantibiotics, display inhibition against a wide range of Gram-positive spore formers. For a review on this topic, the reader is directed to Egan *et al.* (2016). Lacticin 3147 has been shown to display antagonism against the emerging food-borne pathogen *Mycobacterium avium* subspecies *paratuberculosis*, a bacterium associated with Crohn's disease (Carroll *et al.*, 2010), while oral administration of a natural nisin Z producer to rainbow trout has been highlighted as an effective anti-infective agent against the invasive pathogen *Lactococcus garvieae* (Araújo *et al.*, 2015).

4.4 Lantibiotic Bioengineering and Synthetic Engineering

Lantibiotics and traditional antibiotics differ in a variety of ways, particularly with respect to the manner in which they are naturally synthesized. Lantibiotics, like all bacteriocins, are ribosomally synthesized, and, thus, in contrast to classical antibiotics, are the product of a more simple biosynthetic process. This coupled with the fact that the antimicrobial is gene encoded offers the possibility of bioengineering to increase functionality (Cotter *et al.*, 2005a; Perez *et al.*, 2014).

4.4.1 *In vivo* engineering

Despite many beneficial attributes, the potential employment of lantibiotics as novel chemotherapeutic agents or as food biopreservatives in more widespread roles is limited by a number of factors. These include the aforementioned sensitivity to proteolysis and oxidation, and instability and/or insolubility at physiological pHs (Field *et al.*, 2015a). However, because of the ribosomal, gene encoded nature of these peptides and the relative promiscuity of the modification machinary, lantibiotics are amenable to *in vivo* bioengineering strategies to improve on their innate characteristics (Cotter *et al.*, 2005a).

The bioengineering of nisin has yielded an array of variants which exhibit enhanced functionalities in terms of potency or physicochemical characteristics. In particular, the importance of the 'hinge' region of nisin (Fig. 4.2, iv) has often been exploited in bioengineering studies where it has been shown that single amino acid substitutions can lead to increases in the antimicrobial activity of the peptide. A study by Zhou *et al.* (2016) described the creation of hinge variants containing asparagine 20 to lysine (N20K) or methionine 21 to lysine (M21V) changes which displayed activity against Gram-negative strains. The inhibition of clinically relevant Gram-positive pathogens was first demonstrated by Field and co-workers (Field *et al.*, 2008) where the substitiution of lysine (K) for a threonine (T) at position 22 (K22T) showed a marked improvement in activity against the mastitis-associated pathogen *Stretococcus agalactiae*. This was followed by the discovery of a derviative containing a valine (V) in the place of methionine at position 21 with enhanced activity against *L. monocytogenes*, both *in vitro* and *in vivo*, in comparison to nisin A (Field *et al.*, 2010; Campion *et al.*, 2013). The inhibition of this pathogen in a chocolate milk sample by nisin derivatives has also been demonstrated (Rouse *et al.*, 2012). A site saturation mutagenesis study of the nisin A 'hinge' led to the discovery of a number of derivatives displaying increased bioactivity while also providing the blueprint for the rational design of two derivatives, AAA and SAA, both of which exhibited enhanced activity against clinically relevant pathogens (Healy *et al.*, 2013). Away from the hinge region, other studies have shown that the lysine (K) at amino acid position 12 and the serine (S) at position 29 are locations that are amenable to change. A single amino change from lysine to alanine at position 12 (a region between rings B and C) resulted in a peptide with enhanced specific activity against strains of genera *Streptococcus*, *Bacillus*, *Lactococcus*, *Enterococcus* and *Staphylococcus* (Molloy *et al.*, 2013). The first report of lantibiotic derivatives displaying enhanced microbial activity against both Gram-positive and -negative bacteria emerged when a number of derivatives stemming from site saturation mutagenesis of the serine position 29 of the nisin peptide were found to possess enhanced activity against food-associated pathogens, including *E. coli*, *Salmonella enterica* serovar *typhimurium* and *C. sakazakii* (Field *et al.*, 2012). Bioengineered nisin derivatives have also been shown to be effective in controlling biofilm formation from the animal pathogen, *Staphylococcus pseudintermedius* (Field *et al.*, 2015b). The length of the 'hinge' region of nisin has also been shown to be important in terms of bioactivity. A number of derivatives where a single valine,

leucine or isoleucine, or combination thereof, are added after the asparagine at position 20 or derivatives in which the methionine and/or lysine at positions 21 and 22 are removed, display increases in halo size in agar diffusion assays compared to the parent strain (Zhou *et al.*, 2015).

The implemenatation of PCR-based mutagenesis studies have also improved the activity of the two-peptide lantibiotic, lacticin 3147. An alanine-scanning study by Cotter *et al.* (2006a) demonstrated that a number of amino acid residues within both peptides retained bioactivity when substituted by an alanine. However, in that instance, none displayed greater activity than the wild type. It was not until Field *et al.* (2013), where a site saturation approach led to the discovery of a derivative of lacticin 3147 where a subsitution of the histidine for a serine amino acid in the α-peptide (αH22S), that increased specific activity, in this case against the pathogenic *S. aureus* strain, NCDO 1499, was observed. The difficulty in producing enhanced derivatives from a two-peptide system, where both peptides are required to work in synergy, is evidenced by the fact that the αH22S change was only one out of over 200 derivatives created. This remains the only example of improvement in bioactivity of a two-peptide lantibiotic through *in vivo* means.

Previously, the production of enhanced derivatives has also been achieved for mersacidin and nukacin- ISK1 produced by *Bacillus* sp. HILY-84,54738 and *Staphylocccus warneri* ISK1, respectively (Appleyard *et al.*, 2009; Islam *et al.*, 2009). Mutacin 1140, produced by the oral bacterium *Streptococcus mutans* strain JH1140 used to displace disease-causing strains of *S. mutans* from the teeth (Hillman *et al.*, 1998), has been also shown to be amenable to PCR-based mutagenesis systems. In a study by Chen *et al.* (2013), both the bioactivity and the specific activity of a number of the produced derivatives were increased; most notably, a tryptophan for alanine substitution at position 4 led to a four-fold increase in minimum inhibitory concentration (MIC) assays against *S. pneumoniae* ATCC 27336 and a two-fold increase against *C. difficile* UK1. A second derivative, Mu1140_Phe1Ile displayed a two-fold increase against *S. pneumoniae* ATCC 27336 and *S. aureus* ATCC 25923.

Actagardine a single peptide, 19 amino acid lantibiotic produced by *Actinoplanes garbadinensis* (Zimmermann *et al.*, 1995) displays activity against clinical pathogens. An *in trans* site saturation mutagenesis system provided valuable structure/activity relationship data and also led to the creation of a derviative V15F which displayed enhancement in specific activity (MIC) against a number of enterococci and streptococci pathogens (Boakes *et al.*, 2012).

The direct enhancement in the bioactivity of a lantibiotic is not the only feature to which bioengineering strategies can be applied. Studies into physicochemical stability (Liu and Hansen, 1992), influence of the leader peptide (van der Meer *et al.*, 1994), the importance of charged residues for activity (Deegan *et al.*, 2010), the importance of the lanthionine bridges on heat and protease resistance (Suda *et al.*, 2010) and immunity (Draper *et al.*, 2012) have all been investigated by applying various *in vivo* amino acid substitution techniques. Along with these applications, *in vivo* methods of bioengineering can be employed to increase the production of lantibiotics. For example, production of nisin Z (Mulders *et al.*, 1991), was increased from 16,000 au/ml to 25,000 au/ml in cells expressing multi copies of the *nisRK* two component regulatory genes.

In 2006, Cotter *et al.* (2006b) demonstrated that the introduction of extra copies of the biosynthetic machinery along with the regulator LtnR facilitate the overexpression of lacticin 3147. Further bioengineering studies with mutacin 1140 and nukacin ISK-1 led to the creation of derivatives with increased production relative to the parent, from single amino acid modifications (Islam et al., 2009; Chen *et al.*, 2013). *In vivo* engineering approaches have also succeeded in overproducing nisin A through cloning of the biosynthetic genes into a nisin-deficent *L. lactis* host (MG1363),

overexpressing the structural gene with constitute promotors and arrangement of the recombinant pathway on a single circuit (Kong and Lu, 2014). Recently, a system for the *in vivo* introduction of non-canonical amino acids into nisin was demonstrated by (Zhou *et al.*, 2016), with the introduction of tryptophan analogues into the mature peptide structure.

4.4.2 (Semi)Synthetic engineering

A limitation of *in vivo* engineering was its dependancy on the native modification machinary, therefore excluding the incorporation of non-proteinogenic amino acids (Escano and Smith, 2015). The use of solid phase peptide synthesis (SPPS) has allowed for rapid advances in the chemical synthesis of many full length lantibiotics, with lactosin S becoming the first lantibiotic peptide to be produced by such means (Ross *et al.*, 2009). Subsequently, the oxidative stability of lactocin S was improved by replacing the oxidation-prone sulfur residue of lanthionine with diaminopimelate analogues, one of which maintained full biological activity with increased stability (Ross *et al.*, 2012).

One of the stumbling blocks in the use of chemical synthesis has been the difficulty associated with production of overlapping lanthionine rings. This was overcome by Liu *et al.* (2011) through the introduction of Fmoc SPPS technology in the creation of fully active and synergistic α and β lacticin 3147 peptides. Chemical synthesis of lacticin 481, a lantibiotic with three overlapping rings, was achieved in a study by Knerr and van der Donk (2013), while also providing valuable insight into the significance of stereochemistry for the biological activity of the peptide. Analogues of epilanein 15X, a lantibiotic with impressive activity against strains of *S. aureus*, have also been produced through chemical means (Knerr and van der Donk, 2012).

A technique termed *in vitro mutagenesis* (IVM) has been used to describe a procedure where non-proteinogenic amino acids could be introduced by using biosynthetic enzymes (the bifunctional enzyme LctM for lacticin 481) with synthetic substrate analogues (Levengood *et al.*, 2009). This system allowed for the synthesis of analogues containing sarcosine, aminocyclopropanoic acid, D-valine, 4-cyanoaminobutyric acid, homoarginine, *N*-butylglycine, naphthylalanine and homophenylalanine in place of the wild-type amino acids, three of which displayed enhanced bioactivity in agar diffusion assays against *L. lactis* HP. Another approach used for the introduction of non-proteinogenic amino acids into a lantibiotic was achieved in the two component peptide lichenicidin. The biosynthetic machinery for the peptide was heterologously expressed in an auxotrophic *Escherichia coli* strain unable to synthesize metionine. Addition of non-proteinogenic amino acids to the growth media resulted in lichenicidin analogues containing these amino acids in place of methionine (Oldach *et al.*, 2012).

A natural analogue of actagardine, deoxyactagardine B, produced by *Actinoplanes liguriae* NCIMB41362 (Boakes *et al.*, 2010) has also been improved upon through the use of semi-synthetic means to yield the variant NVB302. This analogue has been shown to be equally effective as vancomycin at treating *C. difficile* infections in *in vitro* gut models with less disruption of the *Bacteriodes fragilis* group (Crowther *et al.*, 2013). The use of synthetic technologies has also led to the creation of MU1140-S, an analogue of mu1140 which is currently undergoing pre-clinical trials (Oragenics Inc.)

4.5 Future Outlook and Conclusion

As previously discussed, the gene-encoded origin of lantibiotics offers advantages for bioengineering strategies. Another benefit associated with this feature is the ease with which large-scale *in silico* screens for novel lantibiotics can be carried out (Walsh *et al.*, 2015). Elegant web-based mining tools systems such as Bagel 3 are continuing to aid in the discovery of new lantibiotic gene clusters (van Heel *et al.*, 2013) while the discovery of new lantibiotic modification systems increase the number of targets to search for (Montalbán-López and Kuipers, 2016). Indeed, recently, a novel Class II lantibiotic, pseudomycoicidin was discovered through the combination of a bioinformatics and wet-lab approaches (Basi-Chipalu *et al.*, 2015). However, this is by no means the only approach available with traditional screening methods still being relevant as demonstrated by the discovery of the potent lantibiotic NAI-107 and its structural relative, NAI-97 (Castiglione *et al.*, 2008; Maffioli *et al.*, 2016).

Future applications for existing and newly discovered lantibiotics in biopreservation may lie in their incorporation as a hurdle alongside thermal stress, osmotic inactivation or high pressure systems or through their incorporation into packaging material (Egan *et al.*, 2016; Gálvez *et al.*, 2007). Studies into the use of lantibiotics in concert with natural phenolic compounds have recently reported positive results for the treatment of pathogenic bacteria in milk (Alves *et al.*, 2016). In the clinical space, the use of lantibiotics in synergy with traditional antibiotics has the potential to expand the spectrum of activity of the bacteriocin and extend the life of the antibiotic by means of reduced concentrations.

Ultimately, as the arsenal of unique lantibiotics increases so do the potential uses for these antimicrobials. Through continued development into the large-scale production of these compounds coupled with new engineering strategies to solve structural bottlenecks such as protease sensitivity, the niche for new chemotherapeutics and natural food bio-preservatives can be filled by the lantibiotics.

References

Alkhatib, Z., Lagedroste, M., Fey, I., Kleinschrodt, D., Abts, A. and Smits, S.H. (2014) Lantibiotic immunity: inhibition of nisin mediated pore formation by NisI. *PloS One* 9, e102246.

Allgaier, H., Jung, G., Werner, R.G., Schneider, U. and Zähner, H. (1986) Epidermin: sequencing of a heterodet tetracyclic 21-peptide amide antibiotic. *European Journal of Biochemistry* 160, 9–22.

Alves, F.C., Barbosa, L.N., Andrade, B.F., Albano, M., Furtado, F.B., *et al.* (2016) Short communication: inhibitory activities of the lantibiotic nisin combined with phenolic compounds against *Staphylococcus aureus* and *Listeria monocytogenes* in cow milk. *Journal of Dairy Science* 99, 1831–1836.

Appleyard, A.N., Choi, S., Read, D.M., Lightfoot, A., Boakes, S., *et al.* (2009) Dissecting structural and functional diversity of the lantibiotic mersacidin. *Chemistry and Biology* 16, 490–498.

Araújo, C., Muñoz-Atienza, E., Pérez-Sánchez, T., Poeta, P., Igrejas, *et al.* (2015) Nisin Z production by *Lactococcus lactis* subsp. *cremoris* WA2-67 of aquatic origin as a defense mechanism to protect rainbow trout (*Oncorhynchus mykiss*, Walbaum) against *Lactococcus garvieae*. *Marine Biotechnology* 17, 820–830.

Arnison, P.G., Bibb, M.J., Bierbaum, G., Bowers, A.A., Bugni, T.S., *et al.* (2013) Ribosomally synthesized and post-translationally modified peptide natural products: overview and recommendations for a universal nomenclature. *Natural Product Reports* 30, 108–160.

Ávila, M., Gómez-Torres, N., Hernández, M. and Garde, S. (2014) Inhibitory activity of reuterin, nisin, lysozyme and nitrite against vegetative cells and spores of dairy-related *Clostridium* species. *International Journal of Food Microbiology* 172, 70–75.

Basi-Chipalu, S., Dischinger, J., Josten, M., Szekat, C., Zweynert, A., Sahl, H.-G. and Bierbaum, G. (2015) Pseudomycoicidin, a class II lantibiotic from *Bacillus pseudomycoides*. *Applied and Environmental Microbiology* 81, 3419–3429.

Boakes, S., Appleyard, A.N., Cortés, J. and Dawson, M.J. (2010) Organization of the biosynthetic genes encoding deoxyactagardine B (DAB): a new lantibiotic produced by *Actinoplanes liguriae* NCIMB41362. *The Journal of Antibiotics* 63, 351–358.

Boakes, S., Ayala, T., Herman, M., Appleyard, A.N., Dawson, M.J. and Cortés, J. (2012) Generation of an actagardine A variant library through saturation mutagenesis. *Applied Microbiology and Biotechnology* 95, 1509–1517.

Bowe, W.P., Filip, J.C., Dirienzo, J.M., Volgina, A. and Margolis, D.J. (2006) Inhibition of propionibacterium acnes by bacteriocin-like inhibitory substances (BLIS) produced by *Streptococcus salivarius*. *Journal of Drugs in Dermatology: JDD* 5, 868.

Breukink, E. and De Kruijff, B. (2006) Lipid II as a target for antibiotics. *Nature Reviews Drug Discovery* 5, 321–332.

Brötz, H., Bierbaum, G., Markus, A., Molitor, E. and Sahl, H.-G. (1995) Mode of action of the lantibiotic mersacidin: inhibition of peptidoglycan biosynthesis via a novel mechanism? *Antimicrobial Agents and Chemotherapy* 39, 714–719.

Campion, A., Casey, P.G., Field, D., Cotter, P.D., Hill, C. and Ross, R.P. (2013) In vivo activity of Nisin A and Nisin V against *Listeria monocytogenes* in mice. *BMC Microbiology* 13, 1.

Cao, L., Wu, J., Xie, F., Hu, S. and Mo, Y. (2007) Efficacy of nisin in treatment of clinical mastitis in lactating dairy cows. *Journal of Dairy Science* 90, 3980–3985.

Carroll, J., Draper, L.A., O'Connor, P.M., Coffey, A., Hill, C., *et al.* (2010) Comparison of the activities of the lantibiotics nisin and lacticin 3147 against clinically significant mycobacteria. *International Journal of Antimicrobial Agents* 36, 132–136.

Castiglione, F., Lazzarini, A., Carrano, L., Corti, E., Ciciliato, I., *et al.* (2008) Determining the structure and mode of action of microbisporicin: a potent lantibiotic active against multiresistant pathogens. *Chemistry and Biology* 15, 22–31.

Chen, S., Wilson-Stanford, S., Cromwell, W., Hillman, J.D., Guerrero, A., *et al.* (2013) Site-directed mutations in the lanthipeptide mutacin 1140. *Applied and Environmental Microbiology* 79, 4015–4023.

Cotter, P.D., Hill, C. and Ross, R.P. (2005a) Bacterial lantibiotics: strategies to improve therapeutic potential. *Current Protein and Peptide Science* 6, 61–75.

Cotter, P.D., Hill, C. and Ross, R.P. (2005b) Bacteriocins: developing innate immunity for food. *Nature Reviews Microbiology* 3, 777–788.

Cotter, P.D., Deegan, L.H., Lawton, E.M., Draper, L.A., O'Connor, P.M., Hill, C. and Ross, R.P. (2006a) Complete alanine scanning of the two-component lantibiotic lacticin 3147: generating a blueprint for rational drug design. *Molecular Microbiology* 62, 735–747.

Cotter, P.D., Draper, L.A., Lawton, E.M., McAuliffe, O., Hill, C. and Ross, R.P. (2006b) Overproduction of wild-type and bioengineered derivatives of the lantibiotic lacticin 3147. *Applied and Environmental Microbiology* 72, 4492-4496.

Crowther, G.S., Baines, S.D., Todhunter, S.L., Freeman, J., Chilton, C.H. and Wilcox, M.H. (2013) Evaluation of NVB302 versus vancomycin activity in an in vitro human gut model of *Clostridium difficile* infection. *Journal of Antimicrobial Chemotherapy* 68, 168–176.

Cruz, J. O. C., Iorio, M., Monciardini, P., Simone, M., Brunati, C., *et al.* (2015) Brominated variant of the lantibiotic NAI-107 with enhanced antibacterial potency. *Journal of Natural Products* 78, 2642–2647.

Dal Bello, B., Cocolin, L., Zeppa, G., Field, D., Cotter, P.D. and Hill, C. (2012) Technological characterization of bacteriocin producing *Lactococcus lactis* strains employed to control *Listeria monocytogenes* in cottage cheese. *International Journal of Food Microbiology* 153, 58–65.

Dal Bello, B., Zeppa, G., Bianchi, D.M., Decastelli, L., Traversa, A., *et al.* (2013) Effect of nisin-producing *Lactococcus lactis* starter cultures on the inhibition of two pathogens in ripened cheeses. *International Journal of Dairy Technology* 66, 468–477.

Deegan, L.H., Cotter, P.D., Hill, C. and Ross, P. (2006) Bacteriocins: biological tools for bio-preservation and shelf-life extension. *International Dairy Journal* 16, 1058–1071.

Deegan, L.H., Suda, S., Lawton, E.M., Draper, L.A., Hugenholtz, F., *et al.* (2010) Manipulation of charged residues within the two-peptide lantibiotic lacticin 3147. *Microbial Biotechnology* 3, 222–234.

Delves-Broughton, J., Blackburn, P., Evans, R. and Hugenholtz, J. (1996) Applications of the bacteriocin, nisin. *Antonie Van Leeuwenhoek* 69, 193–202.

Dischinger, J., Basi Chipalu, S. and Bierbaum, G. (2014) Lantibiotics: promising candidates for future applications in health care. *International Journal of Medical Microbiology* 304, 51–62.

Donaldson, S.H. and Galietta, L. (2013) New pulmonary therapies directed at targets other than CFTR. *Cold Spring Harbor Perspectives in Medicine* 3, a009787.

Draper, L.A., Ross, R.P., Hill, C. and Cotter, P.D. (2008) Lantibiotic immunity. *Current Protein and Peptide Science* 9, 39–49.

Draper, L.A., Deegan, L.H., Hill, C., Cotter, P.D. and Ross, R.P. (2012) Insights into lantibiotic immunity provided by bioengineering of LtnI. *Antimicrobial Agents and Chemotherapy* 56, 5122–5133.

Draper, L.A., Cotter, P.D., Hill, C. and Ross, R.P. (2013) The two peptide lantibiotic lacticin 3147 acts synergistically with polymyxin to inhibit Gram negative bacteria. *BMC Microbiology* 13, 1.

Draper, L.A., Cotter, P.D., Hill, C. and Ross, R.P. (2015) Lantibiotic resistance. *Microbiology and Molecular Biology Reviews* 79, 171–191.

Egan, K., Field, D., Rea, M.C., Ross, R.P., Hill, C. and Cotter, P.D. (2016) Bacteriocins: novel solutions to age old spore-related problems? *Frontiers in Microbiology* 7.

Escano, J. and Smith, L. (2015) Multipronged approach for engineering novel peptide analogues of existing lantibiotics. *Expert Opinion on Drug Discovery* 10, 857–870.

Férir, G., Petrova, M.I., Andrei, G., Huskens, D., Hoorelbeke, B., *et al.* (2013) The lantibiotic peptide labyrinthopeptin A1 demonstrates broad anti-HIV and anti-HSV activity with potential for microbicidal applications. *PloS One* 8, e64010.

Field, D., Connor, P.M., Cotter, P.D., Hill, C. and Ross, R.P. (2008) The generation of nisin variants with enhanced activity against specific Gram-positive pathogens. *Molecular Microbiology* 69, 218–230.

Field, D., Quigley, L., O'Connor, P.M., Rea, M.C., Daly, K., *et al.* (2010) Studies with bioengineered Nisin peptides highlight the broad-spectrum potency of Nisin V. *Microbial Biotechnology* 3, 473–486.

Field, D., Begley, M., O'Connor, P.M., Daly, K.M., Hugenholtz, F., *et al.* (2012) Bioengineered nisin A derivatives with enhanced activity against both Gram positive and Gram negative pathogens. *PLoS One* 7, e46884.

Field, D., Molloy, E.M., Iancu, C., Draper, L.A., O'Connor, P.M., Cotter, P.D., Hill, C. and Ross, R.P. (2013) Saturation mutagenesis of selected residues of the α-peptide of the lantibiotic lacticin 3147 yields a derivative with enhanced antimicrobial activity. *Microbial Biotechnology* 6, 564–575.

Field, D., Cotter, P.D., Hill, C. and Ross, R. (2015a) Bioengineering lantibiotics for therapeutic success. *Frontiers in Microbiology* 6.

Field, D., Gaudin, N., Lyons, F., O'Connor, P.M., Cotter, P.D., Hill, C. and Ross, R.P. (2015b) A bioengineered nisin derivative to control biofilms of *Staphylococcus pseudintermedius*. *PloS One* 10, e0119684.

Gálvez, A., Abriouel, H., López, R.L. and Omar, N.B. (2007) Bacteriocin-based strategies for food biopreservation. *International Journal of Food Microbiology* 120, 51–70.

Goto, Y., Li, B., Claesen, J., Shi, Y., Bibb, M.J. and Van Der Donk, W.A. (2010) Discovery of unique lanthionine synthetases reveals new mechanistic and evolutionary insights. *PLoS Biology* 8, e1000339.

Healy, B., Field, D., O'Connor, P.M., Hill, C., Cotter, P.D. and Ross, R.P. (2013) Intensive mutagenesis of the nisin hinge leads to the rational design of enhanced derivatives. *PloS One*, 8, e79563.

Hillman, J., Novák, J., Sagura, E., Gutierrez, J.A., Brooks, T., *et al.* (1998) Genetic and biochemical analysis of mutacin 1140: a lantibiotic from *Streptococcus mutans*. *Infection and Immunity* 66, 2743–2749.

Iftime, D., Jasyk, M., Kulik, A., Imhoff, J.F., Stegmann, E., *et al.* (2015) Streptocollin: a type IV lanthipeptide produced by *Streptomyces collinus* Tü 365. *ChemBioChem* 16, 2615–2623.

Islam, M.R., Shioya, K., Nagao, J., Nishie, M., Jikuya, H., *et al.* (2009) Evaluation of essential and variable residues of nukacin ISK-1 by NNK scanning. *Molecular Microbiology* 72, 1438–1447.

Jabés, D., Brunati, C., Candiani, G., Riva, S., Romanó, G. and Donadio, S. (2011) Efficacy of the new lantibiotic NAI-107 in experimental infections induced by multidrug-resistant Gram-positive pathogens. *Antimicrobial Agents and Chemotherapy* 55, 1671–1676.

Jung, G. (1991). Lantibiotics – ribosomally synthesized biologically active polypeptides containing sulfide bridges and α, β-didehydroamino acids. *Angewandte Chemie International Edition in English* 30, 1051–1068.

Kamarajan, P., Hayami, T., Matte, B., Liu, Y., Danciu, T., *et al.* (2015) Nisin ZP: a bacteriocin and food preservative, inhibits head and neck cancer tumorigenesis and prolongs survival. *PloS One* 10, e0131008.

Karakas Sen, A., Narbad, A., Horn, N., Dodd, H.M., Parr, A.J., Colquhoun, I. and Gasson, M.J. (1999) Post-translational modification of nisin. *European Journal of Biochemistry* 261, 524–532.

Klaenhammer, T.R. (1993) Genetics of bacteriocins produced by lactic acid bacteria. *FEMS Microbiology Reviews* 12, 39–85.

Knerr, P.J. and Van Der Donk, W.A. (2012) Chemical synthesis and biological activity of analogues of the lantibiotic epilancin 15X. *Journal of the American Chemical Society* 134, 7648–7651.

Knerr, P.J. and Van Der Donk, W.A. (2013) Chemical synthesis of the lantibiotic lacticin 481 reveals the importance of lanthionine stereochemistry. *Journal of the American Chemical Society* 135, 7094–7097.

Kong, W. and Lu, T. (2014) Cloning and optimization of a nisin biosynthesis pathway for bacteriocin harvest. *ACS Synthetic Biology* 3, 439–445.

Levengood, M.R., Knerr, P.J., Oman, T.J. and Van Der Donk, W.A. (2009) In vitro mutasynthesis of lantibiotic analogues containing nonproteinogenic amino acids. *Journal of the American Chemical Society* 131, 12024–12025.

Liu, W. and Hansen, J. (1992) Enhancement of the chemical and antimicrobial properties of subtilin by site-directed mutagenesis. *Journal of Biological Chemistry* 267, 25078–25085.

Liu, W., Chan, A.S., Liu, H., Cochrane, S.A. and Vederas, J.C. (2011) Solid supported chemical syntheses of both components of the lantibiotic lacticin 3147. *Journal of the American Chemical Society* 133, 14216–14219.

Lubelski, J., Rink, R., Khusainov, R., Moll, G. and Kuipers, O. (2008) Biosynthesis, immunity, regulation, mode of action and engineering of the model lantibiotic nisin. *Cellular and Molecular Life Sciences* 65, 455–476.

Maffioli, S.I., Cruz, J.C., Monciardini, P., Sosio, M. and Donadio, S. (2016) Advancing cell wall inhibitors towards clinical applications. *Journal of Industrial Microbiology and Biotechnology* 43, 177–184.

Märki, F., Hänni, E., Fredenhagen, A. and Van Oostrum, J. (1991) Mode of action of the lanthionine-containing peptide antibiotics duramycin, duramycin B and C, and cinnamycin as indirect inhibitors of phospholipase A 2. *Biochemical Pharmacology* 42, 2027–2035.

Martin-Visscher, L.A., Yoganathan, S., Sit, C.S., Lohans, C.T. and Vederas, J.C. (2011) The activity of bacteriocins from *Carnobacterium maltaromaticum* UAL307 against Gram-negative bacteria in combination with EDTA treatment. *FEMS Microbiology Letters* 317, 152–159.

Meindl, K., Schmiederer, T., Schneider, K., Reicke, A., Butz, D., *et al.* (2010) Labyrinthopeptins: a new class of carbacyclic lantibiotics. *Angewandte Chemie International Edition* 49, 1151–1154.

Meyer, C., Bierbaum, G., Heidrich, C., Reis, M., Süling, J., Iglesias-Wind, M.I., *et al.* (1995) Nucleotide sequence of the lantibiotic Pep5 biosynthetic gene cluster and functional analysis of PepP and PepC. *European Journal of Biochemistry* 232, 478–489.

Molloy, E.M., Field, D., Cotter, P.D., Hill, C. and Ross, R.P. (2013) Saturation mutagenesis of lysine 12 leads to the identification of derivatives of nisin A with enhanced antimicrobial activity. *PloS One* 8, e58530.

Montalbán-López, M. and Kuipers, O.P. (2016) Posttranslational peptide-modification enzymes in action: key roles for leaders and glutamate. *Cell Chemical Biology* 23, 318–319.

Mota-Meira, M., Lapointe, G., Lacroix, C. and Lavoie, M.C. (2000) MICs of mutacin B-Ny266, nisin A, vancomycin, and oxacillin against bacterial pathogens. *Antimicrobial Agents and Chemotherapy* 44, 24–29.

Mulders, J.W., Boerrigter, I.J., Rollema, H.S., Siezen, R.J. and Vos, W.M. (1991) Identification and characterization of the lantibiotic nisin Z, a natural nisin variant. *European Journal of Biochemistry* 201, 581–584.

Naghmouchi, K., Baah, J., Hober, D., Jouy, E., Rubrecht, C., Sané, F. and Drider, D. (2013) Synergistic effect between colistin and bacteriocins in controlling Gram-negative pathogens and their potential to reduce antibiotic toxicity in mammalian epithelial cells. *Antimicrobial Agents and Chemotherapy* 57, 2719–2725.

Oldach, F., Al Toma, R., Kuthning, A., Caetano, T., Mendo, S., Budisa, N. and Süssmuth, R.D. (2012) Congeneric lantibiotics from ribosomal in vivo peptide synthesis with noncanonical amino acids. *Angewandte Chemie International Edition* 51, 415–418.

Perez, R.H., Zendo, T. and Sonomoto, K. (2014) Novel bacteriocins from lactic acid bacteria (LAB): various structures and applications. *Microbial Cell Factories* 13, 1.

Perin, L.M., Dal Bello, B., Belviso, S., Zeppa, G., De Carvalho, A.F., Cocolin, L. and Nero, L.A. (2015) Microbiota of Minas cheese as influenced by the nisin producer *Lactococcus lactis* subsp. *lactis* GLc05. *International Journal of Food Microbiology* 214, 159–167.

Piper, C., Cotter, P.D., Ross, R.P. and Hill, C. (2009a) Discovery of medically significant lantibiotics. *Current Drug Discovery Technologies* 6, 1–18.

Piper, C., Draper, L.A., Cotter, P.D., Ross, R.P. and Hill, C. (2009b) A comparison of the activities of lacticin 3147 and nisin against drug-resistant *Staphylococcus aureus* and *Enterococcus* species. *Journal of Antimicrobial Chemotherapy* 64, 546–551.

Piper, C., Casey, P.G., Hill, C., Cotter, P.D. and Ross, R.P. (2012) The lantibiotic lacticin 3147 prevents systemic spread of *Staphylococcus aureus* in a murine infection model. *International Journal of Microbiology* 2012: 806230

Plat, A., Kuipers, A., Lange, J.G.D., Moll, G.N. and Rink, R. (2011) Activity and export of engineered Nisin-(1-22) analogs. *Polymers* 3, 1282–1296.

Preet, S., Bharati, S., Panjeta, A., Tewari, R. and Rishi, P. (2015) Effect of nisin and doxorubicin on DMBA-induced skin carcinogenesis – a possible adjunct therapy. *Tumor Biology* 36, 8301–8308.

Qiao, M. and Saris, P.E. (1996) Evidence for a role of NisT in transport of the lantibiotic nisin produced by *Lactococcus lactis* N8. *FEMS Microbiology Letters* 144, 89–93.

Rea, M.C., Clayton, E., O'Connor, P.M., Shanahan, F., Kiely, B., Ross, R.P. and Hill, C. (2007) Antimicrobial activity of lacticin 3147 against clinical *Clostridium difficile* strains. *Journal of Medical Microbiology* 56, 940–946.

Rogers, L. (1928) The inhibiting effect of *Streptococcus lactis* on *Lactobacillus bulgaricus*. *Journal of Bacteriology* 16, 321.

Ross, A.C., Liu, H., Pattabiraman, V.R. and Vederas, J.C. (2009) Synthesis of the lantibiotic lactocin S using peptide cyclizations on solid phase. *Journal of the American Chemical Society* 132, 462–463.

Ross, A.C., McKinnie, S.M. and Vederas, J.C. (2012) The synthesis of active and stable diaminopimelate analogues of the lantibiotic peptide lactocin S. *Journal of the American Chemical Society* 134, 2008–2011.

Rouse, S., Field, D., Daly, K.M., O'Connor, P.M., Cotter, P.D., Hill, C. and Ross, R.P. (2012) Bioengineered nisin derivatives with enhanced activity in complex matrices. *Microbial Biotechnology* 5, 501–508.

Sahl, H.-G. and Bierbaum, G. (1998) Lantibiotics: biosynthesis and biological activities of uniquely modified peptides from Gram-positive bacteria. *Annual Reviews in Microbiology* 52, 41–79.

Saising, J., Dube, L., Ziebandt, A.-K., Voravuthikunchai, S.P., Nega, M. and Götz, F. (2012) Activity of gallidermin on *Staphylococcus aureus* and *Staphylococcus epidermidis* biofilms. *Antimicrobial Agents and Chemotherapy* 56, 5804–5810.

Scheffers, D.-J. and Tol, M.B. (2015) LipidII: Just another brick in the wall? *PLoS Pathogens* 11, e1005213.

Siezen, R.J., Kuipers, O.P. and De Vos, W.M. (1996) Comparison of lantibiotic gene clusters and encoded proteins. *Antonie van Leeuwenhoek* 69, 171–184.

Suda, S., Westerbeek, A., O'Connor, P.M., Ross, R.P., Hill, C. and Cotter, P.D. (2010) Effect of bioengineering lacticin 3147 lanthionine bridges on specific activity and resistance to heat and proteases. *Chemistry and Biology* 17, 1151–1160.

Thomsen, T.T., Mojsoska, B., Cruz, J.C., Donadio, S., Jenssen, H., Løbner-Olesen, A. and Rewitz, K. (2016) The lantibiotic NAI-107 efficiently rescues *Drosophila melanogaster* from infection with methicillin-resistant *Staphylococcus aureus* USA300. *Antimicrobial Agents and Chemotherapy* AAC. 02965-15.

Van Der Meer, J.R., Rollema, H.S., Siezen, R.J., Beerthuyzen, M.M., Kuipers, O.P. and De Vos, W. (1994) Influence of amino acid substitutions in the nisin leader peptide on biosynthesis and secretion of nisin by *Lactococcus lactis*. *Journal of Biological Chemistry* 269, 3555–3562.

Van Heel, A.J., Montalban-Lopez, M. and Kuipers, O.P. (2011) Evaluating the feasibility of lantibiotics as an alternative therapy against bacterial infections in humans. *Expert Opinion on Drug Metabolism and Toxicology* 7, 675–680.

Van Heel, A.J., De Jong, A., Montalban-Lopez, M., Kok, J. and Kuipers, O.P. (2013) BAGEL3: automated identification of genes encoding bacteriocins and (non-)bactericidal posttranslationally modified peptides. *Nucleic Acids Research* 41, W448–W453.

Van Staden, A., Brand, A. and Dicks, L. (2012) Nisin F-loaded brushite bone cement prevented the growth of *Staphylococcus aureus* in vivo. *Journal of Applied Microbiology* 112, 831–840.

Walsh, C.J., Guinane, C.M., Hill, C., Ross, R.P., O'Toole, P.W. and Cotter, P.D. (2015) In silico identification of bacteriocin gene clusters in the gastrointestinal tract, based on the Human Microbiome Project's reference genome database. *BMC Microbiology* 15, 1.

Wiedemann, I., Breukink, E., Van Kraaij, C., Kuipers, O.P., Bierbaum, G., De Kruijff, B. and Sahl, H.-G. (2001) Specific binding of nisin to the peptidoglycan precursor lipid II combines pore formation and inhibition of cell wall biosynthesis for potent antibiotic activity. *Journal of Biological Chemistry* 276, 1772–1779.

Zhou, L., van Heel, A.J. and Kuipers, O.P. (2015) The length of a lantibiotic hinge region has profound influence on antimicrobial activity and host specificity. *Frontiers in Microbiology* 6, 11.

Zhou, L., Shao, J., Li, Q., Van Heel, A.J., De Vries, M.P., Broos, J. and Kuipers, O.P. (2016) Incorporation of tryptophan analogues into the lantibiotic nisin. *Amino Acids* 48, 1309–1318.

Zimmermann, N., Metzger, J.W. and Jung, G. (1995) The tetracyclic lantibiotic actagardine ^{1}H-NMR and ^{13}C-NMR assignments and revised primary structure. *European Journal of Biochemistry* 228, 786–797.

5 Discovery of Novel Antimicrobial Peptides Using Combinatorial Chemistry and High-throughput Screening

Charles G. Starr and William C. Wimley*

Department of Biochemistry SL43, Tulane University Health Sciences Center, New Orleans LA, 70112-2699, USA

Abstract

The field of antimicrobial peptide (AMP) research has now spanned 4 decades in which many hundreds of AMPs have been discovered, designed or engineered. Yet, despite a vast literature, obvious sequence–structure–function relationships are rare, creating a bottleneck in the discovery of novel AMPs. Instead of rigorous structure–function principles, AMP activity may be best addressed using the physical chemistry concept of 'interfacial activity', which does not currently allow for explicit prediction and engineering of AMP activity. In this chapter we address a way to circumvent this engineering bottleneck: combinatorial chemistry and high-throughput screening. Combinatorial methods are first discussed from the perspective of library synthesis techniques for both indexed and non-indexed methods. This is followed by a discussion of available high-throughput screening techniques and the accomplishments to date generated using combinatorial chemistry and high-throughput screening. Lastly, we discuss future directions in the field. Combinatorial chemistry and high-throughput screening are powerful and effective tools for discovering novel antimicrobial peptides. The future of this field holds great promise.

5.1 The Interfacial Activity Model of AMP Activity

Antimicrobial peptides exert their biological activity by first acting on microbial membranes (Steiner *et al.*, 1981; White *et al.*, 1995; Hancock and Sahl, 2006; Wimley, 2010) sometimes followed by additional effects on cytosolic macromolecules (Hancock and Sahl, 2006; Nguyen *et al.*, 2011). Yet, despite decades of intense study, compelling sequence–structure–function relationships for antimicrobial peptides are rarely found and evidence for stable, well-defined transmembrane pores is rarely observed. Recent literature suggests that antimicrobial activity is not dependent on specific amino acid sequences or on specific three-dimensional peptide structures (Hilpert *et al.*, 2005; Jin *et al.*, 2005; Hilpert *et al.*, 2006; Mowery *et al.*, 2007; Rausch *et al.*, 2007). Instead it depends on 'interfacial activity' which we have referred to as 'the ability of a molecule to bind to a

* Corresponding author e-mail: wwimley@tulane.edu

membrane, partition into the membrane–water interface and to alter the packing and organization of the lipids' (Rathinakumar and Wimley, 2008; Rathinakumar *et al.*, 2009; Wimley, 2010) (see Fig. 5.1). Interfacial activity is derived from the appropriate balance of interactions between and among peptides, water and membrane lipids. These interactions depend more on the amino acid composition of a peptide and on its physical chemical properties than on its exact sequence or secondary/tertiary structure (Rathinakumar and Wimley, 2008; Rathinakumar *et al.*, 2009). In support of this idea, Hancock and colleagues showed that a high percentage of random versions of a potent AMP retain good activity and some even have improved activity (Hilpert *et al.*, 2006).

Because few discrete structure–activity relationships have been established, rational

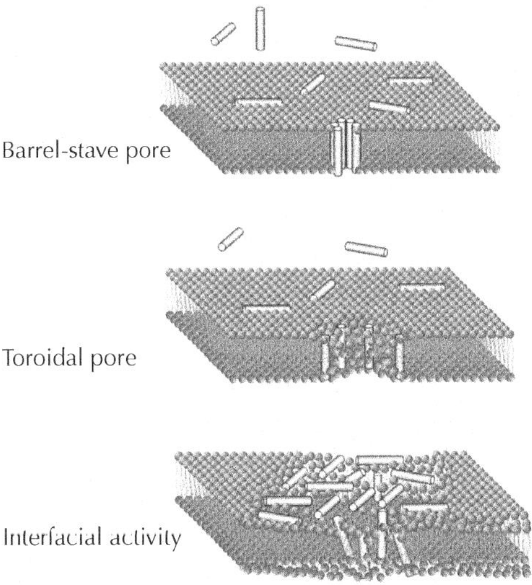

Fig. 5.1. Some schematic models of antimicrobial peptide activity. The literature contains numerous mechanistic models to explain the action of antimicrobial peptides on lipid bilayers. The barrel-stave and toroidal pore models, while commonly referenced, do not explain the experimentally observed actions of most antimicrobial peptides. The interfacial activity model (Rathinakumar and Wimley, 2008) can explain the actions of most AMPs. Most importantly, the interfacial activity model can be used as a basis for designing compositionally-varied combinatorial peptide libraries.

design – the process of designing new peptides based on perceived sequence–structure–function relationships – is rarely successful. Additionally, design based on the principle of interfacial activity is not yet possible because the physicochemical basis of interfacial activity has not been parameterized, especially with respect to target selectivity. In light of these considerations, the use of combinatorial chemistry and high-throughput screening is an especially attractive approach to discovering novel AMPs. To design rational libraries from which the most active sequences can readily be determined by high-throughput screening, one can use the principle of interfacial activity by requiring libraries to contain peptides that adhere to common attributes of known AMPs (e.g. peptide length, amino acid composition, charge, hydrophobicity). In this chapter we explore the design, selection and screening of combinatorial peptide libraries toward the efficient discovery of novel and useful antimicrobial peptides.

5.2 Combinatorial Chemistry Methods

5.2.1 Overview of library synthesis

Almost as soon as the Merrifield method of solid-phase peptide synthesis (Merrifield, 1963) became widely known, combinatorial peptide synthesis was recognized as a natural extension of that chemistry. The usefulness of combinatorial peptide synthesis is derived, in part, from the fact that the chemistry required to make a library is often no more complex than to perform a non-combinatorial synthesis. While some approaches to library synthesis require specialized equipment, others can be performed with the same complement of supplies as a simple, solid-phase peptide synthesis. Combinatorial peptide libraries can be separated into two broad categories: (i) Indexed libraries, in which spatial or chemical indexing allows sequences to be easily identifiable during the course of the screen; (ii) Non-indexed libraries, in which indirect analytical methods, such as Edman sequencing, mass spectrometry or iterative deconvolution must be used to identify active sequences after they have been selected in the screen. In this section we describe some of the more commonly used synthetic approaches to indexed and non-indexed combinatorial peptide library synthesis and discuss their various strengths and weaknesses.

5.2.2 Non-indexed methods

Houghten and colleagues were some of the earliest users of combinatorial chemistry and high-throughput screening to identify novel antimicrobial peptides (Houghten et al., 1991). In this seminal work, they demonstrated the power of combinatorial chemistry by developing peptides for antibody competition assays as well as antimicrobial peptides. For the antimicrobial studies, the first two amino acids of a peptide hexamer were fixed as 'RR' and they followed an iterative screening protocol to determine the most potent complement of residues for the remaining four positions. Briefly, each variable position underwent an iteration of each of the 20 natural amino acids fixed at that position while the remaining positions were occupied by a random mixture of amino acids. Each peptide iteration mixture was assessed for antimicrobial activity and once the residue conferring the most potent peptides was identified at a given position, that amino acid was fixed and the process was repeated with variability at the next position. While this approach requires a large amount of peptide synthesis for deconvolution to identify absolutely the active sequences present in each peptide mixture, and risks the possibility that peptides in the mixture will act synergistically or antagonistically, it is simple and effective and can successfully lead to the discovery of novel, potent antimicrobial peptides. Later, the same group used a more constrained approach to library design in which they used an already established antimicrobial peptide as their template sequence and performed positional scanning, based upon

the predicted α-helical structure of the peptide (Blondelle et al., 1996). In this scanning approach, they used several simple, partially-indexed library design methods in which the peptides screened had fixed residues at the majority of positions (to minimize disruption of the helix) and variable residues in a few positions such that they were modifying either the hydrophobic, hydrophilic, or both faces of the ideal helical structure. Mixtures with the greatest activity were further subdivided by iterative deconvolution that was based on rounds of additional synthesis and testing until a single active sequence was obtained.

An alternate, simpler approach to non-indexed combinatorial peptide libraries can be found in the one-bead:one-sequence methods, also known as split and recombine (Lam et al., 2003). One-bead:one-sequence libraries take advantage of the discrete nature of solid-phase synthesis resins, which are in the form of polymer microbeads of tens to hundreds of microns, and have been used to find novel AMPs (Rathinakumar and Wimley, 2008; Rathinakumar et al., 2009; Rathinakumar and Wimley, 2010). As shown in Figure 5.2, in one-bead:one-sequence libraries, solid-phase synthesis beads are combined into a single vessel when non-variable residue addition is performed and split into separate vessels at combinatorial sites for the addition of varied amino acid residues. Recombination (mixing) of the resin beads into one vessel allows for randomization before the next split. Each bead thus has a unique history of amino acid additions and contains only peptides of a single sequence. Separation of single beads to isolate unique sequences must be performed prior to screening experiments, which requires either manual bead 'picking' or a bead separation technology. Screening can sometimes be accelerated if pools of beads are first screened together, with later deconvolution of the active members (He et al., 2011).

One-bead:one-sequence libraries can be made using beads with densities from 10,000 to 1,000,000 beads per gram of resin. Each bead can theoretically be loaded with 0.1 to 3.5 nmol of peptide, depending on

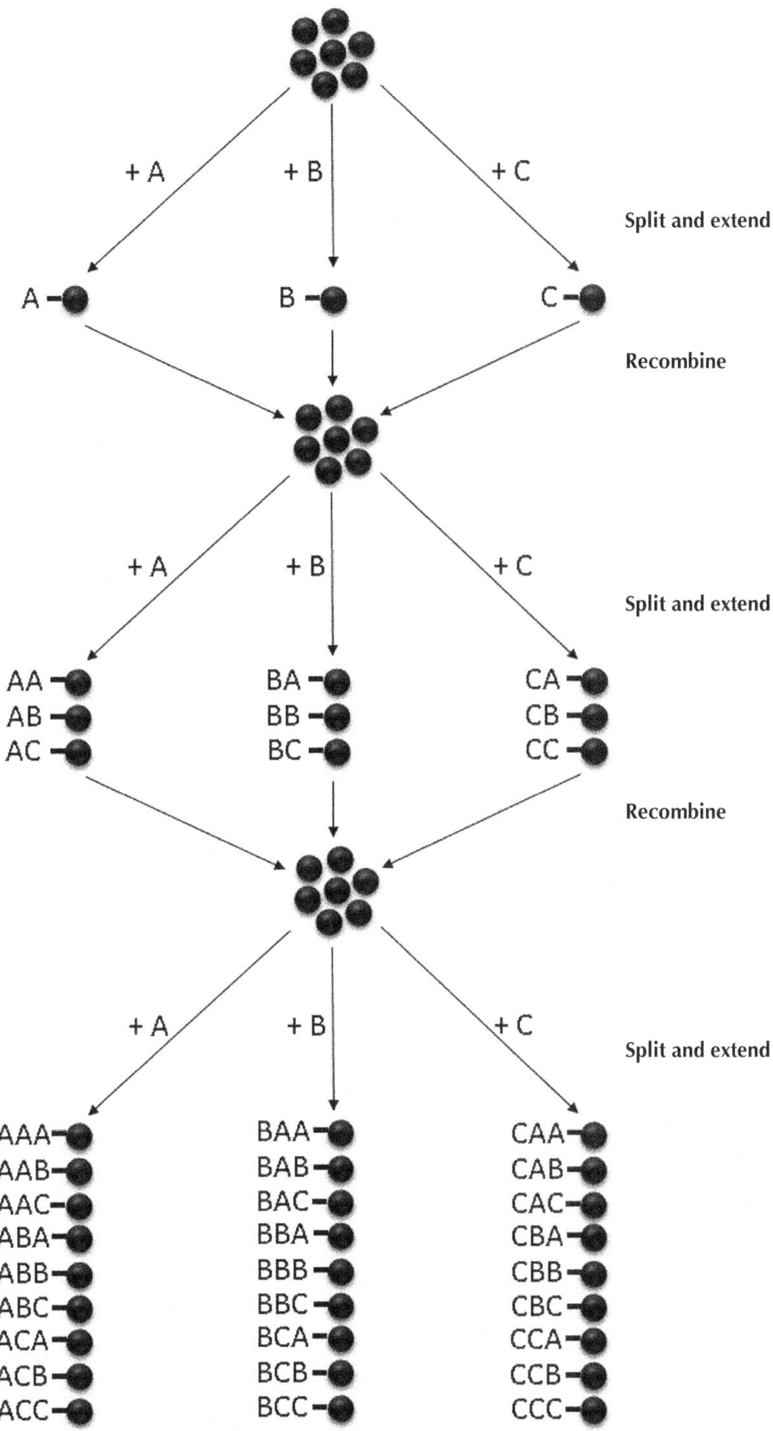

Fig. 5.2. Combinatorial chemistry of the one-bead:one-sequence method of library design. Resin beads are split into pools at each combinatorial site and recombined after each residue is attached. This method generates high sequence variability but requires deconvolution to identify active peptides.

bead size and loading capacity. Bead density (i.e. potential library diversity) is inversely related to the amount of peptide per bead (potential screen complexity) enabling researchers to select beads that provide the needed balance of the two factors. Peptides are often linked to beads by a UV cleavable photolinker for release (Holmes and Jones, 1995) and positive sequences are identified *post facto*, using chemical sequencing, mass spectrometry or deconvolution. In Table 5.1 we show statistics on some commonly used one-bead:one-sequence SPPS resins.

5.2.3 Indexed methods

When the individual members of a library can be identified directly, either by their spatial location or by an easily read coded 'tag' associated with them, the library is 'indexed'. Indexed combinatorial libraries have the advantage of not requiring tedious deconvolution or expensive peptide sequencing, but they can be more complex to construct and are generally more limited in size. One of the first approaches to forming an indexed peptide library was using light-directed synthesis in conjunction with a complex binary masking scheme to synthesize short (<10 residue) and relatively small (1024 member) peptide libraries (Fodor *et al.*, 1991). Another example of a spatially-indexed combinatorial library

method is the SPOT synthesis method (Frank, 1992 and 2002) and its variants in which synthesis is systematically done in rows and columns on a cellulose sheet, followed by cutting of the 'spots' and cleavage into individual solutions. SPOT synthesis can be done with technology as simple as a pipetting robot as described by Hancock and colleagues (Wenschuh *et al.*, 2000; Hilpert *et al.*, 2005; Winkler *et al.*, 2011). Similarly, multi-pin libraries (Geysen *et al.*, 1984; Maeji *et al.*, 1990; Valerio *et al.*, 1994; Saido-Sakanaka *et al.*, 1999) are carried out using multiple pins as solid supports with multiple reaction chambers controlling the chemistry. The size of SPOT and pin libraries depends on a laboratory's inventiveness or investment in synthetic technology, but libraries with hundreds to thousands of members are readily achievable (Ashby *et al.*, 2016).

Although they have not been applied to the search for novel AMPs, powerful techniques for chemical indexing of peptide libraries have also been described. For example, a unique oligonucleotide sequence can be associated with each peptide sequence. In this case, the peptide sequence can be determined by sequencing the oligonucleotide, which is much simpler than sequencing the peptide. Oligonucleotide indexing can be done chemically (Brenner and Lerner, 1992; Needels *et al.*, 1994) or it can be done biologically as in the ribosome display (Mattheakis *et al.*, 1994; Xie *et al.*, 2006) and mRNA display (Keefe and

Table 5.1. Some available synthesis microbeads for one-bead:one-sequence libraries.[a]

Median diameter µm	Typical loading mmol/g	Bead density beads/g	Peptide per bead (nmol) theoretical (actual)	µM conc. (in 100 µl)
90	0.2	1.5×10^6	0.17	1.7
140–170	0.2	520,000	0.5	5
200–250	0.2	160,000	1.5	15
280–320	0.2	65,500	3.5 (1.0)	35 (10)

[a]TentaGel polystyrene with grafted polyethylene glycol (PEG/PS). TentaGel beads made by Rapp-Polymere are commonly used for such libraries because they are especially large and uniformly sized. Bead density, which is inversely proportional to the amount of peptide per bead, ranges from 10^4 to 10^6 beads per gram, an easy benchtop synthesis scale, providing enough peptide for orthogonal screening. In our experience, photolabile linkers allow for release of only a portion of the peptide on the bead so we show the theoretical and measured (actual) release from the largest beads.

Szostak, 2001) techniques. These approaches can produce highly diverse peptide libraries in which a peptide sequence is covalently crosslinked to its own mRNA, for indexing. However, the potential for the tag to interfere with screening assays for the biological activity of AMPs has not yet been tested.

5.3 High-throughput Screening

'High-throughput screening' could mean testing millions of compounds rapidly in massively parallel, automated, robotic applications. On the other hand, in a small academic laboratory, it may only mean screening a few thousand peptides by mostly manual techniques. In either case, high-throughput screening can be defined by the common characteristic of performing selection experiments on molecular libraries at a pace that is orders of magnitude faster than achievable using the traditional approach of single sequence design, synthesis, purification and characterization. As discussed above, combinatorial peptide library synthesis is not, in itself, technically challenging. The real challenge lies in the design of high-throughput screens that efficiently select the most active members from a library. In this section we explore the various approaches that can be used to select antimicrobial peptide sequences in peptide libraries.

5.3.1 Biological assays

The most direct selection method for antimicrobial activity is to screen libraries using living microbes. Broth dilution assays test for the ability of a peptide to inhibit the growth of microbes in a nutrient broth. This method has been used extensively in the discovery and characterization of novel antimicrobial compounds, and as such, many different variations of the protocol have been developed. In order to maintain consistency and comparable results across the literature, it is suggested that researchers adhere to published methods such as those outlined by Hancock and colleagues

(Wiegand *et al.*, 2008). While normally performed using a serially diluted peptide concentration series, this method is easily adapted to library screening and activity assessment at single concentrations. Generally a peptide and a microbe inoculum are incubated overnight in media. Given the long incubation and short doubling time for most microbes, expansion of the inoculum to the opaque stationary phase will occur unless completely inhibited by the peptide. In practice, intermediate results are usually not observed (Rathinakumar and Wimley, 2008; Rausch *et al.*, 2007). Detection of activity can be done photometrically by observing optical density at 600 nm, but even visual inspection will suffice in this experiment because of the binary nature of the result. See Fig. 5.3A for an example of a broth dilution screen in a 96-well plate format. It should be noted that if sterilization is desired, researchers may choose to remove a small amount of inoculum and streak or spot it on an agar plate to assess for the presence of remaining viable colonies. An example of this practice is shown in Fig. 5.3B. Broth dilution screening is readily performed in multiwell plate format and requires a minimum of automation, robotics or specialized detection methods. For more rapid screening, increased sensitivity, and automated throughput one can couple a broth dilution assay with a secondary detection using real-time growth curves.

In addition to using classical optical density measurements to screen for antimicrobial peptides in broth dilution, Hilpert and Hancock have published a broth dilution method that makes use of chemical luminescence to assess antimicrobial activity. The system requires transformation of the bacterial strain of interest with a plasmid containing the luxCDABE (luciferase) cassette. This cassette codes for enzymes that are capable of both synthesizing luminescent substrate and catalysing the light-emitting reaction in the presence of naturally occurring precursors. The energy source for the emission of light is reduced flavin mononucleotide ($FMNH_2$) and as such, unperturbed bacteria emit a strong luminescent signal under normal growing

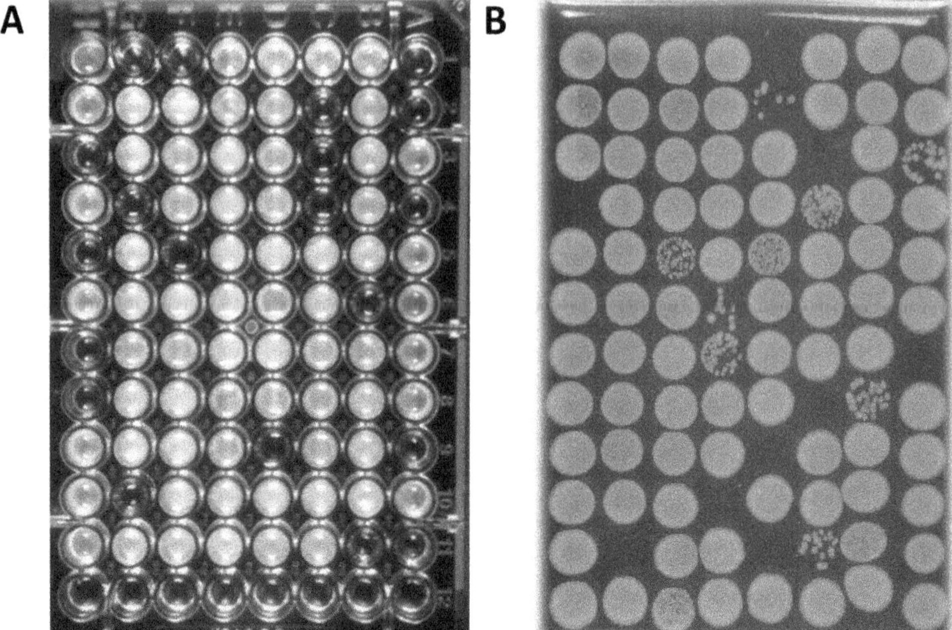

Fig. 5.3.   A. Broth dilution assay as a high-throughput screen. In this example 96-well screen, each well contains a 2.2 µM concentration of one member of a combinatorial peptide library, rich growth medium, and an inoculum of 10³ *Escherichia coli* bacteria. After overnight incubation, wells are either opaque, indicating stationary phase growth, or they are transparent, indicating no growth; i.e. that the bacteria had been sterilized by the peptide. This is a very stringent high-throughput screen which requires no sophisticated equipment to perform. Wells C11 to H11 have no added peptides and wells C12 to H12 have no added bacteria. B. Example of a more quantitative approach to the broth dilution assay. In this experiment, library peptides (one per well) were incubated with *E. coli* (1×10⁵ CFU/ml) in minimal media (1% TSB) for three hours. Following incubation, 10 µl aliquots were removed from each well and spotted on the nutrient agar plate. Several spots are missing from the plate, indicating that the bacteria in that well have been completely sterilized. Additionally, there are a few locations where there are a countable number of colonies in the spot which represent peptides that substantially reduced the population of the well, but were unable to completely sterilize. The plates shown in these figures are from independent experiments.

conditions. When incubated with an antimicrobial peptide, however, intracellular components, including $FMNH_2$ and ATP, are released from the cell due to the loss of membrane integrity. In theory, peptides exhibiting strong lytic activity will cause an almost complete loss of luminescence (Hilpert *et al.*, 2005, 2007). It should be noted that the usefulness of this approach is partially dependent on the AMPs being studied. While most well characterized AMPs have been shown to be membrane active, there is a substantial subset that may act through a variety of alternative mechanisms (Nguyen *et al.*, 2011). In any case,

bacterial cell death will ultimately result in energy depletion and decreased luminescence, but the magnitude and kinetics of the effects may be slower than anticipated and lead to an underestimation of potency.

A second classical antimicrobial activity experiment that can be adapted to high throughput is the agarose diffusion assay (Wiegand *et al.*, 2008) in which peptides are spotted on a thin layer of nutrient agarose seeded with bacteria. Peptides will diffuse into the agarose and active peptides will create a zone of clearance where they inhibit bacterial growth. The area of clearance is proportional to the potency of the peptide.

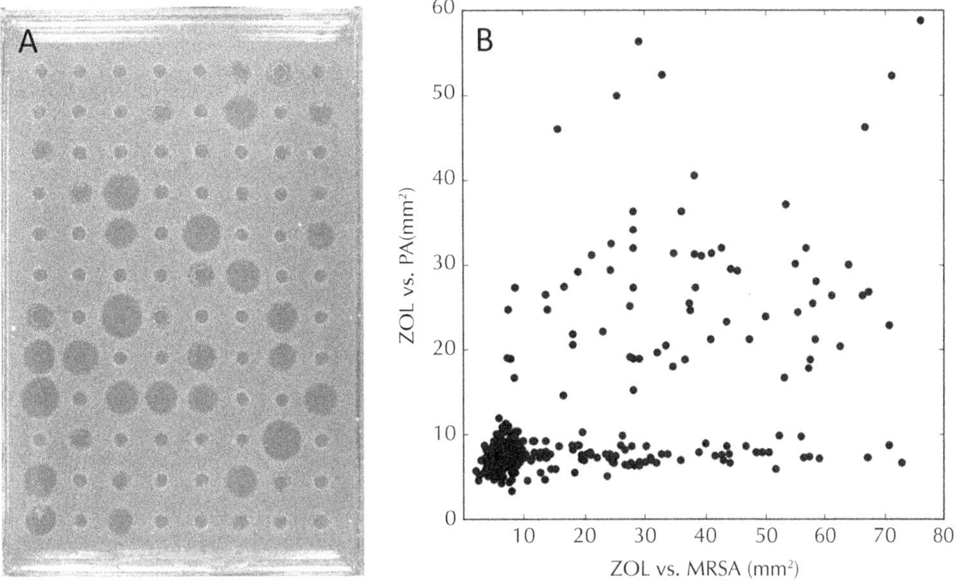

Fig. 5.4. Agarose diffusion approach to antimicrobial peptide library screening. A. The peptides are extracted from synthesis resin in a 96-well microplate. Extracted peptide is transferred to the specially designed 96-well agar plate and allowed to incubate overnight. The zones of inhibition reflect the potency, solubility and ability of the peptide to diffuse through the agarose matrix. B. Distribution of activities for a small screen (500 members) against MRSA and PA (*P. aeruginosa*.)

Our lab has adopted the agarose diffusion assay to accommodate the 96-well plate format commonly used when screening peptide libraries. Briefly, we use a 'one-well' agar plate with the same dimensions as a standard 96-well microplate and use a 96-well plate replicator to create 10 µl wells in the agar. Peptide is easily transferred from the microplate to the agarose plate, which lends itself well to high-throughput screening. Examples of agarose diffusion experiments are shown in Fig. 5.4A. An advantage of agarose diffusion is that the results are semi-quantitative. Assuming equal concentrations, the most potent members of a library can readily be identified from the diameter of the spots (in practice this is not always the case as SPPS resins are prone to inconsistency in peptide release). The distribution of activities for a small library against MRSA and *P. aerugi- nosa* is shown in Fig. 5.4B. In one-bead: one-sequence libraries another possible advantage of agarose diffusion is that peptides do not need to be extracted from the

beads for the assay as they do in a broth dilution assay. This approach was demonstrated by Bicker and colleagues in a study in which direct addition of peptoid-loaded resin to the molten agarose was used to assess antimicrobial potential (Fisher *et al.*, 2016). In this case, the peptoids were attached to the resin via a disulfide linker and the agarose contained a small amount of reducing agent. Once the peptide was added to the agarose, the linker was reduced and the peptoid was free to diffuse into the agar. Positive beads were removed from the agarose and washed to remove any contamination and were then sequenced using an MS/MS based approach.

In our experience, not all peptides diffuse from the beads into the agarose at a useful rate, but this may actually be advantageous because the slowly diffusing peptides are generally the least soluble, thus also the least desirable AMPs. Additionally, we often find that activity in agarose diffusion does not always translate to activity in broth dilution. In contrast, peptides active in broth dilution experiments almost always have activity in agarose diffusion experiments. This inconsistency may be due to the all-or-nothing nature of broth dilution experiments compared to the activity gradient apparent in agarose diffusion experiments.

Recently, an intriguing 'whole animal' high-throughput antimicrobial screen was described (Moy *et al.*, 2009) in which *Caenorhabditis elegans* nematodes in small nutrient chambers were used to test compounds simultaneously for antimicrobial activity and for toxicity towards the nematode.

5.3.2 Non-biological assays

There are countless studies in the literature showing that AMPs interact with and perturb synthetic lipid bilayer membranes as well as bacterial membranes. A typical synthetic bilayer experiment is performed using unilamellar lipid vesicles with an entrapped marker for assaying membrane permeability (Rausch and Wimley, 2001; Rathinakumar and Wimley, 2008). Experimental lipid compositions vary widely between laboratories, but mixtures of anionic and zwitterionic lipids are often used to mimic microbial membranes while phosphatidylcholine (PC) and or PC/cholesterol are used to mimic mammalian membranes. Because cationic/hydrophobic antimicrobial peptides with good interfacial activity are expected to perturb any lipid bilayer membrane to which they bind well enough, the exact anionic lipid content is probably not a crucial factor in vesicle-based characterization of AMPs.

We have developed a vesicle-based high-throughput screen to select for potent vesicle-permeabilizing peptides from combinatorial libraries (Rausch and Wimley, 2001; Rausch *et al.*, 2005; Rathinakumar and Wimley, 2008; Rathinakumar *et al.*, 2009). The high-throughput screen utilizes large unilamellar vesicles with the lanthanide metal terbium (III), Tb^{3+}, entrapped inside and the aromatic chelator dipicolinic acid (DPA) added to the external solution. The Tb-DPA complex, which forms only when the membranes have been permeabilized, is highly fluorescent and can be quantitated. Assays are performed in 96-well plate format and fluorescence is used to rate permeabilization. See Fig. 5.5 for an image of high-throughput screening using this method. By varying the concentration of lipid vesicles added to each well the stringency of the assay can be adjusted to suit the library being studied.

In some cases, researchers may be interested in not only whether a peptide is able to disrupt microbial membranes, but also the nature of the membrane interaction. The assay system described above utilizes Tb^{3+}, a relatively small and irrelevant ion. It is thought that Tb^{3+} and other small ions are able to pass through very small perturbations of the membrane. To study the integrity of the membrane with respect to biologically relevant macromolecules, a different system would need to be used. Such a system was developed by Wiedman and colleagues in a screen for pH-sensitive macromolecular pore-formers (Wiedman *et al.*, 2014). In this assay, a fluorescently-labelled (TAMRA), biotin-tagged, 10 kDa dextran is entrapped in vesicles while a fluorescently-labelled (AF488) streptavidin moiety is added to the external solution. The sizes of both the dextran and streptavidin molecules prohibit leakage of the compound except in the cases of complete vesicle disruption or true pore formation. Because of the unique excitation and emission wavelengths of the fluorophores used and high affinity of biotin for streptavidin, a FRET (Förster resonance energy transfer) pair is formed when dextran leaks into the external environment, indicating that the peptide has had a catastrophic effect on the integrity of the vesicles.

5.3.3 Parallel screening for selection of discrete characteristics

Often, it is desirable to screen a library for peptides with more than a single important characteristic or activity. A simple example

Low Stringency   High Stringency

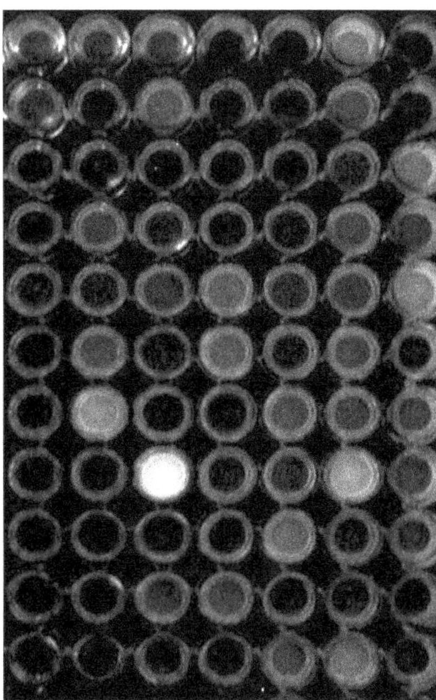

Fig. 5.5. A vesicle-based high-throughput screen for bilayer-permeabilizing peptides. Large unilamellar vesicles containing entrapped Tb^{3+} and external dipicolinic acid are added to each well which also contains about 10 µM of one peptide from a combinatorial library. Permeabilization of the vesicles results in Tb-DPA complex formation which is highly fluorescent. These plates are photographed under UV light. On the right, a lower lipid concentration used for lower stringency screening. On the left higher lipid concentration gives higher stringency. In practice, stringency is altered to provide a desired number or fraction of positive peptides (Rausch *et al.*, 2005).

is the addition of selection for solubility in physiological fluids prior to screening by incubating peptides either directly in such fluids or by creating a buffer system with similar characteristics. In the vesicle-based screen described above, we used a 'premixing' step in which library peptides were added to a buffer and incubated for several hours before the addition of the vesicle test solution. Insoluble peptides will precipitate and will be inactive. By using these two orthogonal screening steps, we select only for peptides that are soluble and have good activity. Another possibility is screening for protease resistance by splitting aliquots of a given peptide solution and subjecting one to degradation and another to a designer anti-microbial assay. Further examples may include but are certainly not limited to: pH sensitivity, eukaryotic cell toxicity or lysis,

biological clearance, eukaryotic cell interactions and activity in the presence of serum proteins. Regardless of the attributes desired, parallel screening for the evaluation of peptide libraries is almost always superior to the use of a single metric. Clever researchers may even find ways to extract multiple datasets from a single assay. Below, we present an approach used by our laboratory to isolate peptides with activity against multiple species of microbes.

Identifying peptides with potent anti-microbial activity against one species of microbe is surprisingly easy. For example, we and others have designed libraries in which more than a quarter of all members have potent antimicrobial activity (Rausch *et al.*, 2007; Rathinakumar and Wimley, 2008; Rathinakumar *et al.*, 2009). A large proportion of random sequence variants of known antimicrobial peptides have also been shown to have good activity (Hilpert *et al.*, 2006) as well as many engineered variants of natural antimicrobial peptides.

Broad-spectrum antimicrobial activity, defined as activity against multiple classes of microbes, is desirable, yet is rarer and more difficult to select than species-specific activity. Selecting directly for broad-spectrum activity using biological screens can be achieved if a single library member is screened in parallel against microbes from multiple classes. This approach requires a complex experiment that reduces the throughput of a screen. However, it has the advantage over other screens that broad-spectrum peptides are identified directly and unambiguously. To test the effectiveness of this approach we have performed parallel multispecies screening using a sample of a one-bead:one-sequence library described in the literature (Rathinakumar and Wimley, 2008; Rathinakumar *et al.*, 2009). We screened in parallel for activity against *Escherochia coli*, a Gram-negative bacteria, *Staphylococcus aureus*, a Gram-positive bacteria and *Cryptococcus neoformans*, a fungus. We found species-specific antimicrobial activity to be surprisingly common while overlapping, broad-spectrum activity is quite rare (see the statistics in Table 5.2). Biological assays have been used successfully to select antimicrobial peptides from combinatorial libraries. But the single-species nature of most experiments and the difficulty in performing multispecies experiments with high throughput are problems that have not yet been overcome.

5.4 Accomplishments

We have constructed Table 5.3 to provide examples of approaches used by different groups in the pursuit of unique antimicrobial peptides. All of the combinatorial synthetic strategies discussed in this chapter have the potential to yield new peptides; and most have been proven at least once in the past. Thus, it is our opinion that the

Table 5.2. Abundance of broad-spectrum AMPs in a combinatorial library.[a]

	# Peptides	Per cent
Total peptides screened	1040	100
Active peptides	175	16.8

Combination of microbes sterilized	# Peptides	Per cent
Only *E. coli*	82	7.9
At least *E. coli*	115	11.1
Only *S. aureus*	54	5.2
At least *S. aureus*	79	7.6
Only *C. neoformans*	3	0.3
At least *C. neoformans*	12	1.2
Only *E. coli* and *S. aureus*	27	2.6
Only *E. coli* and *C. neoformans*	2	0.2
Only *S. aureus* and *C. neoformans*	3	0.3
All three organisms	4	0.4

[a]Spectrum of antimicrobial activity in a one-bead:one-peptide combinatorial peptide library described elsewhere (Rathinakumar and Wimley, 2008; Rathinakumar *et al.*, 2009). Individual peptides were extracted from beads and the solution was divided into into three 96-well plates where the peptide concentration in each well was about 2 μM. Wells were seeded with *E. coli*, a Gram-negative bacteria, *Staph. aureus*, a Gram-positive bacteria, or *Cryptococcus neoformans*, a fungus. Sterilization assays showed that there are many highly active peptides in the library (17%) but that only a small fraction (0.4%) have potent broad-spectrum activity against all three classes of microorganism.

synthesis method should be selected based on the number and diversity of peptides that a lab desires to screen. For example, researchers wanting to make small alterations in a sequence may wish to use SPOT synthesis or the multipin approach to synthesize smaller libraries for which the sequence information is readily retrievable. On the other hand, if large, diverse libraries are desired, the one-bead:one-sequence approach is better-suited even though slightly more work is required to extract the sequence information for active library members. Perhaps more important than the combinatorial technique selected, are the screening conditions. It has been our experience that library screening often yields peptides that behave well under the exact

Table 5.3. Examples of studies that have employed combinatorial chemistry to construct libraries of antimicrobial peptides.[a]

Lead sequence(s)	Target organisms	Library method	Screening method	Reference
YKLLKLLLPKLKGLLFKL-NH2	*S. aureus, P. aeruginosa, C. albicans*	Positional scanning	Broth dilution	Blondelle *et al.*, 1996
KRWRIRVRVIRK-NH2	*P. aeruginosa, E. coli, S. typhimurium, S. aureus, S. epidermidis, C. albicans*	SPOT synthesis	Broth dilution	Hilpert *et al.*, 2006
RRWRIVVIRVRR-NH2	*P. aeruginosa, E. coli, S. typhimurium, S. aureus, S. epidermidis, E. faecalis, C. albicans*	SPOT synthesis	Luminescent broth dilution	Hilpert *et al.*, 2005
RRWWCR-NH2	*S. aureus*	Iterative soluble combinatorial library	Broth dilution	Houghten *et al.*, 1991
RRGWALRLVLAY-NH2	*S. aureus, E. coli, P. aeruginosa, C. neoformans*	One-bead:one-sequence	Synthetic vesicles	Rathinakumar and Wimley, 2008
RRGWNLALTLTYGRR-NH2	*S. aureus, E. coli, C. neoformans*	One-bead:one-sequence	Broth dilution	Rathinakumar and Wimley, 2010
KVLKVLKVLKVLKVL	*B. subtilis, S. aureus, E. coli*	Ribosome display	Synthetic model membrane	Xie *et al.*, 2006
LCAAHCLAIGRR-NH2	*S. aureus, E. coli, P. aeruginosa*	Multi-pin	Broth dilution	Saido-Sakanaka, 1999
c(kVOrnLfThiYOrnLq)	*E. coli, B. subtilis*	One-bead:one-sequence	Agar diffusion	Fluxá *et al.*, 2011

[a]Far from exhaustive, this list is meant to provide examples of some of the techniques described in this chapter and serve as a starting point for researchers wishing to learn more about the these approaches.

conditions of the screen, but perform differently/poorly when the conditions are altered or the target organism is changed. Parameterization and assay development with well-characterized control compounds is a critical step in study design before screening even begins. If this step is executed properly, combinatorial library screening is an immensely powerful tool that will almost certainly lead to the development of novel antimicrobial peptides.

5.4.1 Beyond high-throughput screening

Identification of potential antimicrobial peptides using high-throughput screening is only the first step in the pipeline towards therapeutic antimicrobial peptides. It is possible, perhaps even likely, that researchers will gain insight into what makes peptides from their libraries active through screening and sequencing. This may allow for fine-tuning of activity through small sequence alterations or even by the building of consensus sequences, if enough information is available. Once a panel of the most promising peptides has been chosen, selected peptides must be tested for broad-spectrum activity against multiple classes of microbes. Peptides must also be tested for their lytic or toxic effects on mammalian cells. Experimentally, these latter effects are quantitated by measuring lysis of mammalian red blood cells (RBC), lysis of mammalian nucleated cells, or by measuring cytotoxicity against living mammalian cells. Other important factors include stability and activity in serum and the ability to diffuse and distribute into the appropriate tissues, as the ultimate goal is moving towards testing in animal models and eventually human clinical trials. Beyond activity and biological relevance, an effective scheme for the large-scale synthesis of AMPs must be established. SPPS is an efficient and cost-effective method in the laboratory setting, but in order to develop drugs for use on a large scale, new methods must be developed and employed.

5.5 Future Directions

Combinatorial chemistry and high-throughput screening are powerful and effective tools for discovering novel antimicrobial peptides. The future holds great promise as advances in technology drive increases in throughput. However, throughput is probably not the critical factor in the discovery of therapeutically useful antimicrobial peptides. Even libraries smaller than 10,000 members contain potent, broad-spectrum antimicrobial peptides which can be identified with manual screening (Rausch *et al.*, 2005; Rathinakumar and Wimley, 2008). Perhaps more importantly, improvements in our understanding of AMP mechanisms of action will drive improvements in library design leading to peptides that are more effective. We can also look forward in the near future to multiply orthogonal high-throughput screens that select in parallel for (or against) other factors that determine the true therapeutic effectiveness of a potential antibiotic drug. For example, future screens could include selection based on membrane permeabilization, bioactivity, solubility, bioavailability, pharmacokinetics, cytotoxicity, susceptibility to acquired resistance, and other factors. We envision a multiply orthogonal high-throughput pipeline strategy for the development of novel antimicrobial peptides which uses high-throughput screening to select active peptides from rationally designed libraries, followed by focused bioactivity, formulation and toxicity assays to select the most promising candidates for clinical testing.

References

Ashby, M., Petkova, A., Gani, J., Mikut, R. and Hilpert, K. (2016) Use of peptide libraries for identification and optimization of novel antimicrobial peptides. *Current Topics in Medicinal Chemistry* 17, 537–553. DOI: 10.2174/1568026616666160713125555

Blondelle, S.E., Takahashi, E., Houghten, R.A. and Pérez-Payá, E. (1996) Rapid identification of compounds with enhanced antimicrobial activity by using conformationally defined combinatorial libraries. *Biochemical Journal* 313,141–147.

Brenner, S. and Lerner, R.A. (1992) Encoded combinatorial chemistry. *Proceedings of the National Academy of Sciences of the United States of America* 89, 5381–5383.

Fisher, K.J., Turkett, J.A., Corson, A.E. and Bicker, K.L. (2016) Peptoid library agar diffusion (PLAD) assay for the high-throughput identification of antimicrobial peptoids. *ACS Combinatorial Science* 18, 287–291.

Fluxá, V.S., Maillard, N., Page, M.G. and Reymond, J.L. (2011) Bead diffusion assay for discovering antimicrobial cyclic peptides. *Chemical Communications* 47, 1434–1436.

Fodor, S.P.A., Read, J.L., Pirrung, M.C., Strayer, L., Lu, A.T. and Solas, D. (1991) Light-directed, spatially addressable parallel chemical synthesis. *Science* 251, 767–773.

Frank, R. (1992) Sport-synthesis: an easy technique for the positionally addressable, parallel chemical synthesis on a membrane support. *Tetrahedron* 48, 9217–9232.

Frank, R. (2002) The SPOT-synthesis technique: synthetic peptide arrays on membrane supports: principles and applications. *Journal of Immunological Methods* 267, 13–26.

Geysen, H.M., Meloen, R.H. and Barteling, S.J. (1984) Use of peptide synthesis to probe viral antigens for eptitopes to a resolution of a single amino acid. *Proceedings of the National Academy of Sciences of the United States of America* 81, 3998–4002.

Hancock, R.E. and Sahl, H.G. (2006) Antimicrobial and host-defense peptides as new anti-infective therapeutic strategies. *Nature Biotechnology* 24, 1551–1557.

He, L., Hoffmann, A.R., Serano, C., Hristova, K. and Wimley, W.C. (2011) High-throughput selection of transmembrane sequences that enhance receptor tyrosine kinase activation. *Journal of Molecular Biology* 412, 43–54.

Hilpert, K., Volkmer-Engert, R., Walter, T. and Hancock, R.E. (2005) High-throughput generation of small antibacterial peptides with improved activity. *Nature Biotechnology* 23, 1008–1012.

Hilpert, K., Elliott, M.R., Volkmer-Engert, R., Henklein, P., Donini, O., *et al.* (2006) Sequence requirements and an optimization strategy for short antimicrobial peptides. *Chemical Biology* 13, 1101–1107.

Hilpert, K., Winkler, D.F. and Hancock, R.E. (2007) Peptide arrays on cellulose support: SPOT synthesis: a time and cost efficient method for synthesis of large numbers of peptides in a parallel and addressable fashion. *Nature Protocols* 2, 1333–1349.

Holmes, C.P. and Jones, D.G. (1995) Reagents for combinatorial organic synthesis: development of a new o-Nitrobenzyl Photolabile Linker for solid phase synthesis. *Journal of Organic Chemistry* 60, 2318–2319.

Houghten, R.A., Pinilla, C., Blondelle, S.E., Appel, J.R., Dooley, C.T. and Cuervo, J.H. (1991) Generation and use of synthetic peptide libraries for basic research and drug discovery. *Nature* 354, 84–86.

Jin, Y., Hammer, J., Pate, M., Zhang, Y., Zhu, F., Zmuda, E. and Blazyk, J. (2005) Antimicrobial activities and structures of two linear cationic peptide families with various amphipathic beta-sheet and alpha-helical potentials. *Antimicrobial Agents and Chemotherapy* 49, 4957–4964.

Keefe, A.D. and Szostak, J.W. (2001) Functional proteins from a random-sequence library. *Nature* 410, 715–718.

Lam, K.S., Lehman, A.L., Song, A., Doan, N., Enstrom, A.M., Maxwell, J. and Liu, R. (2003) Synthesis and screening of 'one-bead one-compound' combinatorial peptide libraries. *Methods in Enzymology* 369, 298–322.

Maeji, N.J., Bray, A.M., and Geysen, H.M. (1990) Multi-pin peptide synthesis strategy for T cell determinant analysis. *Journal of Immunological Methods* 134, 23–33.

Mattheakis, L.C., Bhatt, R.R. and Dower, W.J. (1994) An in vitro polysome display system for identifying ligands from very large peptide libraries. *Proceedings of the National Academy of Sciences of the United States of America* 91, 9022–9026.

Merrifield, R.B. (1963) Solid phase peptide synthesis. I. The synthesis of a tetrapeptide. *Journal of the American Chemical Society* 85, 2149–2154.

Mowery, B.P., Lee, S.E., Kissounko, D.A., Epand, R.F., Epand, R.M., Weisblum, B., Stahl, S.S., *et al.* (2007) Mimicry of antimicrobial host-defense peptides by random copolymers. *Journal of the American Chemical Society* 129, 15474–15476.

Moy, T.I., Conery, A.L., Larkins-Ford, J., Wu, G., Mazitschek, R., *et al.* (2009) High-throughput screen for novel antimicrobials using a whole animal infection model. *ACS Chemical Biology* 4, 527–533.

Needels, M.C., Jones, D.G., Tate, E.H., Heinkel, G.L., Kochersperger, L.M., *et al.* (1994) Generation and screening of an oligonucleotide-encoded synthetic peptide library. *Proceedings of the National Academy of Sciences of the United States of America* 90, 10700–10704.

Nguyen, L.T., Haney, E.F. and Vogel H.J. (2011) The expanding scope of antimicrobial peptide structures and their modes of action. *Trends in Biotechnology* 29, 464–472.

Rathinakumar, R. and Wimley, W.C. (2010) High-throughput discovery of broad-spectrum peptide antibiotics. *FASEB Journal* 24, 3232–3238.

Rathinakumar, R. and Wimley, W.C. (2008) Biomolecular engineering by combinatorial design and high-throughput screening: small, soluble peptides that permeabilize membranes. *Journal of the American Chemical Society* 130, 9849–9858.

Rathinakumar, R., Walkenhorst, W.F. and Wimley, W.C. (2009) Broad-spectrum antimicrobial peptides by rational combinatorial design and high-throughput screening: the importance of interfacial activity. *Journal of the American Chemical Society* 131, 7609–7617.

Rausch, J.M. and Wimley, W.C. (2001) A high-throughput screen for identifying transmembrane pore-forming peptides. *Analytical Biochemistry* 293, 258–263.

Rausch, J.M., Marks, J.R. and Wimley, W.C. (2005) Rational combinatorial design of pore-forming beta-sheet peptides. *Proceedings of the National Academy of Sciences of the United States of America* 102, 10511–10515.

Rausch, J.M., Marks, J.R., Rathinakumar, R. and Wimley, W.C. (2007) Beta-sheet pore-forming peptides selected from a rational combinatorial library: mechanism of pore formation in lipid vesicles and activity in biological membranes. *Biochemistry* 46, 12124–12139.

Saido-Sakanaka, H., Ishibashi ,J., Sagisaka, A., Momotani, E. and Tamakawa, M. (1999) Synthesis and characterization of bactericidal oligopeptides designed on the basis of an insect anti-bacterial peptide. *Biochemical Journal* 338, 29–33.

Steiner, H., Hultmark, D., Engstrom, A., Bennich, H. and Boman, H.G. (1981) Sequence and specificity of two antibacterial proteins involved in insect immunity. *Nature* 292, 246–248.

Valerio, R.M., Bray, A.M. and Maeji, N.J. (1994) Multiple peptide synthesis on acid-labile handle derivatized polyethylene supports. *International Journal of Peptide and Protein Research* 44, 158–165.

Wenschuh, H., Volkmer-Engert, R., Schmidt, M., Schulz, M., Schneider-Mergener, J. and Reineke U. (2000) Coherent membrane supports for parallel microsynthesis and screening of bioactive peptides. *Biopolymers* 55, 188–206.

White, S.H., Wimley, W.C. and Selsted, M.E. (1995) Structure, function, and membrane integration of defensins. *Current Opinion in Structural Biology* 5, 521–527.

Wiedman, G., Fuselier, T., He, J., Searson, P.C., Hristova, K. and Wimley, W.C. (2014) Highly efficient macromolecule-sized poration of lipid bilayers by a synthetically evolved peptide. *Journal of the American Chemical Society* 136, 4724–4731.

Wiegand, I., Hilpert, K. and Hancock, R.E. (2008) Agar and broth dilution methods to determine the minimal inhibitory concentration (MIC) of antimicrobial substances. *Nature Protocols* 3, 163–175.

Wimley, W.C. (2010) Describing the mechanism of antimicrobial peptide action with the interfacial activity model. *ACS Chemical Biology* 5, 905–917.

Winkler, D.F.H., Andresen, H. and Hilpert, K. (2011) SPOT synthesis as a tool to study protein-protein interactions. *Methods in Molecular Biology* 723, 105–127.

Xie, Q., Matsunaga, S., Wen, Z., Niimi, S., Kumano, M., Sakakibara, Y. and Machida, S. (2006) *In vitro* system for high-throughput screening of random peptide libraries for antimicrobial peptides that recognize bacterial membranes. *Journal of Peptide Science* 12, 643–652.

6 Prediction and Design of Antimicrobial Peptides: Methods and Applications to Genomes and Proteomes

Guangshun Wang*

*Department of Pathology and Microbiology, College of Medicine,
University of Nebraska Medical Center, Omaha, NE 68198-6495, USA*

Abstract

The growing antibiotic resistance issue requires the search for novel antimicrobial agents. Antimicrobial peptides (AMPs) are potent innate defence molecules that constitute useful templates for antimicrobial design. The establishment of databases facilitates the development of computer algorithms for peptide prediction. Most of the predictions are made based on the mature peptide sequences. These methods range from the simple rule-based to the more sophisticated machine learning. A shortcoming of these methods is that they all depend on the completeness of the representative templates used to train the programs. There are also, however, other methods that make predictions based on the conserved genes outside of the AMP gene box. The applications of these prediction methods to genomes and proteomes followed by experimental validation further accelerate the pace of peptide discovery. A combined use of genomic and proteomic approaches allows a more complete mapping of potential AMPs in a single organism. This chapter also discusses the major approaches for peptide design, including library screening, sequence shuffling, hybridization and *de novo* design. Database filtering technology has been developed and can be enhanced to design peptides with desired activity, structure and pharmaceutical parameters.

The classic method for discovering natural antimicrobial peptides (AMPs) is to isolate them from natural sources chromatographically. This important method played an essential role in shaping our current view on AMPs in terms of biological source, amino acid sequence, 3D structure and antimicrobial activity (Chapter 1). Because such identification is demanding and costly, there is a strong desire to discover AMPs by different approaches: computer-based prediction and design. The prediction of AMPs commenced in the 1990s. In 1995, the only human cathelicidin in the human genome was discovered based on sequence alignment of the unknown with the known conserved pre-peptide domain (Agerberth *et al.*, 1995). Similarly, Schutte *et al.* (2002) reported the identification of dozens of human defensins. In 2004, defensins were also predicted from the chicken (Lynn *et al.*, 2004). In the same year, the γ-core motif was also discovered and used to identify

---

* Corresponding author e-mail: gwang@unmc.edu

potential new candidates (Yount and Yeaman, 2004). More efficient genomic and proteomic methods were also developed and applied to peptide identification (Coquet *et al.*, 2016; Li *et al.*, 2007; Yang *et al.*, 2012). These methods involve the use of the conserved features in the AMPs.

An automatic computer-aided prediction requires the development of algorithms for pattern recognition and training data sets that enable the program to distinguish the positive from the negative. Around 1997, Tossi and colleagues decided to register AMP information into the antimicrobial sequence database (Tossi and Sandri, 2002). A significant advance in database development was made during 2003–2004 (Brahmachary *et al.*, 2004; Wang and Wang, 2004; Whitmore and Wallace, 2004). In particular, the antimicrobial peptide database (APD) became more popular (Wang and Wang, 2004), especially after its expansion during 2007–2009 (Wang *et al.*, 2009). This database is convenient to use and has a powerful search engine. Since then, 15 additional databases have been constructed

with varying scopes (Table 6.1). These databases can be accessed via the links of the APD (http://aps.unmc.edu/AP/links.php) and a comparison of them has been discussed (Wang, 2015a). According to the APD3, over 2700 natural AMPs have been discovered and characterized (Wang *et al.*, 2016). A careful registration of AMP information into databases laid the foundation for developing AMP prediction methods. The APD first programmed an interface for rule-based peptide predictions (Wang and Wang, 2004). This database has stimulated the development of a variety of peptide prediction and design approaches. This chapter first summarizes peptide prediction and design strategies before featuring genomic and proteomic predictions of AMPs in both prokaryotic and eukaryotic life domains.

6.1 Antimicrobial Peptide Prediction

The prediction of AMPs is a non-trivial problem due to diversity in sequence,

Table 6.1. Online accessible databases dedicated to antimicrobial peptides.[a]

Year	Database	Website	Content
2004	Peptaibols	http://www.cryst.bbk.ac.uk/peptaibol/home.shtml	Fungal AMPs
2004	APD	http://aps.unmc.edu/AP/	AMPs
2004	DAMPD	http://apps.sanbi.ac.za/dampd/	AMPs
2006	Cybase	http://www.cybase.org.au	Cyclic polypeptides
2007	BACTIBASE	http://bactibase.pfba-lab-tun.org/main.php	Bacteriocins
2007	Defensins	http://defensins.bii.a-star.edu.sg/	Defensins
2009	PhytAMP	http://phytamp.pfba-lab-tun.org/main.php	Plant AMPs
2010	CAMP	http://www.bicnirrh.res.in/antimicrobial	AMPs + predicted
2012	YADAMP	http://yadamp.unisa.it/	Helical AMPs
2012	DADP	http://split4.pmfst.hr/dadp/	Frog AMPs
2012	THIOBASE	http://db-mml.sjtu.edu.cn/THIOBASE/	Thiopeptides
2012	EnzyBase[b]	http://biotechlab.fudan.edu.cn/database/EnzyBase/home.php	Lytic enzymes
2013	LAMP[b]	http://biotechlab.fudan.edu.cn/database/lamp/	AMPs with links
2014	MilkAMP	http://milkampdb.org/home.php	Milk peptides
2014	DBAASP	http://dbaasp.org/home.xhtml	AMPs + synthetic
2015	BaAMPs	http://www.baamps.it/	Antibiofilms
2016	DRAMP	http://dramp.cpu-bioinfor.org/	AMPs + patent
2016	ANTISTAPHYBASE[b]	https://www.antistaphybase.com/	Anti-Staph AMPs

[a]Taken from the APD website http://aps.unmc.edu/AP (Accessed November 2016). [b]These databases currently not available (accessed August 2017).

structure and function. The similarity between the trained peptides (known to have antimicrobial activity) and the unknown sequences constitutes the basis for prediction. To train the computer program, a set of negative sequences is also generated based on the assumption that these sequences do not possess antimicrobial activity. The AMP prediction methods fall into five categories depending on the type of information used in the computer programs (Table 6.2). The first method is the most common and involves only the amino acid sequence information of mature peptides (i.e. AMPs). The second method utilizes the highly conserved amino acid sequences of propeptides of AMPs. The third method uses both propeptides and mature peptides. The fourth method makes predictions on the basis of the homologous sequences of post-translational modification enzymes or AMP transporters. Lastly, bacteriocins are identified by considering the genetic information related to the AMP expression, processing, transport and self-immunity. These methods are described in the following five sections.

6.1.1 Prediction based on mature peptides

Peptide sequence motifs

By examining disulfide-containing AMPs such as defensins, Yeaman and colleagues identified a well-conserved 'GXC' sequence motif (Yount and Yeaman, 2004). This motif is common in defensins, ranging from plants, bacteria and fungi to animals. In the 3D structures of the peptides, this sequence motif forms a 'γ-core'. Applications of this signature model led to the discovery of previously unidentified AMPs such as brazzein (see Chapter 1) and charybdotoxin that are active against bacteria and *Candida albicans*. Structural motif-based prediction has also been performed at the gene level. Based on the conserved six-cysteine motif in β-defensins and by combining the HMMER and BLAST analysis tools, Schutte *et al.* (2002) mapped 28 new human and 43 new mouse β-defensin genes in five syntenic chromosomal regions. HMMER (http://hmmer.org/) is a bioinformatics tool based on hidden Markov models (HMM). These genes were missed in previous annotations of human and mouse genomes. Future studies will elucidate when, where and why particular defensins are expressed or suppressed.

Database parameter-based prediction

The prediction protocol in the APD has been updated. It now makes prediction based on the peptide parameter space defined in the APD (Wang, 2015b). Thus, the program will calculate peptide parameters for the input sequence, including peptide length, charge, hydrophobic residues content and amino acid composition. If the calculated properties of an input sequence fall within the parameter space defined in the APD database, the program will classify the sequence into one of the three possible AMP classes (β-sheet, amino acid rich, or α-helix). Subsequently, the prediction interface performs sequence alignment to

Table 6.2. Classification of methods for prediction of antimicrobial peptides.

Prediction method	Mature peptide	Propeptide	Modification enzymes	Peptide transporter	Other modules
I	Y				
II		Y			
III	Y	Y			
IVa			Y		
IVb				Y	
IVc			Y	Y	Y
V	Y		Y		

identify AMPs most similar to the input sequence (Wang and Wang, 2004). Future programming will also consider distinct amino acid signatures. See the amino acid content of AMPs from bacteria (BacP), plants (PlaP), and animals (AmpP) in Table 6.3. If the properties of the peptide are outside the defined parameter ranges in the database, it will be rejected.

Machine-learning methods

Various machine-learning methods have been programmed to predict AMPs (Table 6.4). Neural networks handle information in a way similar to the human brain. Artificial neural networks (ANN) are a powerful machine-learning tool, which are insensitive to noise and correlated inputs. ANN can be trained using carefully registered known AMP data and perform predictions based on the extracted rules. The support vector machine (SVM) approach includes a set of related supervised learning methods used for classification and regression. In conjugation with peptide terminal sequence analysis, Lata *et al.* (2007) reported an accuracy of 88% for ANN and 92% for the SVM method. By including new peptide entries and source information annotated in the APD2, the overall prediction accuracy reached 98.95% (Lata *et al.*, 2010). Some other machine-learning algorithms have also been programmed in the CAMP (Waghu *et al.*, 2016). Interestingly, a better machine-learning prediction using conditional random fields (CRF) was achieved using the core antimicrobial sequences (Chang *et al.*, 2015). Interestingly, the abundant amino acids found in these core sequences

Table 6.3. Amino acid properties useful for AMP prediction and design.

AA[a]	AA[b]	Residue mass	BacP (%)[c]	PlaP (%)[d]	AmpP (%)[e]	AAOF[f]	PV[g]	AASI[h]
I	Ile	113.16	6.16	4.19	7.86	**0.810**	**0.198**	1.97
V	Val	99.13	6.63	4.42	6.87	**0.769**	**0.200**	2.37
L	Leu	113.16	6.14	3.33	**14.5**	**0.877**	0.246	1.74
F	Phe	147.18	3.03	2.92	4.77	0.685	0.246	1.53
C	Cys	103.14	5.63	**16.6**	4.01	0.550	**0.165**	1.73
M	Met	131.20	1.52	0.69	1.51	0.288	0.265	**2.50**
A	Ala	71.08	**10.23**	4.11	**10.82**	**0.777**	0.307	1.89
W	Trp	186.21	3.35	1.44	0.62	0.352	**0.172**	2.00
Y	Tyr	163.18	3.28	3.63	0.44	0.386	**0.185**	2.01
G	Gly	57.05	**13.55**	**11.27**	12.13	**0.911**	0.265	**2.67**
P	Pro	97.12	3.07	5.71	3.01	0.602	0.327	0.22
T	Thr	101.11	6.71	6.26	3.9	0.634	0.242	2.18
S	Ser	87.08	7.8	7.58	5.61	**0.768**	0.281	2.14
Q	Gln	128.13	2.36	2.68	1.46	0.408	0.248	**3.05**
N	Asn	114.10	5.51	5.17	3.09	0.611	0.240	2.33
E	Glu	129.12	2.06	3.71	1.71	0.460	0.449	**3.14**
D	Asp	115.09	2.18	2.51	2.18	0.450	0.479	**3.13**
H	His	137.14	1.75	1.69	1.08	0.365	0.202	**3.00**
K	Lys	128.17	6.56	6.31	**12.87**	**0.860**	**0.111**	2.28
R	Arg	156.19	2.4	5.68	1.48	0.547	**0.106**	1.91

[a]Amino acid in the single-letter code. [b]Amino acid in the three-letter code. [c,d,e]Amino acid percentage calculated from 269 bacterial AMPs (BacP), 332 plant AMPs (PlaP), and 1017 amphibian AMPs (AmpP), respectively (Wang *et al.*, 2016). [f]Amino acid occurrence frequency (AAOF) in the 2722 AMPs in the APD3. For instance, 2114 AMP contains A, the occurrence frequency is 2114/2722 = 0.777 (Wang G., unpublished). [g]Bactericidal propensity value (PV) (Torrent *et al.*, 2009). [h]Amino acid selectivity index (Juretić *et al.*, 2009). Some outstanding values are in bold.

corresponded well to the findings obtained from the APD (Wang and Wang, 2004; Wang *et al.*, 2016).

For a more quantitative structure–activity relationship (QSAR) evaluation, a clean activity data set for AMPs is required. In this context,'clean' means that the antimicrobial activity data should be obtained under the same conditions (e.g. same lab, bacterial assay method, strain, plate reading method and data processing). Some laboratories have compiled or generated such an activity data set for a large number of AMPs against the same target bacterial strain. These data sets are then utilized to train the program to predict the activity of new candidate sequences (Cherkasov *et al.*, 2009; Juretić *et al.*, 2009). The establishment of the method for rapid synthesis of small peptides in laboratories laid a solid foundation for designing new peptides and testing their efficacies (Merrifield *et al.*, 1995).

AMPs are known to possess multiple functions. The iAMP-2L program is a two level multiple label classifier for identification of AMPs. The program first predicts, based on the sequence information alone, whether the peptide is antimicrobial (success rate 86%) (Xiao *et al.*, 2013). If antimicrobial properties are predicted, iAMP-2L will then predict whether the input sequence possesses other functions such as anticancer, antifungal and antiviral (66% success rate) based on the annotations in the APD2 database (Wang *et al.*, 2009).

Bacteria frequently live together as communities (i.e. biofilms), which are more challenging to treat than planktonic bacteria. Importantly, AMPs can also have anti-biofilm activity, ranging from inhibition of bacterial surface attachment and growth to disruption of preformed biofilms. A prediction tool has been programmed for antibiofilm peptides (Sharma *et al.*, 2016) based on a small number of antibiofilm peptides selected from BaAMPs, a database for biofilm active peptides (Di Luca *et al.*, 2015).

6.1.2 Prediction based on highly conserved propeptide sequences

Since the discovery of the first cathelicidin peptide in 1988, over 100 such peptides have been identified (Chapter 2). The main strategy (Table 6.2) is derived from the

Table 6.4. Select websites for prediction of antimicrobial peptides.[a]

Resource	Website	Algorithms	Scope
APD	http://aps.unmc.edu/AP/prediction/prediction_main.php	Peptide parameter space	AMPs
AntiBP[b]	http://www.imtech.res.in/raghava/antibp2/	SVM, QM, or ANN	AMPs
CAMP	http://www.camp.bicnirrh.res.in/predict/	SVM, RF, ANN, DA	AMPs
iAMP-2L	http://www.jci-bioinfo.cn/iAMP-2L	Two layer prediction	AMPs with multiple functions
AMPA	http://tcoffee.crg.cat/apps/ampa/do	AA propensity index	Protein sequence scanning
CyPred	http://biomine.cs.vcu.edu/servers/CyPred/	Peptide features (e.g., composition, motifs, structure, charge)	Cyclic peptides
AMPer[b]	http://marray.cmdr.ubc.ca/cgi-bin/amp.pl	Peptide sequence clustering	AMPs
BAGLE	http://bagel.molgenrug.nl/	HMM for peptides, and genomic context	bacteriocins
BOA	https://github.com/idoerg/BOA	Genomic context	Bacteriocins
AntiSMASH	http://antismash.secondarymetabolites.org	Genomic context	Synthetic gene clusters
dPABBs	http://ab-openlab.csir.res.in/abp/antibiofilm	Machine learning	Anti-biofilm peptides

[a]Based on the APD website (http://aps.unmc.edu/AP/links.php). [b]These databases currently not available (accessed August 2017).

observation that the amino acid sequences of the propeptides (the cathelin domains) are highly conserved, while those of the antimicrobial regions are more variable (Zanetti, 2005). In analogy to swine cathelicidin PR-39, human cathelicidin was predicted as FALL-39, a 39 amino acid peptide (Agerberth *et al.*, 1995). This predicted form only slightly differs from the two isolated forms: 37-residue LL-37 isolated from human neutrophils and 38-residue ALL-38 from the reproductive system (Sørenson *et al.* 2001; 2003). Such analyses reveal that humans and mice have only one cathelicidin gene, whereas horses, cattle, sheep, goats and pigs have multiple copies (Zanetti, 2005).

The use of this strategy is not limited to cathelicidins. For instance, the precursors of ranid antimicrobial peptides also possess a common and highly conserved proregion, usually acidic and terminated at a typical processing signal LysArg. This finding was utilized as a basis for identifying peptides at a large scale in amphibians (Li *et al.*, 2007; Yang *et al.*, 2012). However, not all the sequences predicted in this manner are antimicrobial. Future studies will determine whether these peptides are expressed for other functions or work together to be antimicrobial.

6.1.3 Prediction based on both propeptides and mature peptides

In the AMPer prediction model, Fjell *et al.* (2007) considered both propeptide sequences and mature peptides (Method III in Table 6.2). This may be a direct outcome from the use of the AMSDb data set, which contains both mature and propeptides (Tossi and Sandri, 2002). The basic idea is to classify the peptides in the database into multiple groups (or clusters) and then calculate their property profiles as a basis for subsequent prediction. The authors identified 146 clusters for mature peptides and 40 clusters for propeptides (186 clusters in total). The mutual overlap between the matched pairs should be greater than 90%. In this manner, they identified an additional

229 mature peptides from the 230,133 peptides collected in the Swiss-Prot database. Most of these peptides could be associated with known activity data in the literature. This tool achieved a high prediction accuracy of 99%. However, it is not clear how many more clusters can be found based on the most recent collection of naturally occurring AMPs (Wang *et al.*, 2016), and whether there is any room to make the prediction even better.

6.1.4 Prediction based on the processing enzymes or transporters

It has been illustrated that sequence similarities among polypeptide modification enzymes such as LanM are useful in identifying novel lantibiotics. Because this approach does not utilize polypeptide information of either AMPs or their precursors, it can be regarded as a fourth method (Method IVa in Table 6.2). Both haloduracin and lichenicidin were identified using this approach (McClerren *et al.*, 2006; Begley *et al.*, 2009). O'Sullivan *et al.* (2011) identified 124 LanM homologues from genomesequenced microbes and 11 additional such genes from metagenomics data sets, further expanding the reservoir for lantibiotics.

Other gene elements in the biosynthetic machinery can also be used. Using homologous sequences of a conserved lantibiotic transporter LanT, Singh and Sareen (2014) identified 54 bacterial strains containing LanT homologues (Method IVb in Table 6.2). A further analysis of 24 clusters led to the identification of two LanM genes in 8 clusters and a single LanM gene in 13 clusters. Thus, 87% of predictions might also have been identified based on a search of homologous LanM genes. Thus, these approaches complement each other.

Recently Morton *et al.* (2015) further advanced this type of prediction by utilizing more conserved genes in the cluster that encodes various proteins required for the modification, transport, and self-immunity of bacteriocins. This protocol is called Bactericin Operon and gene block Associator

(BOA) (Table 6.2, method IVc). This program included seven known bacteriocin-associated gene blocks, including circular peptide AS-48, microcin J25, nisin A, streptolysin S, salivaricin A, and thiocillin (thiopeptides). Of note is that the transporter gene block is most widely present in such clusters. BOA does not depend on the less conserved bacteriocin portion for prediction, and so in principle, it enables the identification of new bacterial AMPs with structure and sequence distinct from the existing bacteriocins. In total, the authors predicted bacteriocin gene blocks for 2773 genomes. If verified, this prediction will dramatically increase the total number of known bacteriocins (272 in APD3, Wang *et al.*, 2016; 228 in BACTIBASE2, Hammami *et al.*, 2010). A database BactPepDB has been established to house predicted bacteriocins (<80 aa) (Rey *et al.*, 2014).

6.1.5 Genomic context-based prediction

A possible reason for missing AMPs during gene annotations is the small size of their open reading frames (ORFs). BAGEL (BActeriocin GEnome mining tooL) is a program for detecting bacteriocins in bacterial genomes (De Jong *et al.*, 2006). To improve the detection of the small ORFs for bacteriocins, this program includes a few published prediction tools, such as Glimmer/RBSfinder, Zcurve and GeneMark. In addition, the program also considers the existence of gene clusters that encode proteins for processing, modification, transport, regulation and/or immunity of bacteriocins. Finally, the program compares the candidate with those in the knowledge-based bacteriocin database. Because this approach is of integrated nature and differs from all other methods discussed above, it can be named 'genomic context-based prediction' (Method V in Table 6.2). Recently, the program has been further advanced to version 3 (van Heel *et al.*, 2013). The major new feature is that the program is less dependent on ORF predictions by using DNA nucleotide sequences as input. In addition, BAGEL3

has extended the prediction to other gene clusters with or without antimicrobial activity. Both BOA and BAGEL are gene context-based prediction methods. The main difference is that BOA does not consider the peptide portion.

There are other developments on the same lines. For example, Weber *et al.* (2015) developed antiSMASH (version 3), a more general program for identification of synthetic gene clusters for *anti*biotics as well as *Secondary Metabolites*. In particular, ClusterFinder was integrated to improve the detection capability for gene clusters. This program should also be useful to locate new bacteriocins (Table 6.4).

6.1.6 Applications to genomes and proteomes

Identification of potential AMPs from eukaryotic genomes

Data mining for novel AMPs has also been applied to sequenced eukaryotic genomes. Lynn *et al.* (2004) identified nine novel AMPs from chicken by homology searching of clustered expressed sequences tags (ESTs) using BLAST and the more sensitive hidden Markov model. Amaral *et al.* (2012) searched potential AMPs from the transcriptome of a pathogenic fungus *Paracoccidioides brasiliensis* and the human genome. Based on peptide length, total charge surface, and hydrophobic moment, they identified ~100 potential peptides. Four peptide candidates were synthesized and P1 and P2 showed weak antifungal activities (MIC 80–130 μM). Yan *et al.* (2013) used a refined procedure (i.e. QSAR) to screen one million protein fragments from the human genome. They obtained four candidates with slightly better antibacterial activity (MIC 10–60 μg/ml). These peptides may add to the known repository of human AMPs (Wang, 2014). Kim *et al.* (2016) predicted 86 potential AMPs based on a *de novo* analysis of the American cockroach transcriptome (*Periplaneta americana*). Of the 21 tested, 11 candidates showed strong activity against yeast and bacteria. Likewise, the same group discovered 10 active peptides from 17 selected transcripts of the centipede *Scolopendra subspinipes mutilans* (Yoo *et al.*, 2014). It is proposed that possible plant disulfide-bonded peptides are underpredicted (Silverstein *et al.*, 2007). However, whether they are antimicrobial remain to be established. Slavokhotova *et al.* (2015) were able to predict almost all known plant AMP families (Table 1.3, Chapter 1) in the transcriptome of a single plant species using programs developed in-house, leading to a total of 166 predicted AMPs.

Identification of potential AMPs from proteomes

Similarly, one can also identify potential AMPs by a proteome approach. The basis for this is that most AMPs are released from proteins through enzyme cleavage. Torrent *et al.* (2009) developed a theoretical method to spot active regions in proteins based on the antimicrobial activity data obtained for bactenecin 2A. A bactericidal propensity index (PV value) was calculated for each amino acid (Table 6.3). The PV values for residues Arg, Lys, Cys, Trp, Tyr and Ile are smaller than 0.2 and are favoured in short AMPs such as a 12-mer bactenecin 2A (sequence RLARIVVIRVAR-NH$_2$). A potentially active region should have a low PC value on average. This method achieved a prediction accuracy of 85%. This tool may be used to scan all the protein sequences. By training machine learning algorithms, Mooney *et al.* (2013) developed a more general tool PeptideLocator for predicting bioactive peptides from proteins, including antimicrobial peptides, cytokines, hormones, toxins, venoms and growth factors.

Brand *et al.* (2012) used the software Kamal to filter potential AMPs from the proteome of plant soybean *Glycine max*. Two peptides were found to have *in vitro* antibacterial activity against the plant pathogen *X. axonopodis pv. Glycines*. In addition, plants transformed with a vector encoding the identified peptide showed resistance to Asian rust. Using machine-learning algorithms, a large-scale scanning of 33,877 proteins of 2112 plant species led to 15,174,905 predicted AMPs (5 to 100 amino acids) in the C-PAmP database. On average, 448 are predicted from each protein and 7185 AMPs are predicted for each species (Niarchou *et al.*, 2013). These are the highest predictions made to date and provide an example for overprediction.

While the above protocols handle linear sequences, CyPred predicts whether a given polypeptide is cyclic (i.e. a peptide bond between the termini). The authors identified ~3500 putative cyclic proteins from the 642 fully sequenced proteomes from bacteria, archaea and eukaryotes (Kedarisetti *et al.*, 2014).

It can be more effective to predict potential peptides at both genetic and protein levels. Hellinger *et al.* (2015) combined transcriptome and proteome mining to identify 164 unique cyclotides from a single plant *Viola tricolor*. Among them, 108 were identified from the genome, 127 from mass signals deconvolution, and 82 were found by tandem mass spectrometry (MS/MS). The common peptides discovered by any two methods varied from 17 to 54 and only 11 peptides were detected by all three methods. This study enriched our view on cyclotides. It suggested that the number of cyclotides per *Viola* species could be higher than previously estimated (10 by Simonsen *et al.* 2005 and 53 by Zhang *et al.*, 2015). This remarkable achievement laid the foundation for complete deciphering of the mechanism of cyclotide biosynthesis. Future development of this technology may lead to a much better understanding of the relationships between cyclotide expression, plant disease and crop yield.

6.2 Database-aided Peptide Design and Improvement

6.2.1 Anti-HIV and anti-MRSA peptide screening

Database screening

Because effective human immunodeficiency virus (HIV) vaccines are not yet available, topical microbicides that prevent the sexual transmission of HIV-1 are urgently needed (Turpin, 2002; Buckheit *et al.*, 2010). Naturally occurring AMPs also show inhibitory activities against HIV. Examples are insect melittin and cecropins, amphibian AMPs, mammalian cathelicidins, defensins and plant cyclotides (Wachinger *et al.*, 1998; Jenssen *et al.*, 2006; Ireland *et al.*, 2008; Lehrer and Wu, 2012; Wang, 2012; VanCompernolle *et al.*, 2015).

Because less than 5% of the AMPs in the APD are known to be HIV inhibitory, we hypothesize that a large number of AMPs with a variety of sequences in our database (Wang *et al.*, 2009) contain useful templates for developing novel agents that prevent HIV transmission. To test the hypothesis, we have recently conducted a peptide screen against HIV type 1 (HIV-1). In total, 30 natural peptides were selected from the APD by considering peptide length, charge, cysteine content, toxicity to mammalian cells and uniqueness of the candidate sequences (Wang *et al.*, 2010). The well accepted and highly standardized cytopathic effects (CPE) inhibition assay in CEM-SS cells was utilized to evaluate efficacy and toxicity of candidate peptides. The therapeutic index (TI) is defined as the ratio of TC_{50}/EC_{50}, where EC_{50} is the concentration for 50% inhibition of viral replication and TC_{50} is the concentration for 50%

reduction in cell viability. We found that 11 peptides displayed an EC_{50} less than 10 μM. The top four most potent anti-HIV peptides are ascaphin-8, DASamP1, DASamP5 and ponericin L2 (EC_{50} 0.63–1.4 μM).

Surprisingly, the total deaths from methicillin-resistant *Staphylococcus aureus* (MRSA) are now comparable to those from HIV-1. To identify potent anti-MRSA peptides, we also evaluated antibacterial activity of these 30 peptides against *S. aureus* USA300. The four most active peptides are Ascaphin-8, DASamP1, Lycotoxin I and Piscidin 1 (MIC 3.1 μM) (Menousek *et al.*, 2012). Thus, the most potent four anti-MRSA peptides are overlapping but not identical to anti-HIV AMPs (Wang, 2013).

Human cathelicidin LL-37 is HIV-1 inhibitory (Bergman *et al.*, 2007). Since this peptide is relatively long, it is useful to identify the major HIV-1 inhibitory regions of LL-37 (Wang *et al.*, 2008). While FK-13 is the smallest anti-HIV region, GI-20 possesses the highest TI (Table 6.5). Likewise, BMAP-18, which corresponds to the N-terminal 18-resiudes of BMAP-27, is found to have a TI value greater than 20. A recent study found similar TI for select amphibian peptides (VanCompernolle *et al.*, 2015).

While KR-12 is the smallest antibacterial peptide of human LL-37 (Wang, 2008), it lost activity against HIV-1. Also,

Table 6.5. Select HIV-1 inhibitory peptides identified from the APD.[a]

Name	Peptide sequence	EC_{50} (μM)	TC_{50} (μM)	TI
KR-12	KRIVQRIKDFLR-NH$_2$	>63.5	>63.5	–
FK-13	FKRIVQRIKDFLR-NH$_2$	3.4	10.4	3.1
Retro-FK13	RLFDKIRQVIRKF-NH$_2$	>58.1	33.7	–
GF-17	GFKRIVQRIKDFLRNLV-NH$_2$	0.98	8.9	9.1
GF-17d1	GFKRIVQRIKDFLRNLV-NH$_2$	>47.5	22.7	–
GF-17d2	GFKRIVQRIKDFLRNLV-NH$_2$	>47.5	>47.5	–
GI-20	GIKEFKRIVQRIKDFLRNLV-NH$_2$	1.08	22.7	21
BMAP-18	GRFKRFRKKFKKLFKKIS	0.35	8.45	24.1
GLK-19	GLKKLLGKLLKKLGKLLLK	>47.5	25.1	–
GLR-19	GLRRLLGRLLRRLGRLLLR	4.4	25.7	5.8
DRS S9	GLRSKIWLWVLLMIWQESNKFKKM	31.6	>32.9	–
DRS S9r3	GLRSRIWLWVLLMIWQFSNRFKRM	1.25	>32.1	>25.7

[a]Adapted from Wang *et al.* (2008; 2010).

incorporation of one or two D-amino acids into GF-17 kept its antibacterial activity but not anti-HIV property (Table 6.5). These results underscore different length and structural requirements for designing antibacterial and anti-HIV peptides. One important reason for this could be the difference in molecular targets: membranes in the case of bacteria (Wang *et al.*, 2012), but reverse transcriptase in the case of HIV-1 (Wong *et al.*, 2011).

Database-aided enhancement of anti-HIV activity

A database analysis reveals that the average Lys and Arg contents of AMPs vary in different activity groups. Antiviral peptides in the APD possess the highest Arg content (Wang, 2010). Indeed, we succeeded in converting HIV-1 inactive peptide GLK-19 to a HIV-1 inhibitory peptide GLR-19 (Table 6.5) after substituting the Lys residues with Arg. Similarly, while frog DRS S9 showed a poor HIV-inhibitory activity, an arginine mutant (DRS S9r3) displayed a high TI of ~26 (Table 6.5) (Wang *et al.*, 2010). Chen *et al.* (2012) also found an increase in potency by increasing the arginine number in the scorpion peptide BmKn2. These examples suggest that the increase in arginine is a useful strategy for enhancing the anti-HIV efficacy of peptides.

6.2.2 Sequence shuffling and the combinatorial library approach

Sequence reversal influences the activity of AMPs. Merrifield *et al.* (1995) found that the hybrid peptide became less antimicrobial after sequence reversal. The LL-37-derived core antimicrobial peptide (FK-13) is active against both *Escherichia coli* and HIV. After sequence reversal, retro-FK13 retained its bactericidal activity against *E. coli* (Li *et al.*, 2006b), but lost its HIV inhibitory activity (Table 6.5). These examples indicate that the sequence order of AMPs determines their activity spectrum. Sequence reversal, however, is only a special case of sequence shuffling or

rearrangement, since the latter can produce numerous new sequences with a constant amino acid composition.

To evaluate the effect of sequence shuffling on anti-HIV-1 activity, we created some new peptides based on an aurein 1.2 analogue, where Phe13 of aurein 1.2 was mutated to Trp13 (sequence: GLFDIIKKI-AESW). The peptides were generated by rearranging the 13 amino acid residues of aurein1.2F13W based on the known helical AMP models. Among the eight peptides synthesized, two displayed reduced TIs, three showed little variation, and two showed improved TIs. Hence, sequence shuffling provides a useful approach for generating better HIV inhibitory peptides (Wang *et al.*, 2010).

A more general approach is to construct a combinatorial library (Chapter 5), where the amino acid residues at all or selected positions of a peptide can be varied and optimized. For example, Monroc *et al.* (2006b) demonstrated that the TIs of cyclic peptides against plant pathogenic bacteria are improved using a combinatorial library approach.

6.2.3 The hybrid approach and grammar-based peptide design

A classic approach for generating new templates is the hybrid method where parts of amino acid sequences from two or more AMPs with desired properties are merged to produce new peptides. Merrifield *et al.* (1995) synthesized various peptide hybrids based on a cecropin and a melittin to help elucidate the structure–activity relationship of AMPs. Their studies uncovered the modular nature of AMPs. This useful approach is still employed today to optimize the desired properties of the designer peptides (Wei *et al.*, 2016). A large-scale hybrid version is described below.

Loose *et al.* (2006) have derived a linguistic model based on the original 525 natural AMPs collected in the original APD (Wang and Wang, 2004). In the linguistic model, natural peptide sequences are treated as sentences and the amino acids are regarded as words. From the 525 AMPs, the authors identified 684 regular grammars with the aid of the Teiresias pattern discovery tool. These 'grammars' are in essence the simple rules that define the AMP 'language'. Each 'grammar' consists of a string of ten amino acids. The authors generated a library of synthetic peptides with 20 amino acids each by combining two grammars (or building blocks) in each case. To find new candidates, the authors selected a subset of peptides that are dissimilar to natural templates. Using this approach, they identified D28 and D51 that showed antibacterial activity against both Gram-positive and Gram-negative bacteria. Although it is difficult to predict the success rate of this approach, the 'grammar' approach is likely to generate new hybrid AMPs not yet found in nature. With the increase in natural AMPs in the APD (Wang *et al.*, 2016), more 'building blocks' may be identified to generate many more new AMPs.

6.2.4 *De novo* and database-aided peptide design

In the reductionist method, few amino acids were utilized in peptide design: two for helical peptides and five for β-sheet proteins (Villain *et al.*, 2000). A prototype helix design only involved two amino acids (Lys and Leu), which represent positively charged and hydrophobic components, respectively, required to form an amphipathic model. Such peptides are referred to as LK peptides. Among a series of peptides constructed, 14- or 15-residue peptides in the amphipathic helix pattern were found to be most active against bacteria (Blondelle and Houghten, 1992). Shorter peptides are inactive and longer peptides tend to be haemolytic. Wang *et al.* (2009) found that a 12-residue LK-peptide was inactive. Kang *et al.* (2008) were able to obtain a highly active LK-peptide with merely 11 residues only after including an excellent membrane anchor Trp (Chapter 10). These results agree with our observation that the shortest

helical peptides are of 10–12 residues (Wang *et al.*, 2005; Wang, 2008; Wang *et al.*, 2008). Consistent with this, Monroc *et al.* (2006a) revealed that the linear form of *de novo* designed peptides of 4–10 residues displayed no antimicrobial activity. However, cyclization enhanced the hydrophobicity of the peptides and rendered them antibacterial. Indeed, small cyclic AMPs exist in nature. An investigation of the APD revealed that the shortest cyclic peptides contain six residues. These bacterial circular peptides, such as baceridin, also contain D-amino acids to facilitate the formation of a circular structure (Niggemann *et al.*, 2014).

Wang *et al.* (2009) developed a database approach for peptide design. Amino acids such as Gly, Leu and Lys are frequently occurring in amphibian AMPs (AmpP >10% in Table 6.3). This finding sheds light on the biological significance of the earlier choices of Leu and Lys for *de novo* peptide design above. Using these three residues, Wang designed a GLK peptide. When commonly occurring motifs are chosen, the likelihood of the peptide to be antimicrobial increases. In addition, the motifs are assembled by following the amphipathic pattern. GLK-19 (Table 6.5) is active against *E. coli* K12 (Wang *et al.*, 2009). This idea has been advanced by developing a database filtering technology (Mishra and Wang, 2012). This approach involves two stages: (i) identification of peptide templates with desired activity (antibacterial, antiviral, antioxidant, etc); (ii) derivation of sequence and structural parameters from the templates for peptide design. Because *S. aureus* is a common pathogen for skin infections in the United States, we aimed to design anti-MRSA peptides. Thus, peptides active against Gram-positive bacteria are utilized as templates for deriving critical peptide parameters (e.g., length, charge and structure) by following the most probable principle in each step. Interestingly, DFTamP1, the first anti-MRSA peptide designed based on the database filtering technology, consists of more hydrophobic amino acids (65%) and few positively charged amino acids (one Lys only). DFTamP1 is highly potent in killing MRSA (MIC 3.1 μM) by targeting membranes, but is not active against Gram-negative bacteria. We refer to this database approach as *ab initio* design since it differs from other *de novo* approaches. We further prove that this database-derived design concept can be applied to the synthesis of small molecule mimics. In our mimics, each molecular component is regarded as an equivalent of one amino acid. A new class of synthetic bis-indole diimidazolines resembles DFTamP1 in terms of both composition and activity spectrum. Further details of this study can be found in our recent article (Dong *et al.*, 2017).

The significance of the abundance of glycines in natural AMPs (11.7% in Table 6.3) is yet to be illustrated. Juretić *et al.* (2009) arrived at an amino acid selectivity index (AASI) based on TIs and amino acid occurrences in peptides (Table 6.3). One of the peptides, adepanin-1 (sequence GIGKH-VGKALKGLKGLLKGLGES), showed the highest TI. Interestingly, this peptide is also rich in glycine, leucine and lysine residues (74%). The seven glycine residues in adepanin-1 could be important for peptide selectivity because LK-peptides, consisting only of Leu and Lys, are known to be cytotoxic to human cells (Braunstein *et al.*, 2004). To further test this idea, Gellman and colleagues inserted a glycine-like unit into binary polymers, leading to more cell selective peptide mimics (Chakraborty *et al.*, 2014).

One can conceive two different amphipathic models in constructing the defence peptides. In both the 'grammar'-based and '*ab initio*' approaches, the amphipathic segregation is along the peptide backbone, which is the classic amphipathic helix model (Tossi *et al.*, 2000). Our choice of the classic model in designing DFTamP1 is based on the fact that there are no AMPs in the APD that are composed of a string of four leucines (LLLL) or more. Duval *et al.* (2009) designed a two-segment amphipathic structure (i.e. hydrophobic aa in one segment and hydrophilic aa in another segment). The peptide was found to be active against both Gram-positive and Gram-negative bacteria, indicating the feasibility of an alternative peptide design as previously demonstrated by Glukhov *et al.* (2008). It is of outstanding interest to note that dermaseptin S9 (DRS S9 in Table 6.5), a natural AMP isolated from the South American hylid frog (Lequin *et al.*, 2006), possesses such an amphipathic structure. Hence, there are examples in nature for both amphipathic models, although the classic amphipathic model dominates.

6.3 Computational Design of Novel AMPs

Recently, advances have also been made in computer-aided screening and identification of short peptide antibiotics (Cherkasov *et al.*, 2009). This was made feasible as a consequence of technical innovations in large-scale peptide synthesis using the SPOT arrays as well as activity evaluation based on luminescence assays (Cherkasov *et al.*, 2009). It is necessary to build biased peptide libraries that are rich in residues Trp, Arg and Lys and do not contain Glu, Asp, Cys and Pro, because active candidates are absent in 200 randomly synthesized peptides.

The goal of this computational approach is to correlate peptide sequence with activity by various models. For example, Cherkasov *et al.* (2009) used the ANN approach and QSAR with 44 descriptors. These descriptors are usually calculated based on the peptide sequence, with each term dealing with one aspect of the peptide property that is proportional to peptide antimicrobial activity. While hydrophobicity is a measure of peptide tendency to stay away from water, hydrophilicity is a measure of peptide tendency to be in water. The term amphipathicity refers to a peptide with both hydrophobic and hydrophilic elements and tend to be segregated when bound to membranes. There are also other descriptors for charge and peptide length. It is clear that such descriptors are not unique and can be overlapping. Further refinements of these descriptors may improve the prediction accuracy of such computational approaches.

This program was trained using 1400 peptides with measured activities against *Pseudomonas aeruginosa*. Remarkably, the protocol successfully predicted 94% of the most active candidates from the 100,000 peptides *in silico*. This program is useful for predicting short linear AMPs with activity against *P. aeruginosa*. It is interesting to note that those highly active 9-mer peptides are rich in tryptophans, whereas those poorly active candidates contain only one Trp or none. This approach nicely illustrates the feasibility of discovery of novel AMPs from a computer-generated virtual library.

6.4 Prediction Based on Biophysical Approaches

Understanding the mechanism of the peptide action via biophysical studies may provide a basis for AMP prediction, especially when the sequence motif is considered. It may be reasonable to predict that many Pro-rich AMPs, if not all, target ribosomes (see Chapters 9 and 10). However, many AMPs are proposed to target bacterial membranes. Before a general sequence motif is identified, one can also use biophysical measurements to make predictions. Deciding which measurement to use for AMP prediction is not always trivial. In fact, there may not be a single peptide parameter that can predict or design an AMP reliably. Wang *et al.* (2005) found that the peptide antibacterial activity did not correlate with helicity, charge, amphipathicity, the size of the hydrophobic surface, or transfer free energy of the peptide. A membrane-perturbation potential proposed based on the 3D structure of peptides appears to explain peptide activity. In this model, a broad hydrophobic surface bordered by basic charges is most effective in perturbing bacterial membranes. Besides the peptide, bacterial membranes may also be utilized to predict peptide activity (Papo and Shai, 2003). For instance, the peptide most potent to *E. coli* also

generated an isotropic peak in the ^{31}P NMR spectrum, implying micellization (Wang *et al.*, 2005). Epand found lipid clustering only in bacterial membranes with a combination of anionic and zwitterionic lipids, but not in bacterial membranes that are largely anionic (Epand *et al.*, 2008). Nevertheless, these experiment-based approaches are much slower than computational approaches because they require a combined use of both peptide samples and instruments to obtain the desired measurements. As a consequence, such biophysical predictions are not as popular as sequence-based *in silico* predictions.

6.5 Concluding Remarks

The antibiotic resistance issue has made it necessary to search for alternative antimicrobial agents. The interest in AMPs persists mainly because of the potency of these compounds (Jenssen *et al.*, 2006; Wang *et al.*, 2015; Zasloff, 2002). During the past decade, a variety of prediction programs have been developed and refined. Although the extent of information used in each program varies (Table 6.2), the majority of predictions are based on mining the information encoded in the amino acid sequence of mature AMPs. A well-registered data set in the APD (Wang *et al.*, 2016) has facilitated the programming of such predictors (Lata *et al.*, 2010; Xiao *et al.*, 2013). However, our knowledge on the known AMP templates is not yet complete, leading to insufficient training of the current prediction programs. That is why the existing machine-learning programs could fail when a newly discovered and unique AMP sequence is tested (Wang *et al.*, 2015). A significant advance has been made in predicting bacteriocins (Morton *et al.*, 2015). Such an elegant gene context-based approach is built on the conserved genes outside the variable AMP box. We anticipate that a large number of naturally occurring bacteriocins will be characterized in the near future. Similar efforts will be rapidly expanded into other genomes to accelerate the pace of AMP discovery.

These methods, together with continued isolation from natural sources, will further expand the repository of natural AMPs for prediction and design.

A useful peptide template against a particular pathogen can be identified by screening natural or artificial peptide libraries. Sequence truncation, mutation, shuffling and hybridization of naturally occurring AMPs can generate new peptides and may help improve peptide properties. While building novel peptides using minimal types of amino acids (e.g. Leu and Lys) is the classic *de novo* approach, a database filtering technology has also been demonstrated (Mishra and Wang, 2012). This general approach can be advanced to build new peptides with desired properties, structurally and pharmaceutically. With the adoption of a unified peptide classification scheme in the APD (Chapter 1), different types of templates can be chosen. The continued peptide design work will not only deepen our knowledge of antimicrobial peptides but also enrich the peptide space.

Prediction or design of a potent peptide is only the beginning of the game. There are more hurdles to overcome for therapeutic use. It is imperative to achieve an acceptable therapeutic index, production cost and bioavailability. The major strategy for reducing peptide cytotoxicity is to decrease peptide hydrophobicity (Wang, 2010). Peptide stability can be enhanced by incorporating D-amino acids or cyclization based on 3D structure (Chapter 10). Peptides may be chemically synthesized or heterologously expressed in a variety of systems (e.g., bacteria, yeasts and plants). With the advancement of biotechnology, we have reason to believe that therapeutic peptides can be produced at an affordable price. However, a large-scale production of therapeutic peptides may not always be necessary. In the future, a particular quantity of a designer medicine will be produced on demand for a specific patient (i.e. personalized medicine). Then, peptide therapeutics will prevail for its desired properties such as specificity in targeting and adjustable lifetime in human bodies.

Acknowledgements

This study is supported by the NIAID/NIH grants R01 AI105147 to GW.

Chapter editor: Amram Mor.

References

Agerberth, B., Gunne, H., Odeberg, J., Kogner, P., Boman, H.G. and Gudmundsson, G.H. (1995) FALL-39, a putative human peptide antibiotic, is cysteine-free and expressed in bone marrow and testis. *Proceedings of the National Acadamy of Sciences of the United States of America* 92, 195–199.

Amaral, A.C., Silva, O.N., Mundim, N.C., de Carvalho, M.J., Migliolo, L., *et al.* (2012) Predicting antimicrobial peptides from eukaryotic genomes: *in silico* strategies to develop antibiotics. *Peptides* 37, 301–308.

Begley, M., Cotter, P.D., Hill, C. and Ross, R.P. (2009) Identification of a novel two-peptide lantibiotic, lichenicidin, following rational genome mining for LanM proteins. *Applied and Environmental Microbiology* 75, 5451–5460.

Bergman, P., Walter-Jallow, L., Broliden, K., Agerberth, B. and Soderlund, J. (2007) The antimicrobial peptide LL-37 inhibits HIV-1 replication. *Current HIV Research* 5, 410–415.

Blondelle, S.E. and Houghten, R.A. (1992) Design of model amphipathic peptides having potent antimicrobial activities. *Biochemistry* 31, 12688–12694.

Brahmachary, M., Krishnan, S.P., Koh, J.L., Khan, A.M., Seah, S.H., *et al.* (2004) ANTIMIC: a database of antimicrobial sequences. *Nucleic Acids Research* 32 (database issue), D586–D589.

Brand, G.D., Magalhaes, M.T., Tinoco, M.L., Aragao, F.J., Nicoli, J., Kelly, S.M., *et al.* (2012) Probing protein sequences as sources for encrypted antimicrobial peptides. *PLoS One* 7, e45848.

Braunstein, A., Papo, N. and Shai, Y. (2004) *In vitro* activity and potency of an intravenously injected antimicrobial peptide and its DL amino acid analog in mice infected with bacteria. *Antimicrobial Agents and Chemotherapy* 48, 3127–3129.

Buckheit, R.W., Jr, Watson, K.M., Morrow, K.M. and Ham, A.S. (2010) Development of topical micro-bicides to prevent the sexual transmission of HIV. *Antiviral Research* 85, 142–158.

Chakraborty, S., Liu, R., Hayouka, Z., Chen, X., Ehrhardt, J., *et al.* (2014) Ternary nylon-3 copolymers as host-defense peptide mimics: beyond hydrophobic and cationic subunits. *Journal of the American Chemical Society* 136, 14530–14535.

Chang, K.Y., Lin, T.P., Shih, L.Y. and Wang, C.K. (2015) Analysis and prediction of the critical regions of antimicrobial peptides based on conditional random fields. *PLoS One* 10, e0119490.

Chen, Y., Cao, L., Zhong, M., Zhang, Y., Han, C., *et al.* (2012) Anti-HIV-1 activity of a new scorpion venom peptide derivative Kn2-7. *PLoS One* 7, e34947.

Cherkasov, A., Hilpert, K., Jenssen, H., Fjell, C.D., Waldbrook, M., *et al.* (2009) Use of artificial intelligence in the design of small peptide antibiotics effective against a broad spectrum of highly antibiotic-resistant superbugs. *ACS Chemical Biology* 4, 65–74.

Coquet, L., Kolodziejek, J., Jouenne, T., Nowotny, N., King, J.D. and Conlon, J.M. (2016) Peptidomic analysis of the extensive array of host-defense peptides in skin secretions of the dodecaploid frog *Xenopus ruwenzoriensis* (Pipidae). *Comparative Biochemistry and Physiology. Part D, Genomics & Proteomics* 19, 18–24.

De Jong, A., van Hijum, S.A., Bijlsma, J.J., Kok, J. and Kuipers, O.P. (2006) BAGEL: a web-based bacteriocin genome mining tool. *Nucleic Acids Research* 34 (web server issue), W273–W279.

Di Luca, M., Maccari, G., Maisetta, G. and Batoni, G. (2015) BaAMPs: the database of biofilm-active antimicrobial peptides. *Biofouling* 31, 193–199.

Dong, Y., Lushnikova, T., Golla, R.M., Wang, X. and Wang, G. (2017) Small molecule mimics of DFTamP1: a database designed anti-Staphylococcal peptide. *Bioorganic & Medicinal Chemistry*, in press.

Duval, E., Zatylny, C., Laurencin, M., Baudy-Floc'h, M. and Henry, J. (2009) KKKKPLFGLFFGLF: a cationic peptide designed to exert antibacterial activity. *Peptides* 30, 1608–1612.

Epand, R.M., Rotem, S., Mor, A., Berno, B. and Epand, R.F. (2008) Bacterial membranes as predictors of antimicrobial potency. *Journal of the American Chemical Society* 130, 14346–14352.

Fjell, C.D., Hancock, R.E. and Cherkasov, A. (2007) AMPer: a database and an automated discovery tool for antimicrobial peptides. *Bioinformatics* 23, 1148–1155.

Glukhov, E., Burrows, L.L. and Deber, C.M. (2008) Membrane interactions of designed cationic antimicrobial peptides: the two thresholds. *Biopolymers* 89, 360–371.

Hammami, R., Zouhir, A., Le Lay, C., Ben Hamida, J. and Fliss, I. (2010) BACTIBASE second release: a database and tool platform for bacteriocin characterization. *BMC Microbiology* 10, 22.

Hellinger, R., Koehbach, J., Soltis, D.E., Carpenter, E.J., Wong, G.K. and Gruber, C.W. (2015) Peptidomics of circular cysteine-rich plant peptides: analysis of the diversity of cyclotides from *Viola tricolor* by transcriptome and proteome mining. *Journal of Proteome Research* 14, 4851–6482.

Ireland, D.C., Wang, C.K., Wilson, J.A., Gustafson, K.R. and Craik, D.J. (2008) Cyclotides as natural anti-HIV agents. *Biopolymers* 90, 51–60.

Jenssen, H., Hamill, P. and Hancock, R.E. (2006) Peptide antimicrobial agents. *Clinical Microbiology Reviews* 19, 491–511.

Juretić, D., Vukicević, D., Ilić, N., Antcheva, N. and Tossi, A. (2009) Computational design of highly selective antimicrobial peptides. *The Journal of Chemical Information and Modeling* 49, 2873–2882.

Kang, S.J., Won, H.S., Choi, W.S. and Lee, B.J. (2008) De novo generation of antimicrobial LK peptides with a single tryptophan at the critical amphipathic interface. *Journal of Peptide Science* 15, 583–588.

Kedarisetti, P., Mizianty, M.J., Kaas, Q., Craik, D.J. and Kurgan, L. (2014) Prediction and characterization of cyclic proteins from sequences in three domains of life. *Biochimica et Biophysica Acta* 1844, 181–190.

Kim, I.W., Lee, J.H., Subramaniyam, S., Yun, E.Y., Kim, I., Park, J. and Hwang, J.S. (2016) *De novo* transcriptome analysis and detection of antimicrobial peptides of the American cockroach *Periplaneta americana* (Linnaeus). *PLoS One* 11, e0155304.

Lata, S., Sharma, B.K. and Raghava, G.P.S. (2007) Analysis and prediction of antibacterial peptides. *BMC Bioinformatics* 8, 263.

Lata, S., Mishra, N.K. and Raghava, G.P.S. (2010) AntiBP2: improved version of antibacterial peptide prediction. BMC *Bioinformatics* 11, S19.

Lehrer, R.I. and Wu, L. (2012) α-defensins in human innate immunity. *Immunology Reviews* 245, 84–112.

Lequin, O., Ladram, A., Chabbert, L., Bruston, F., Convert, O., *et al.* (2006) Dermaseptin S9: an alpha-helical antimicrobial peptide with a hydrophobic core and cationic termini. *Biochemistry* 45, 468–480.

Li, J., Xu, X., Xu, C., Zhou, W., Zhang, K., *et al.* (2007) Anti-infection peptidomics of amphibian skin. *Molecular & Cellular Proteomics* 6, 882–894.

Li, X., Li, Y., Han, H., Miller, D.W. and Wang, G. (2006a) Solution structures of human LL-37 fragments and NMR-based identification of a minimal membrane-targeting antimicrobial and anticancer region. *Journal of the American Chemical Society* 128, 5776–5785.

Li. X., Li, Y., Peterkofsky, A. and Wang, G. (2006b) NMR studies of aurein 1.2 analogs. *Biochimica et Biophysica Acta* 1758, 1203–1214.

Loose, C., Jensen, K., Rigoutsos, I. and Stephanopoulos, G. (2006) A linguistic model for the rational design of antimicrobial peptides. *Nature* 443, 867–869.

Lynn, D.J., Higgs, R., Gaines, S., Tierney, J., James, T., Lloyd, A.T., Fares, M.A., Mulcahy, G. and O'Farrelly, C. (2004) Bioinformatic discovery and initial characterisation of nine novel antimicrobial peptide genes in the chicken. *Immunogenetics* 56, 170–177.

McClerren, A.L., Cooper, L.E., Quan, C., Thomas, P.M., Kelleher, N.L. and van der Donk, W.A. (2006) Discovery and *in vitro* biosynthesis of haloduracin: a two-component lantibiotic. *Proceedings of the National Academy of Sciences of the United States of America* 103, 17243–17248.

Menousek, J., Mishra, B., Hanke, M.L., Heim, C.E., Kielian, T. and Wang, G. (2012) Database screening and *in vivo* efficacy of antimicrobial peptides against methicillin-resistant *Staphylococcus aureus* USA300. *International Journal of Antimicrobial Agents* 39, 402–406.

Merrifield, R.B., Juvvadi, P., Andreu, D., Ubach, J., Boman, A. and Boman, H.G. (1995) Retro and retroenantio analogs of cecropin-melittin hybrids. *Proceedings of the National Academy of Sciences of the United States of America* 92, 3449–3453.

Mishra, B. and Wang, G. (2012) *Ab initio* design of potent anti-MRSA peptides based on database filtering technology. *Journal of the American Chemical Society* 134, 12426–12429.

Monroc, S., Badosa, E., Feliu, L., Planas, M., Montesinos, E. and Bardají, E. (2006a) *De novo* designed cyclic cationic peptides as inhibitors of plant pathogenic bacteria. *Peptides* 27, 2567–2574.

Monroc, S., Badosa, E., Besalu, E., Planas, M., Bardají, E., Montesinos, E. and Feliu, L. (2006b) Improvement of cyclic decapeptides against plant pathogenic bacteria using a combinatorial chemistry approach. *Peptides* 27, 2575–2584.

Mooney, C., Haslam, N.J., Holton, T.A., Pollastri, G. and Shields, D.C. (2013) PeptideLocator: prediction of bioactive peptides in protein sequences. *Bioinformatics* 29, 1120–1126.

Morton, J.T., Freed, S.D., Lee, S.W. and Friedberg, I. (2015) A large scale prediction of bacteriocin gene blocks suggests a wide functional spectrum for bacteriocins. *BMC Bioinformatics* 16, 381.

Niarchou, A., Alexandridou, A., Athanasiadis, E. and Spyrou, G. (2013) C-PAmP: large scale analysis and database construction containing high scoring computationally predicted antimicrobial peptides for 44 of all the available plant species. *PLoS One* 8, e79728.

Niggemann, J., Bozko, P., Bruns, N., Wodtke, A., Gieseler, M.T., *et al.* (2014) Baceridin, a cyclic hexapeptide from an Epiphytic Bacillus strain, inhibits the proteasome. *ChemBioChem* 15, 1021–1029.

O'Sullivan, O., Begley, M., Ross, R.P., Cotter, P.D. and Hill, C. (2011) Further identification of novel lantibiotic operons using LanM-based genome mining. *Probiotics and Antimicrobial Proteins* 3, 27–40.

Papo, N. and Shai, Y. (2003) Can we predict biological activity of antimicrobial peptides from their interactions with model phospholipid membranes? *Peptides* 24, 1693–1703.

Rey, J., Deschavanne, P. and Tuffery, P. (2014) BactPepDB: a database of predicted peptides from an exhaustive survey of complete prokaryote genomes. *Database* 2014, pii:bau106.

Schutte, B.C., Mitros, J.P., Bartlett, J.A., Walters, J.D., Jia, H.P., *et al.* (2002) Discovery of five conserved β-defensin gene clusters using computational search strategy. *Proceedings of the National Academy of Sciences of the United States of America* 99, 2129–2133.

Sharma, A., Gupta, P., Kumar, R. and Bhardwaj, A. (2016) dPABBs: a novel *in silico* approach for predicting and designing anti-biofilm peptides. *Scientific Reports* 6, 21839.

Silverstein, K.A., Moskal, W.A. Jr, Wu, H.C., Underwood, B.A., Graham, M.A., Town, C.D. and VandenBosch, K.A. (2007) Small cysteine-rich peptides resembling antimicrobial peptides have been under-predicted in plants. *Plant Journal* 51, 262–280.

Simonsen, S.M., Sando, L., Ireland, D.C., Colgrave, M.L., Bharathi, R., Goransson, U. and Craik, D.J. (2005) A continent of plant defense peptide diversity: cyclotides in Australian *Hybanthus* (Violaceae). *The Plant Cell* 17, 3176–3189.

Singh, M. and Sareen, D. (2014) Novel LanT associated lantibiotic clusters identified by genome database mining. *PLoS One* 9, e91352.

Slavokhotova, A.A., Shelenkov, A.A. and Odintsova, T.I. (2015) Prediction of *Leymus arenarius* (L.) antimicrobial peptides based on de novo transcriptome assembly. *Plant Molecular Biology* 89, 203–214.

Sørensen, O.E., Follin, P., Johnsen, A.J., Calafat, J., Tjabringa, G.S., Hiemstra, P.S. and Borregaard, N. (2001) Human cathelicidin, hCAP-18, is processed to the antimicrobial peptide LL-37 by extracellular cleavage with proteinase 3. *Blood* 97, 3951–3959.

Sørensen, O.E., Gram, L., Johnsen, A.J., Andersson, E., Bangsboll, S., Tjabringa, G.S., Hiemstra, P.S., Malm, J., Egesten, A. and Borregaard, N. (2003) Processing of seminal plasma hCAP-18 to ALL-38 by gastricsin: a novel mechanism of generating antimicrobial peptides in vagina. *Journal of Biological Chemistry* 278, 28540–28546.

Torrent, M., Nogués, V.M. and Boix, E. (2009) A theoretical approach to spot active regions in antimicrobial proteins. *BMC Bioinformatics* 10, 373.

Tossi, A. and Sandri, L. (2002) Molecular diversity in gene-coded, cationic antimicrobial polypeptides. *Current Pharmaceutical Design* 8, 743–761.

Tossi, A., Sandri, L. and Giangaspero, A. (2000) Amphipathic, alpha-helical antimicrobial peptides. *Biopolymers* 55, 4–30.

Turpin, J.A. (2002) Considerations and development of topical microbicides to inhibit the sexual transmission of HIV. *Expert Opinion on Investigational Drugs* 11, 1077–1097.

van Heel, A.J., de Jong, A., Montalbán-López, M., Kok, J. and Kuipers, O.P. (2013) BAGEL3: automated identification of genes encoding bacteriocins and (non-)bactericidal posttranslationally modified peptides. *Nucleic Acids Research* 41 (web server issue), W448–W453.

VanCompernolle, S.E., Smith, P.B., Bowie, J.H., Tyler, M.J., Unutmaz, D. and Rollins-Smith, L.A. (2015) Inhibition of HIV infection by caerin 1 antimicrobial peptides. *Peptides* 71, 296–303.

Villain, M., Jackson, P.L., Manion, M.K., Dong, W.J., Su, Z., *et al.* (2000) *De novo* design of peptides targeted to the EF hands of calmodulin. *Journal of Biological Chemistry* 275, 2676–2685.

Wachinger, M., Klenschmidt, A. Winder, D., *et al.* (1998) Antimicrobial peptides melittin and cecropin inhibit replication of human immunodeficiency virus 1 by suppressing viral gene expression. *Journal of General Virology* 79, 731–740.

Waghu, F.H., Barai, R.S., Gurung, P. and Idicula-Thomas, S. (2016) CAMPR3: a database on sequences, structures and signatures of antimicrobial peptides. *Nucleic Acids Research* 44, D1094–D1097.

Wang, G. (2008) Structures of human host defense cathelicidin LL-37 and its smallest antimicrobial peptide KR-12 in lipid micelles. *Journal of Biological Chemistry* 283, 32637–32643.

Wang, G. (ed.) (2010) *Antimicrobial Peptides: Discovery, Design and Novel Therapeutic Strategies.* CABI, Oxford, UK.

Wang, G. (2012) Natural antimicrobial peptides as promising anti-HIV candidates. *Current Topics in Peptide & Protein Research* 13, 93–110.

Wang, G. (2013) Database-guided discovery of potent peptides to combat HIV-1 or superbugs. *Pharmaceuticals* 6, 728–758.

Wang, G. (2014) Human antimicrobial peptides and proteins. *Pharmaceuticals* 7, 545–594.

Wang, G. (2015a) Database resources dedicated to antimicrobial peptides. In: Chen, C.-Y., Yan, X. and Jackson, C.R. (eds) *Antimicrobial Resistance and Food Safety: Methods and Techniques.* Academic Press, Boston, MA, pp. 365–384.

Wang, G. (2015b) Improved methods for classification, prediction, and design of antimicrobial peptides. *Methods in Molecular Biology* 1268, 43–66.

Wang, G., Li, Y. and Li, X. (2005) Correlation of three-dimensional structures with the antibacterial activity of a group of peptides designed based on a non-toxic bacterial membrane anchor. *Journal of Biological Chemistry* 280, 5803–5811.

Wang, G., Watson, K.M. and Buckheit, R.W., Jr. (2008) Anti-human immunodeficiency virus type 1 activities of antimicrobial peptides derived from human and bovine cathelicidins. *Antimicrobial Agents and Chemotherapy* 52, 3438–3440.

Wang, G., Li, X. and Wang, Z. (2009) APD2: the updated antimicrobial peptide database and its application in peptide design. *Nucleic Acids Research* 37, D933–D937.

Wang, G., Watson, K.M., Peterkofsky, A. and Buckheit, R.W., Jr. (2010) Identification of novel human immunodeficiency virus type 1 inhibitory peptides based on the antimicrobial peptide database. *Antimicrobial Agents and Chemotherapy* 54, 1343–1346.

Wang, G., Epand, R.F., Mishra, B., Lushnikova, T., Thomas, V.C., Bayles, K.W. and Epand, R. (2012) Decoding the functional roles of cationic side chains of the major antimicrobial region of human cathelicidin LL-37. *Antimicrobial Agents and Chemotherapy* 56, 845–856.

Wang, G., Mishra, B., Lau, K., Lushnikova, T., Golla, R. and Wang, X. (2015) Antimicrobial peptides in 2014. *Pharmaceuticals* 8, 123–150.

Wang, G., Li, X. and Wang, Z. (2016) APD3: the antimicrobial peptide database as a tool for research and education. *Nucleic Acids Research* 44, D1087–1093.

Wang, Z. and Wang, G. (2004) APD: the antimicrobial peptide database. *Nucleic Acids Research* 32, D590–D592.

Weber, T., Blin, K., Duddela, S., Krug, D., Kim, H.U., *et al.* (2015) antiSMASH 3.0-a comprehensive resource for the genome mining of biosynthetic gene clusters. *Nucleic Acids Research* 43, W237–W243.

Wei, X.B., Wu, R.J., Si, D.Y., Liao, X.D., Zhang, L.L. and Zhang, R.J. (2016) Novel hybrid peptide cecropin A (1-8)-LL37 (17-30) with potential antibacterial activity. *International Journal of Molecular Sciences* 17, pii: E983.

Whitmore, L. and Wallace, B.A. (2004) The peptaibol database: a database for sequences and structures of naturally occurring peptaibols. *Nucleic Acids Research* 32, D593–D594.

Wong, J.H., Legowska, A., Rolka, K., Ng, T.B., Hui, M., *et al.* (2011) Effects of cathelicidin and its fragments on three key enzymes of HIV-1. *Peptides* 32, 1117–1122.

Xiao, X., Wang, P., Lin, W.Z., Jia, J.H. and Chou, K.C. (2013) iAMP-2L: a two-level multi-label classifier for identifying antimicrobial peptides and their functional types. *Anaytical Biochemistry* 436, 168–177.

Yan, L., Yan, Y., Liu, H. and Lv, Q. (2013) Stepwise identification of potent antimicrobial peptides from human genome. *Biosystems* 113, 1–8.

Yang, X., Lee, W.H. and Zhang, Y. (2012) Extremely abundant antimicrobial peptides existed in the skins of nine kinds of Chinese odorous frogs. *Journal of Proteome Research* 11, 306–319.

Yoo, W.G., Lee, J.H., Shin, Y., Shim, J.Y., Jung, M., *et al.* (2014) Antimicrobial peptides in the centipede *Scolopendra subspinipes mutilans*. *Functional and Integrative Genomics* 14, 275–283.

Yount, N.Y. and Yeaman, M.R. (2004) Multidimensional signatures in antimicrobial peptides. *Proceedings of the National Academy of Sciences of the United States of America* 101, 7363–7368.

Zanetti, M. (2005) The role of cathelicidins in the innate host defenses of mammals. *Current Issues in Molecular Biology* 7, 179–196.

Zasloff, M. (2002) Antimicrobial peptides of multicellular organisms. *Nature* 415, 389–395.

Zhang, J., Li, J., Huang, Z., Yang, B., Zhang, X., *et al.* (2015) Transcriptomic screening for cyclotides and other cysteine-rich proteins in the metallophyte *Viola baoshanensis*. *Journal of Plant Physiology* 178, 17–26.

7   Antimicrobial Peptides: Multiple Mechanisms against a Variety of Targets

Li-av Segev-Zarko[1], Maria Luisa Mangoni[2] and Yechiel Shai[1,*]

[1]Department of Biomolecular Sciences, The Weizmann Institute of Science Rehovot, 76100 Israel; [2]Department of Biochemical Sciences, La Sapienza University, Via degli Apuli, 9-00185 Rome, Italy

Abstract

Antimicrobial peptides (AMPs) are small molecules that are produced by all life forms ranging from prokaryotes to humans. They are an essential part of the innate immune system and serve as the first line of defence mainly against pathogenic bacteria. Although Gram-negative and Gram-positive bacteria are the most studied targets for AMPs, other targets have been investigated, such as fungi, viruses, cancer or the prevention of undesirable inflammatory responses. There is no common specific structure, nor length that AMPs share. They exhibit different lengths, charges and secondary structures. All the above allow diversity in their mechanism of activity and it is not uncommon to find peptides that act with more than one mechanism. During the past few decades, numerous studies have been dedicated to identify new natural AMPs, sequence them and study their structure and function parallel to designing and synthesizing *de-novo* ones. Most of those peptides work as a non-specific defensive mechanism and target the bacterial cytoplasmic membrane, causing membrane disruption and cell death. However, specific targets were also found. Overall, it is believed that bacterial killing is the result of a multi-hit mechanism.

Antimicrobial peptides (AMPs) are small biopolymers that can be found in all life forms across the evolutionary spectrum ranging from prokaryotes to humans. They are an essential part of the innate immune system as a non-specific defensive mechanism, and serve as the first line of defence mainly against pathogenic bacteria (Boman, 1995; Lehrer and Ganz, 1999; Hancock and Scott, 2000). In higher organisms, AMPs are stored in phagocytes in large quantities and released when required to neutralize invading microorganisms (Rietschel *et al.*, 1996). The immediate response is crucial in order to stop the potential microbial proliferation (Boman, 1991; Boman, 1995; Hoffmann *et al.*, 1999; Lehrer and Ganz, 1999; Devine and Hancock, 2002; Hoffmann and Reichhart, 2002; Lehrer and Ganz, 2002; Zasloff, 2002). Although Gram-negative and Gram-positive bacteria are the most studied targets for AMPs, other targets have been investigated (Scott *et al.*, 2002), such as fungi, viruses (Hancock and Diamond, 2000), cancer (Gaspar *et al.*, 2013) or the prevention of undesirable inflammatory responses. Another reported activity of AMPs is that of

* Corresponding author e-mail: yechiel.shai@weizmann.ac.il

immunomodulators (McPhee *et al.*, 2005) that can stimulate the production of chemokines or enhance chemotaxis for leukocytes (Bowdish *et al.*, 2005a; Xhindoli *et al.*, 2016). There is no common specific structure or length that AMPs share. Some are linear α-helices, others adopt β-sheet structures, while AMPs with no distinct secondary structure are also found (Shai, 1999). It is common to find natural AMPs rich in specific amino acids such as His, Arg, Pro and Trp (Scocchi *et al.*, 2011), or some synthetic ones that are made up of only two amino acids (Papo *et al.*, 2002; Reddy *et al.*, 2004). All the above allow diversity in their mechanism of activity and it is not uncommon to find peptides that act with more than one mechanism (Epand *et al.*, 2016).

Multi-drug-resistant bacteria are a growing problem worldwide. Since the discovery of penicillin by Fleming (1929), the emergence of resistant pathogenic strains has grown alarmingly due to the extreme use of antibiotics. This has led to an urgent need to find new drugs for treating numerous infections.

In the search for new therapeutics, AMPs are studied as a promising strategy to fight both Gram-positive and Gram-negative pathogenic bacteria. During the past few decades, numerous studies have been dedicated to identify new natural AMPs, sequence them and study their structure and function (see Chapter 1). Most of those peptides target the bacterial cytoplasmic membrane, causing membrane disruption and cell death (Shai, 2002). However, specific targets were also found. For example, recent studies identified a peptide activity at non-lethal concentrations against inner components of bacterial cells (Guilhelmelli *et al.*, 2013; also see Chapter 9). A summary of selected mechanisms of activity discussed in this chapter are listed in Table 7.1, alongside the peptides' targets. Overall, it is believed that the actual killing of bacteria is the result of a multi-hit mechanism (Epand *et al.*, 2016).

7.1 Target Selectivity of Antimicrobial Peptides

Antimicrobial peptides can be divided into two major classes according to their functionality (i) *non cell-selective cytolytic peptides* – peptides that target both mammalian cells and microorganisms, for example melittin (Rathinakumar *et al.*, 2009) and pardaxin (Shai *et al.*, 1990); (ii) *cell-selective cytolytic peptides* – peptides that target Gram-positive and Gram-negative bacteria, fungi and viruses or only some, but are not active against mammalian cells at similar concentrations. For example magainin (Zasloff, 1987) and cecropin (Steiner *et al.*, 1981). Cell-specific peptides are either receptor-mediated or share several common features that allow them to target bacteria and fungi without causing mammalian cell damage. Receptor-mediated peptides are a small group of peptides such as nisin (Breukink and de Kruijff, 1999) and lactococcin (Diep *et al.*, 2007). They include a receptor binding domain and pore forming domain, and are active at nanomolar concentrations (Holo *et al.*, 1991). The other larger group of non-receptor mediated peptides can vary in their biophysical

Table 7.1. Various mechanisms explaining the activity of antimicrobial peptides and their cell targets.

Mechanism of activity	Target
Membrane disruption	Bacteria, fungi, virus, tumour cells
Nucleic acid synthesis	Bacteria
Biosynthesis of the cell wall	Bacteria, fungi
Gene expression and regulation	Bacteria, virus, tumour cells
Receptor binding	Bacteria, virus, tumour cells
Induction of the host immune system	Bacteria, tumour cells

properties, size (generally short with 15–50 amino acids), positive charge due to the presence of basic amino acids mainly lysine and arginine (ranging from +2 to +9) and hydrophobic (Oren and Shai, 1998; Lehrer and Ganz, 1999). Studies suggest that the extent of hydrophobicity and the distribution of the positively charged amino acids allow cell specificity against bacteria (Dathe *et al.*, 1996; Tossi *et al.*, 2000). The outer surfaces of both Gram-negative and Gram-positive bacteria are negatively charged due to the lipopolysaccharides (LPS) and lipoteichoic acid (LTA), respectively (Silhavy *et al.*, 2010). Moreover, the outer leaflets of the bacterial plasma membranes contain a high fraction of anionic phospholipids such as phosphatidylglycerol (PG). Although the outer surface of mammalian cells comprises negatively charged components such as sialic acid, the distribution of anionic phospholipids in their plasma membranes is different from that in bacteria. The outer leaflet of mammalian cells contains mainly zwitterionic phospholipids (Glukhov *et al.*, 2005). Hence, the net positive charge of AMPs allows them to favour binding to the negatively charged bacterial outer surface (Shai, 1999).

7.2 Membrane-lytic Antimicrobial Peptides

Many studies have been conducted to decipher the mechanism of membrane-lytic AMPs. Two main mechanisms of membrane disruption are illustrated in Fig. 7.1, the barrel-stave and carpet mechanisms. Most of the naturally occurring AMPs possess a distinct secondary structure when bound to a membrane, which is considered essential for their lytic activity against both Gram-negative and Gram-positive bacteria (Takahashi *et al.*, 2010). An amphipathic secondary structure of α-helix, β-sheet or both is essential for the barrel-stave model

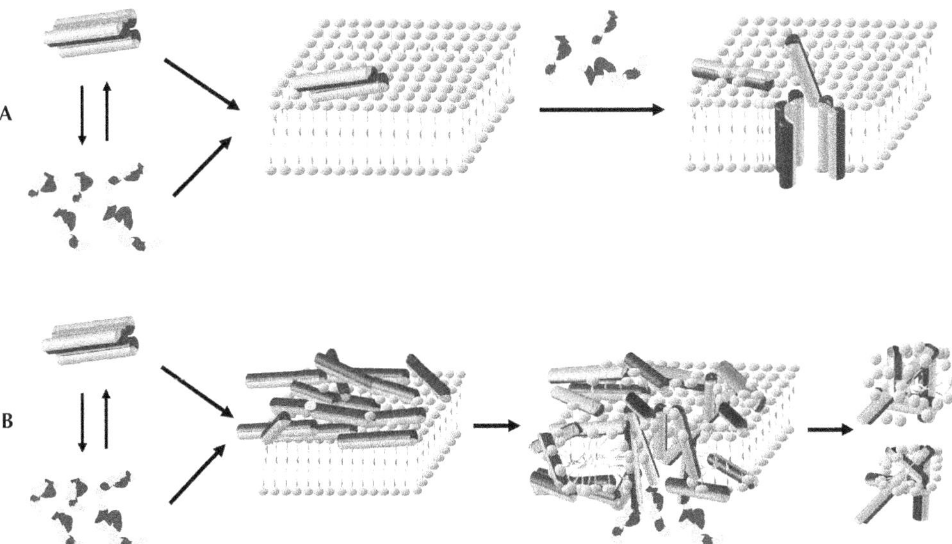

Fig. 7.1. Illustration of the barrel stave (A) and carpet (B) models of membrane lytic AMPs. (A) Peptides arrive at the bacterial membrane as monomers or oligomers. They then penetrate the lipid bilayer where they interact with each other and recruit additional peptides. Finally, they acquire a stable state and form a barrel-like pore. (B) Peptides arrive at the bacterial membrane as monomers or oligomers due to electrostatic forces. Their hydrophobic areas are facing the membrane and their hydrophilic areas are facing the solvent. When reaching a threshold concentration, the membrane is permeated, disrupting the bacterial protective phospholipids bilayer. Darker tone: hydrophobic surface; lighter tone: hydrophilic surface (Shai, 2002)

(Ehrenstein and Lecar, 1977). In this model peptides organize to form a permeation pathway. First, peptides bind to the bacterial membrane, then insert into the lipid bilayer where they interact with each other, acquire a stable state and form a barrel-like pore (Cruciani *et al.*, 1992; Rapaport and Shai, 1992; Hilchie *et al.*, 2011). Doing so, they allow ion leakage from the cytosol, thus disrupting the energy metabolism of the bacteria (Christensen *et al.*, 1988). The weakness of this model is the need for a very hydrophobic peptide to interact with the membrane core. The possible result of this is an interaction with zwitterionic membranes, resulting in non-cell selective cytolytic peptides (Shai, 2002). A second model is the 'carpet-like' mechanism. In this model, there is no need for a specific secondary structure since the peptides integrate within the membrane in a detergent-like manner. The positively charged amino acids of the peptides electrostatically interact with the negatively charged phospholipid of the bacterial membrane until a threshold concentration is reached. Then the hydrophobic residues face the hydrophobic core of the membrane, disrupting the bacterial protective phospholipids bilayer (Pouny and Shai, 1992). This allows uncontrolled transport of ions to the cytosol and cell death (Shai, 2002). Additional/alternative models include (i) 'toroidal pores' where the peptide and lipid head groups of the target membrane line together in the pore (Ludtke *et al.*, 1996; Sengupta *et al.*, 2008); (ii) 'channel aggregates' where the hydrophobic peptides aggregate in the hydrophobic core of the target membrane (Rozek *et al.*, 2000) and (iii) clustering of anionic lipids where peptides induce anionic lipid clustering against bacteria sensitive to lipid clustering agents (Wadhwani *et al.*, 2012).

7.3 Intracellular Targets of Antimicrobial Peptides

Recent evidence indicates that AMPs can promote cell damage by traversing the bacterial outer and inner membranes and interact with one or more intracellular targets such as DNA and RNA. This can interfere with proteins and cell wall synthesis (Patrzykat *et al.*, 2002; Brogden, 2005; Straus and Hancock, 2006). Some AMPs, for example buforin II and indolicidin, were shown to bind DNA and RNA and inhibit nucleic acid synthesis (Park *et al.*, 1998; del Castillo *et al.*, 2001; Nan *et al.*, 2009). Their mode of action is not fully understood but it is reasonable to assume that the positively charged amino acids of the peptides electrostatically interact with the phosphate groups of the nucleic acids (Park *et al.*, 1998; Uyterhoeven *et al.*, 2008) or other synthesized proteins (Xiong *et al.*, 2002).

All the above suggest that AMPs can target bacteria and promote cell death in one or more cooperative mechanisms (Zhang *et al.*, 2000), depending on the bacteria localization and growth phase (Yeaman and Yount, 2003).

7.4 LPS and LTA Neutralization by Antimicrobial Peptides

LPS, also termed endotoxin, is the major component of the outer membrane of Gram-negative bacteria (Ginsburg, 2002; Raetz and Whitfield, 2002; De Castro *et al.*, 2012). These negatively charged molecules consist of a lipid A, a preserved lipophilic component anchored to the outer membrane and surface-exposed polysaccharides, or oligosaccharides. The saccharide portion is diverse in length and composition among the different Gram-negative bacteria species (Alexander and Rietschel, 2001). LTA is the major constituent of the outer surface of Gram-positive bacteria. Its physiochemical properties are similar to those of LPS. It is also an anionic molecule consisting of a diacylglycerol moiety anchored in the peptidoglycan substratum. The surface-exposed, polyanionic, 1-3-linked polyglycerophosphate portion is also diverse in its subunit composition among the different Gram-positive bacteria species (Percy and Grundling, 2014).

Peptidoglycan is the main component in the outer leaflet of Gram-positive bacteria. It also appears in Gram-negative bacteria, combined with LPS but is not found in eukaryotic cells (Vollmer and Bertsche, 2008). Peptidoglycan forms a closed shell (sacculus) designed to be both strong and elastic to protect the cell membrane against antimicrobial agents, support turgor pressure and control the bacterial shape. Therefore studying its structural arrangement is crucial to understanding bacterial physiology and virulence, and to the development of new antibacterial agents. Very recently, an advanced atomic force microscopy technique (PeakForce tapping) was used to investigate peptidoglycan in live streptococcus from a net-like mega-architecture to single strands (Dover *et al.*, 2015). This structural investigation was accompanied by high-resolution mapping of cell wall mechanical properties. The data showed that the cell wall mechanics are affected by turgor pressure and peptidoglycan degradation globally, and by cell geometry and peptidoglycan arrangement locally. Since peptidoglycan in live bacteria is under stretching forces, the technique allowed the first direct visualization of single strands in their native context (Dover *et al.*, 2015). Another interesting peptidoglycan target of AMPs is lipid II. This is an important precursor of peptidoglycan synthesis (de Kruijff *et al.*, 2008; Yount and Yeaman, 2013). Binding of AMPs to proteins participating in the biosynthesis of peptidoglycan, LPS or LTA leads to cell death (Muller *et al.*, 2012; Yount and Yeaman, 2013). An example is the human β-defensin 3 which inhibits cell wall biosynthesis. Impaired biosynthesis machinery was observed when the peptide binds lipid II-rich sites of cell wall biosynthesis (Sass *et al.*, 2010).

Following treatment against bacterial infection, there is a release of LPS or LTA to the bloodstream. LPS then binds LPS-binding protein (LBP) present in the blood, which transfers it to immune cell CD14 receptor. This complex initiates intracellular signalling reactions, which mediate the production of inflammatory cytokines (Hancock and Diamond, 2000). The immune system response to LPS is mainly mediated via Toll-like receptor 4 (TLR4) but also TLR2 (Kimbrell *et al.*, 2008). LTA induces a pro-inflammatory reaction mainly in a TLR2 dependent manner but also through TLR4 (Takeuchi *et al.*, 1999). It is critical to prevent LPS and LTA-receptor binding since it hyperstimulates the immune system. Systemic inflammation may result in sepsis, develop to septic shock and lead to multiple organ failure and death. Beside their ability to kill bacteria, several AMPs were also shown to inhibit the pro-inflammatory process (Bowdish *et al.*, 2005b; Rosenfeld *et al.*, 2006; Scott and Hancock, 2000).

Several proposed mechanisms of LPS neutralization are: (i) preventing LPS–LBP interaction by direct binding to LPS (Scott *et al.*, 2000; Rosenfeld *et al.*, 2006; Rosenfeld *et al.*, 2008;); (ii) preventing LPS–TLR interaction by direct binding to the TLR signalling complex (Nagaoka *et al.*, 2001; Rosenfeld *et al.*, 2006; Rosenfeld *et al.*, 2008); (iii) inhibiting NFκB translocation into the nucleus; (iv) triggering the MAPK pathways, influencing inflammatory genes expression (Mookherjee *et al.*, 2006). Some LPS neutralizing peptides can also inhibit LTA pro-inflammatory activities. The proposed mechanisms are similar to those against LPS: (i) neutralization of LTA by high-density lipoproteins (HDL) (Grunfeld *et al.*, 1999), probably due to direct binding to the anionic LTA via electrostatic and hydrophobic interactions (David, 2001); (ii) direct interaction with TLRs which in return prevents cytokine production by macrophages (Scott *et al.*, 1999).

7.5 Antibiofilm Antimicrobial Peptides

In nature, bacteria hardly ever appear in their single cell form but in multicellular colonies also known as biofilms. Recently, studies have focused on AMPs antibiofilm activity but their mechanism of biofilm prevention and degradation is not fully understood.

Many Gram-negative and Gram-positive bacteria live as biofilms to cope with unfavourable surroundings. Biofilms start from (i) a planktonic stage, (ii) initial adhesion to surfaces (organic or inorganic), and (iii) formation of sessile micro-colonies that secrete extracellular polymeric substance (EPS) (An and Friedman, 1998). Biofilms are highly resistant to antimicrobial agents (Costerton *et al.*, 1999). Their resistance is obtained by several factors: (i) high frequency of mutation caused by horizontal gene transmission and also by oxidative stress; (ii) maintenance of a stationary-like growth due to nutrient depletion; (iii) secretion of EPS (Hoiby *et al.*, 2001; Hall-Stoodley and Stoodley, 2009). The biofilm EPS constitutes up to 90% of the biofilm dry mass and is composed of polysaccharide, DNA and protein (Wingender *et al.*, 2001; Keller and Surette, 2006). It acts as a barrier and protects embedded bacteria from desiccation, oxidizing or charged biocides, metallic cations, ultraviolet radiation and many protozoan grazers (Flemming and Wingender, 2010). It also protects bacteria from some antibiotics and host immune defences by delaying, repulsing or degrading them (by enzymes) (Mah and O'Toole, 2001). Several membrane-active AMPs, for example the human cathelicidin LL-37, histatin and nisin, are potent against biofilms. Different mechanisms of activity have been proposed (Overhage *et al.*, 2008; Chennupati *et al.*, 2009) including direct killing of sessile bacteria and prevention of bacterial attachment to polymers through modulation of adhesion-related genes, primarily those for fimbria and flagella assembly (Fogaca *et al.*, 2010; Kapoor *et al.*, 2011; Luca *et al.*, 2013). Moreover, it has been shown that a group of *de-novo* designed AMPs can act as coating agents that cover biomaterial surfaces, the bacterial surface or both, thereby reducing bacterial attachment and biofilm formation (Segev-Zarko *et al.*, 2015).

Another challenge of AMPs in the fight against biofilms is to eradicate them once they are already formed (Jorge *et al.*, 2012). The peptides need to penetrate the protective layer of the EPS and to affect bacteria in a stationary-like phase. Two possible mechanisms for reducing the total biofilm biomass are (i) by direct killing of embedded bacteria (Overhage *et al.*, 2008) or (ii) detachment of live bacteria in a yet unknown mechanism (Segev-Zarko *et al.*, 2015).

7.6 Antifungal Antimicrobial Peptides

In the past decade, the frequency of opportunistic fungal infections has increased dramatically and has become a central cause of morbidity and mortality. The growing resistance of fungi to existing drugs has generated the urgent need for finding new therapeutics for numerous infections. Since fungi and mammalian cells are both eukaryotic, it is hard to find a selective treatment that will damage the first without targeting the second. Still, there are two decisive differences between the mammalian and fungal cell surface: (i) in fungi, the plasma membrane outer leaflet is negatively charged while in most mammalian cells it is mainly zwitterionic; (ii) fungal cells contain a rigid cell wall that is quite different from the mammalian flexible glycocalyx layer (Tada *et al.*, 2013). Indeed, so far several AMPs which are active mainly on fungi but less or not at all on bacteria or mammalian cells have been found (Hoffmann and Reichhart, 2002). Examples include the bacillomycin F (Mhammedi *et al.*, 1982), histatin (Raj *et al.*, 1994) and defensins (Andreu and Rivas, 1998). Several known modes of action for antifungal peptides are: (i) direct membrane lysis (van der Weerden *et al.*, 2013); (ii) inhibition of cell wall synthesis, mainly components such as (1,3)-β-D-glucan or chitin (Bouffard *et al.*, 1994); and (iii) interaction with fungal mitochondria in a manner very similar to bacteria (Helmerhorst *et al.*, 1999).

7.7 Anticancer Antimicrobial Peptides

Cancer is defined by an uncontrolled growth and spread of abnormal cells. It is a major cause of death of millions of people worldwide (Ferlay *et al.*, 2010). Alongside the optional treatments available today such as surgery and chemotherapy that present a risk of reappearance of the disease (Harris *et al.*, 2013), the alternatives (e.g. DNA-alkylating agents, hormone agonists and antagonists, and anti-metabolites) are insufficiently selective. Therefore, they are also toxic towards healthy cells (Kalyanaraman *et al.*, 2002; Al-Benna *et al.*, 2011).

Since AMPs are small proteins that can penetrate tissue with sufficient selectivity against healthy mammalian cells, they are a good therapeutic option. Several AMPs with anticancer activity are magainins (Jacob and Zasloff, 1994), defensins (Lichtenstein *et al.*, 1986), melittin (Winder *et al.*, 1998), and others (Makovitzki *et al.*, 2009; Papo *et al.*, 2004; Papo *et al.*, 2006). The mechanism of anticancer peptides is still not fully known but several options have been suggested (Papo and Shai, 2005). One possible mechanism is cell death by membrane disruption. As opposed to the normal mammalian cell membranes, which are zwitterionic, cancerous cells are slightly negatively charged due to anionic molecules present on their membrane, such as phosphatidylserine, O-glycosylated mucins, sialylated gangliosides and heparin sulfate (Schweizer, 2009). The electrostatic interactions between the cationic peptides and the anionic cells allow targeted selectivity and membrane disruption through the 'barrel stave' or 'carpet' mechanisms (Oren and Shai, 1998; van Zoggel *et al.*, 2012). Anticancer peptides may also disrupt the mitochondrial membrane causing it to swell, release cytochrome c and ultimately cause apoptosis (Mai *et al.*, 2001).

Other possible non-membrane-lytic mechanisms are: (i) blocking receptors expressed on angiogenic endothelial cells, thus blocking angiogenesis and disturbing the formation of the vasculature that allows the tumour to prosper (Arap *et al.*, 1998; Lee *et al.*, 2011; Rosca *et al.*, 2011); (ii) blocking Toll-like receptors expressed on various solid tumours but not on normal cells in the same organs, hence preventing tumours from modifying their microenvironment, thus exposing them to the immune system cells (Sato *et al.*, 2009); (iii) interference

with necrosis or apoptosis pathways which is reflected in shrinking or swelling cells, blebbing of the membrane, chromatin compression and cytoplasmic vacuoles (Elmore, 2007; Feliu *et al.*, 2010; Wang *et al.*, 2013; Xu *et al.*, 2013); (iv) targeting hormonal receptors by mimicking them, their agonists and antagonists, affecting hormone regulated genes (Kampa *et al.*, 2011; Leuschner and Hansel, 2005); (v) induction of the host immune cells against the tumorous cells, for example recruitment and activation of dendritic or macrophage cells (Wang *et al.*, 2009); (vi) protein–protein interactions with intracellular molecules known to have a central function in malignant cells and affecting their regulation (Patra *et al.*, 2012; Rerole *et al.*, 2011).

7.8 Antiviral Antimicrobial Peptides

Most viral diseases lack an effective treatment. Together with the emergence of antiviral drug resistance and high costs of existing treatments there is a need to develop new therapeutic options. Since AMPs mode of action comprises multiple targets like membrane interactions and receptor targeting, they are considered as good candidates for antiviral treatment. The mode of action of antiviral AMPs includes targeting the virus itself or the host cells (Bahar and Ren, 2013).

AMP–virus interactions were shown to occur: (i) on the virus envelope, where AMP integration may cause membrane instability therefore blocking its ability to infect the host cells (Sitaram and Nagaraj, 1999); (ii) with the virus glycoproteins, hence preventing the virus from interacting with its target cells (Yasin *et al.*, 2004). Besides direct interaction with the virus, AMPs can also block its spread by interacting with the host cells. For example, this can occur by (i) competing with the virus on receptor binding of the host cells, hence preventing cell infection (Song *et al.*, 2001); (ii) penetrating the host cells and interacting with cytoplasmic organelles, causing changes in gene expression and blocking cell-to-cell infection (Sinha *et al.*, 2003).

7.9 Antimicrobial Peptide Modification and How It Affects the Mode of Action

7.9.1 Lipopeptides

Lipopeptides are compounds formed by conjugation of peptides to a lipid tail or other lipophilic compound (Robbel and Marahiel, 2010; Arnusch *et al.*, 2012; Meena and Kanwar, 2015). Lipopeptides were investigated as antimicrobial agents and their biophysical properties were characterized to better understand their mode of action. There are naturally occurring lipopeptides like polymyxin A (Jones, 1949) and daptomycin (Robbel and Marahiel, 2010) but also synthetic ones formed to improve the efficiency of AMPs (Makovitzki *et al.*, 2006).

It is known that hydrophobicity is a key feature of AMPs. Incorporation of acyl chains having different lengths allows us to manipulate the level of lipopeptide hydrophobicity. Increased hydrophobicity enhances lipopeptides oligomerization, and hence improves permeability into the bacterial membrane. This leads to transient leakage of ions and other cytoplasmic molecules, leading to cell death (Avrahami and Shai, 2004; Tam *et al.*, 2005; Mangoni and Shai, 2011). In some cases, lipopeptide oligomerization was shown to involve ion binding (Muraih *et al.*, 2011). Alongside membrane disruption, lipopeptides were also shown to act via other mechanisms against both multidrug-resistant bacteria and fungi (Denning, 2002; Chu-Kung *et al.*, 2004). Inhibition of fungi cell wall formation by interacting with ribosomal subunits, ATPase binding on the mitochondrial membrane and inhibition of protein synthesis were all shown to be improved in peptides conjugated to acyl chains (Bosso, 2005; Qi *et al.*, 2010; Yao *et al.*, 2012).

The drawback of increased hydrophobicity and oligomerization is reduced specificity and higher toxicity against host cells alongside reduced activity against bacterial membranes (Shai, 1999; Hancock and Diamond, 2000).

7.9.2 Modification of amino acid content

There are several strategies to modify AMPs to get better activity against a variety of pathogenic targets (Bahar and Ren, 2013; Pearson *et al.*, 2016). Reducing the content of amino acids like prolines, with low propensity to form α-helical structures, improves peptide activity (Zhang *et al.*, 1999). Another approach is adding positively charged amino acids to the sequence. It reduces AMP cytotoxicity against eukaryotic cells and improves their attraction to bacterial membranes (Nell *et al.*, 2006; Goblyos *et al.*, 2013). Including D-amino acids in AMP sequences reduces their susceptibility to protease degradation and increases their selectivity towards bacteria versus mammalian cells (Oren *et al.*, 1997; Oren *et al.*, 1999). Proteases are found in human serum but are also produced by bacteria as part of their resistance mechanism (Mah and O'Toole, 2001). Complete L- to D-amino acid substitution is known to improve peptide resistance to protease degradation (Carmona *et al.*, 2013) and reduce haemolytic activity, but usually also reduces antibacterial activity (Dean *et al.*, 2011; Otvos *et al.*, 2000).

Studies have shown that partial substitution of L- to D-amino acids forms non-haemolytic, protease-resistant peptides (Papo *et al.*, 2002). Since D-amino acids are enantiomers of their L-form, the peptide's secondary structure is changed, typically to an unstructured form. Peptide oligomerization on bacterial membranes is a crucial step in the 'carpet' mechanism discussed above. Still, high self-assembly in solution can hinder the ability of AMPs to reach the bacterial membrane. Secondary structure alternation reduces their tendency to self-assemble and allows structural flexibility (Hara *et al.*, 2001; Liu *et al.*, 2009) without affecting their antibacterial activity (Papo and Shai, 2004; Segev-Zarko *et al.*, 2015).

7.10 Conclusion

AMPs/lipopeptides differ in length, amino-acid sequence and diversity of amino-acid composition, as well as having multiple common (e.g. the phospholipid membrane) and non-common targets. All of the above allow diversity in their mechanisms of action leading to their ability to target various microorganisms. Nevertheless, it is believed that the actual killing of each microorganism is the result of a multi-hit mechanism. Importantly, AMP mechanisms of antibiofilm activity have yet to be fully understood. Further work in this area and in elucidating their biophysical features might enable us in the future to engineer peptides such that various microorganisms will not develop resistance to them, making them highly effective.

Acknowledgements

This study was supported by The Pasteur-Weizmann Foundation, Israel Science Foundation (ISF) and the German-Israel Foundation (GIF).

References

Al-Benna, S., Shai, Y., Jacobsen, F. and Steinstraesser, L. (2011) Oncolytic activities of host defense peptides. *International Journal of Molecular Sciences* 12, 8027–8051.

Alexander, C. and Rietschel, E.T. (2001) Bacterial lipopolysaccharides and innate immunity. *Journal of Endotoxin Research* 7, 167–202.

An, Y.H. and Friedman, R.J. (1998) Concise review of mechanisms of bacterial adhesion to biomaterial surfaces. *Journal of Biomedical Materials Research* 43, 338–348.

Andreu, D. and Rivas, L. (1998) Animal antimicrobial peptides: an overview. *Biopolymers* 47, 415–433.

Arap, W., Pasqualini, R. and Ruoslahti, E. (1998) Cancer treatment by targeted drug delivery to tumor vasculature in a mouse model. *Science* 279, 377–380.

Arnusch, C.J., Ulm, H., Josten, M., Shadkchan, Y. and Osherov, N., *et al.* (2012) Ultrashort peptide bioconjugates are exclusively antifungal agents and synergize with cyclodextrin and amphotericin B. *Antimicrobial Agents and Chemotherapy* 56, 1–9.

Avrahami, D. and Shai, Y. (2004) A new group of antifungal and antibacterial lipopeptides derived from non-membrane active peptides conjugated to palmitic acid. *Journal of Biological Chemistry* 279, 12277–12285.

Bahar, A.A. and Ren, D. (2013) Antimicrobial peptides. *Pharmaceuticals* 6, 1543–1575.

Boman, H.G. (1991) Antibacterial peptides: key components needed in immunity. *Cell* 65, 205–207.

Boman, H.G. (1995) Peptide antibiotics and their role in innate immunity. *Annual Review of Immunology* 13, 61–92.

Bosso, J.A. (2005) The antimicrobial armamentarium: evaluating current and future treatment options. *Pharmacotherapy* 25, 55S–62S.

Bouffard, F.A., Zambias, R.A., Dropinski, J.F., Balkovec, J.M., Hammond, M.L., *et al.* (1994) Synthesis and antifungal activity of novel cationic pneumocandin B(o) derivatives. *Journal of Medicinal Chemistry* 37, 222–225.

Bowdish, D.M., Davidson, D. J. and Hancock, R.E. (2005a) A re-evaluation of the role of host defence peptides in mammalian immunity. *Current Protein & Peptide Science* 6, 35–51.

Bowdish, D.M., Davidson, D.J., Scott, M.G. and Hancock, R.E. (2005b) Immunomodulatory activities of small host defense peptides. *Antimicrobial Agents and Chemotherapy* 49, 1727–1732.

Breukink, E. and De Kruijff, B. (1999) The lantibiotic nisin: a special case or not? *Biochimica et Biophysica Acta* 1462, 223–234.

Brogden, K.A. (2005) Antimicrobial peptides: pore formers or metabolic inhibitors in bacteria? *Nature Reviews Microbiology* 3, 238–250.

Carmona, G., Rodriguez, A., Juarez, D., Corzo, G. and Villegas, E. (2013) Improved protease stability of the antimicrobial peptide Pin2 substituted with D-amino acids. *Protein Journal* 32, 456–466.

Chennupati, S.K., Chiu, A.G., Tamashiro, E., Banks, C.A., Cohen, M. B., *et al.* (2009) Effects of an LL-37-derived antimicrobial peptide in an animal model of biofilm *Pseudomonas sinusitis*. *American Journal of Rhinology & Allergy* 23, 46–51.

Christensen, B., Fink, J., Merrifield, R.B. and Mauzerall, D. (1988) Channel-forming properties of cecropins and related model compounds incorporated into planar lipid membranes. *Proceedings of the National Academy of Sciences of the United States of America* 85, 5072–5076.

Chu-Kung, A.F., Bozzelli, K.N., Lockwood, N.A., Haseman, J.R., Mayo, K.H. and Tirrell, M.V. (2004) Promotion of peptide antimicrobial activity by fatty acid conjugation. *Bioconjugate Chemistry* 15, 530–535.

Costerton, J.W., Stewart, P.S. and Greenberg, E.P. (1999) Bacterial biofilms: a common cause of persistent infections. *Science* 284, 1318–1322.

Cruciani, R.A., Barker, J.L., Durell, S.R., Raghunathan, G., Guy, H.R., Zasloff, M. and Stanley, E.F. (1992) Magainin 2, a natural antibiotic from frog skin, forms ion channels in lipid bilayer membranes. *European Journal of Pharmacology* 226, 287–296.

Dathe, M., Schumann, M., Wieprecht, T., Winkler, A., Beyermann, M., *et al.* (1996) Peptide helicity and membrane surface charge modulate the balance of electrostatic and hydrophobic interactions with lipid bilayers and biological membranes. *Biochemistry* 35, 12612–12622.

David, S.A. (2001) Towards a rational development of anti-endotoxin agents: novel approaches to sequestration of bacterial endotoxins with small molecules. *Journal of Molecular Recognition* 14, 370–387.

De Castro, C., Holst, O., Lanzetta, R., Parrilli, M. and Molinaro, A. (2012) Bacterial lipopolysaccharides in plant and mammalian innate immunity. *Protein & Peptide Letters* 19, 1040–1044.

De Kruijff, B., Van Dam, V. and Breukink, E. (2008) Lipid II: a central component in bacterial cell wall synthesis and a target for antibiotics. *Prostaglandins, Leukotrienes and Essential Fatty Acids* 79, 117–121.

Dean, S.N., Bishop, B.M. and Van Hoek, M.L. (2011). Susceptibility of *Pseudomonas aeruginosa* biofilm to alpha-helical peptides: D-enantiomer of LL-37. *Frontiers in Microbiology* 2, 128.

Del Castillo, F.J., Del Castillo, I. and Moreno, F. (2001) Construction and characterization of mutations at codon 751 of the *Escherichia coli* gyrB gene that confer resistance to the antimicrobial peptide microcin B17 and alter the activity of DNA gyrase. *Journal of Bacteriology* 183, 2137–2140.

Denning, D.W. (2002) Echinocandins: a new class of antifungal. *Journal of Antimicrobial Chemotherapy* 49, 889–891.

Devine, D.A. and Hancock, R.E. (2002) Cationic peptides: distribution and mechanisms of resistance. *Current Pharmaceutical Design* 8, 703–714.

Diep, D.B., Skaugen, M., Salehian, Z., Holo, H. and Nes, I.F. (2007) Common mechanisms of target cell recognition and immunity for class II bacteriocins. *Proceedings of the National Academy of Sciences of the United States of America* 104, 2384–2389.

Dover, R.S., Bitler, A., Shimoni, E., Trieu-Cuot, P. and Shai, Y. (2015) Multiparametric AFM reveals turgor-responsive net-like peptidoglycan architecture in live streptococci. *Nature Communications* 6, 7193.

Ehrenstein, G. and Lecar, H. (1977) Electrically gated ionic channels in lipid bilayers. *Quarterly Reviews of Biophysics* 10, 1–34.

Elmore, S. (2007) Apoptosis: a review of programmed cell death. *Toxicological Pathology* 35, 495–516.

Epand, R.M., Walker, C., Epand, R.F. and Magarvey, N.A. (2016) Molecular mechanisms of membrane targeting antibiotics. *Biochimica et Biophysica Acta* 1858, 980–987.

Feliu, L., Oliveras, G., Cirac, A.D., Besalu, E., Roses, C., *et al.* (2010) Antimicrobial cyclic decapeptides with anticancer activity. *Peptides* 31, 2017–2026.

Ferlay, J., Shin, H.R., Bray, F., Forman, D., Mathers, C. and Parkin, D.M. (2010) Estimates of worldwide burden of cancer in 2008: GLOBOCAN 2008. *International Journal of Cancer* 127, 2893–2917.

Fleming, A.G. (1929) Responsibilities and opportunities of the private practitioner in preventive medicine. *Canadian Medical Association Journal* 20, 11–13.

Flemming, H.C. and Wingender, J. (2010) The biofilm matrix. *Nature Reviews Microbiology* 8, 623–633.

Fogaca, A.C., Zaini, P.A., Wulff, N.A., Da Silva, P.I., Fazio, M.A., *et al.* (2010) Effects of the antimicrobial peptide gomesin on the global gene expression profile: virulence and biofilm formation of *Xylella fastidiosa*. *FEMS Microbiology Letters* 306, 152–159.

Gaspar, D., Veiga, A.S. and Castanho, M.A. (2013) From antimicrobial to anticancer peptides: a review. *Frontiers in Microbiology* 4, 294.

Ginsburg, I. (2002) Role of lipoteichoic acid in infection and inflammation. *Lancet Infectious Diseases* 2, 171–179.

Glukhov, E., Stark, M., Burrows, L.L. and Deber, C.M. (2005) Basis for selectivity of cationic antimicrobial peptides for bacterial versus mammalian membranes. *Journal of Biological Chemistry* 280, 33960–33967.

Goblyos, A., Schimmel, K.J., Valentijn, A.R., Fathers, L.M., Cordfunke, R.A., *et al.* (2013) Development of a nose cream containing the synthetic antimicrobial peptide P60.4Ac for eradication of methicillin-resistant *Staphylococcus aureus* carriage. *Journal of Pharmaceutical Science* 102, 3539–3544.

Grunfeld, C., Marshall, M., Shigenaga, J.K., Moser, A.H., Tobias, P. and Feingold, K.R. (1999) Lipoproteins inhibit macrophage activation by lipoteichoic acid. *Journal of Lipid Research* 40, 245–252.

Guilhelmelli, F., Vilela, N., Albuquerque, P., Derengowski Lda, S., Silva-Pereira, I. and Kyaw, C.M. (2013) Antibiotic development challenges: the various mechanisms of action of antimicrobial peptides and of bacterial resistance. *Frontiers in Microbiology* 4, 353.

Hall-Stoodley, L. and Stoodley, P. (2009) Evolving concepts in biofilm infections. *Cellular Microbiology* 11, 1034–1043.

Hancock, R.E. and Diamond, G. (2000) The role of cationic antimicrobial peptides in innate host defences. *Trends in Microbiology* 8, 402–410.

Hancock, R.E. and Scott, M.G. (2000) The role of antimicrobial peptides in animal defenses. *Proceedings of the National Academy of Sciences of the United States of America* 97, 8856–8861.

Hara, T., Kodama, H., Kondo, M., Wakamatsu, K., Takeda, A., Tachi, T. and Matsuzaki, K. (2001) Effects of peptide dimerization on pore formation: antiparallel disulfide–dimerized magainin 2 analogue. *Biopolymers* 58, 437–446.

Harris, F., Dennison, S.R., Singh, J. and Phoenix, D.A. (2013) On the selectivity and efficacy of defense peptides with respect to cancer cells. *Medicinal Research Reviews* 33, 190–234.

Helmerhorst, E.J., Breeuwer, P., Van't Hof, W., Walgreen-Weterings, E., Oomen, L.C., *et al.* (1999) The cellular target of histatin 5 on *Candida albicans* is the energized mitochondrion. *Journal of Biological Chemistry* 274, 7286–7291.

Hilchie, A.L., Doucette, C.D., Pinto, D.M., Patrzykat, A., Douglas, S. and Hoskin, D.W. (2011) Pleurocidin-family cationic antimicrobial peptides are cytolytic for breast carcinoma cells and prevent growth of tumor xenografts. *Breast Cancer Research* 13, R102.

Hoffmann, J.A. and Reichhart, J.M. (2002) Drosophila innate immunity: an evolutionary perspective. *Nature Immunology* 3, 121–126.

Hoffmann, J.A., Kafatos, F.C., Janeway, C.A. and Ezekowitz, R.A. (1999) Phylogenetic perspectives in innate immunity. *Science* 284, 1313–1318.

Hoiby, N., Krogh Johansen, H., Moser, C., Song, Z., Ciofu, O. and Kharazmi, A. (2001) *Pseudomonas aeruginosa* and the *in vitro* and *in vivo* biofilm mode of growth. *Microbes and Infection* 3, 23–35.

Holo, H., Nilssen, O. and Nes, I.F. (1991) Lactococcin A, a new bacteriocin from *Lactococcus lactis* subsp. *cremoris*: isolation and characterization of the protein and its gene. *Journal of Bacteriology* 173, 3879–3887.

Jacob, L. and Zasloff, M. (1994) Potential therapeutic applications of magainins and other antimicrobial agents of animal origin. *Ciba Foundation Symposium* 186, 197–216; discussion pp. 216–23.

Jones, T.S. (1949) Chemical evidence for the multiplicity of the antibiotics produced by *Bacillus polymyxa*. *Annals of the New York Academy of Science* 51, 909–916.

Jorge, P., Lourenco, A. and Pereira, M.O. (2012) New trends in peptide-based anti-biofilm strategies: a review of recent achievements and bioinformatic approaches. *Biofouling* 28, 1033–1061.

Kalyanaraman, B., Joseph, J., Kalivendi, S., Wang, S., Konorev, E. and Kotamraju, S. (2002) Doxorubicin-induced apoptosis: implications in cardiotoxicity. *Molecular and Cellular Biochemistry* 234–235(1–2), 119–124.

Kampa, M., Pelekanou, V., Gallo, D., Notas, G., Troullinaki, M., *et al.* (2011) ERalpha17p, an ERalpha P295-T311 fragment, modifies the migration of breast cancer cells through actin cytoskeleton rearrangements. *Journal of Cellular Biochemistry* 112, 3786–3796.

Kapoor, R., Wadman, M.W., Dohm, M.T., Czyzewski, A.M., Spormann, A.M. and Barron, A.E. (2011) Antimicrobial peptoids are effective against *Pseudomonas aeruginosa* biofilms. *Antimicrobial Agents and Chemotherapy* 55, 3054–3057.

Keller, L. and Surette, M.G. (2006) Communication in bacteria: an ecological and evolutionary perspective. *Nature Reviews Microbiology* 4, 249–258.

Kimbrell, M.R., Warshakoon, H., Cromer, J.R., Malladi, S., Hood, J.D., *et al.* (2008) Comparison of the immunostimulatory and proinflammatory activities of candidate Gram-positive endotoxins, lipoteichoic acid, peptidoglycan, and lipopeptides, in murine and human cells. *Immunology Letters* 118, 132–141.

Lee, E., Rosca, E.V., Pandey, N.B. and Popel, A.S. (2011) Small peptides derived from somatotropin domain-containing proteins inhibit blood and lymphatic endothelial cell proliferation, migration, adhesion and tube formation. *International Journal of Biochemistry & Cell Biology* 43, 1812–1821.

Lehrer, R.I. and Ganz, T. (1999) Antimicrobial peptides in mammalian and insect host defence. *Current Opinion in Immunology* 11, 23–27.

Lehrer, R.I. and Ganz, T. (2002) Cathelicidins: a family of endogenous antimicrobial peptides. *Current Opinion in Hematology* 9, 18–22.

Leuschner, C. and Hansel, W. (2005) Targeting breast and prostate cancers through their hormone receptors. *Biology of Reproduction* 73, 860–865.

Lichtenstein, A., Ganz, T., Selsted, M.E. and Lehrer, R.I. (1986) *In vitro* tumor cell cytolysis mediated by peptide defensins of human and rabbit granulocytes. *Blood* 68, 1407–1410.

Liu, L., Xu, K., Wang, H., Tan, P.K., Fan, W., Venkatraman, S.S., Li, L. and Yang, Y.Y. (2009) Self-assembled cationic peptide nanoparticles as an efficient antimicrobial agent. *Nature Nanotechnology* 4, 457–463.

Luca, V., Stringaro, A., Colone, M., Pini, A. and Mangoni, M.L. (2013) Esculentin(1-21), an amphibian skin membrane-active peptide with potent activity on both planktonic and biofilm cells of the bacterial pathogen *Pseudomonas aeruginosa*. *Cellular and Molecular Life Sciences* 70, 2773–2786.

Ludtke, S.J., He, K., Heller, W.T., Harroun, T.A., Yang, L. and Huang, H.W. (1996) Membrane pores induced by magainin. *Biochemistry* 35, 13723–13728.

Mah, T.F. and O'Toole, G.A. (2001) Mechanisms of biofilm resistance to antimicrobial agents. *Trends in Microbiology* 9, 34–39.

Mai, J.C., Mi, Z., Kim, S.H., Ng, B. and Robbins, P.D. (2001) A proapoptotic peptide for the treatment of solid tumors. *Cancer Research* 61, 7709–7712.

Makovitzki, A., Avrahami, D. and Shai, Y. (2006) Ultrashort antibacterial and antifungal lipopeptides. *Proceedings of the National Academy of Sciences of the United States of America* 103, 15997–16002.

Makovitzki, A., Fink, A. and Shai, Y. (2009) Suppression of human solid tumor growth in mice by intratumor and systemic inoculation of histidine-rich and pH-dependent host defense-like lytic peptides. *Cancer Research* 69, 3458–3463.

Mangoni, M.L. and Shai, Y. (2011) Short native antimicrobial peptides and engineered ultrashort lipopeptides: similarities and differences in cell specificities and modes of action. *Cellular and Molecular Life Sciences* 68, 2267–2280.

McPhee, J.B., Scott, M.G. and Hancock, R.E. (2005) Design of host defence peptides for antimicrobial and immunity enhancing activities. *Combinatorial Chemistry & High Throughput Screening* 8, 257–272.

Meena, K.R. and Kanwar, S.S. (2015) Lipopeptides as the antifungal and antibacterial agents: applications in food safety and therapeutics. *Biomedical Research International* 2015, 4730–4750.

Mhammedi, A., Peypoux, F., Besson, F. and Michel, G. (1982) Bacillomycin F, a new antibiotic of iturin group: isolation and characterization. *Journal of Antibiotics* 35, 306–311.

Mookherjee, N., Brown, K.L., Bowdish, D.M., Doria, S., Falsafi, R., *et al.* (2006) Modulation of the TLR-mediated inflammatory response by the endogenous human host defense peptide LL-37. *Journal of Immunology* 176, 2455–2464.

Muller, A., Ulm, H., Reder–Christ, K., Sahl, H.G. and Schneider, T. (2012) Interaction of type A lantibiotics with undecaprenol-bound cell envelope precursors. *Microbial Drug Resistance* 18, 261–270.

Muraih, J.K., Pearson, A., Silverman, J. and Palmer, M. (2011) Oligomerization of daptomycin on membranes. *Biochimica et Biophysica Acta* 1808, 1154–1160.

Nagaoka, I., Hirota, S., Niyonsaba, F., Hirata, M., Adachi, Y., Tamura, H. and Heumann, D. (2001) Cathelicidin family of antibacterial peptides CAP18 and CAP11 inhibit the expression of TNF-alpha by blocking the binding of LPS to CD14(+) cells. *Journal of Immunology* 167, 3329–3338.

Nan, Y.H., Park, K.H., Park, Y., Jeon, Y.J., Kim, Y., *et al.* (2009) Investigating the effects of positive charge and hydrophobicity on the cell selectivity: mechanism of action and anti-inflammatory activity of a Trp-rich antimicrobial peptide indolicidin. *FEMS Microbiology Letters* 292, 134–140.

Nell, M.J., Tjabringa, G.S., Wafelman, A.R., Verrijk, R., Hiemstra, P.S., *et al.* (2006) Development of novel LL-37 derived antimicrobial peptides with LPS and LTA neutralizing and antimicrobial activities for therapeutic application. *Peptides* 27, 649–660.

Oren, Z. and Shai, Y. (1998) Mode of action of linear amphipathic alpha-helical antimicrobial peptides. *Biopolymers* 47, 451–463.

Oren, Z., Hong, J. and Shai, Y. (1997) A repertoire of novel antibacterial diastereomeric peptides with selective cytolytic activity. *Journal of Biological Chemistry* 272, 14643–14649.

Oren, Z., Hong, J. and Shai, Y. (1999) A comparative study on the structure and function of a cytolytic alpha-helical peptide and its antimicrobial beta-sheet diastereomer. *European Journal of Biochemistry* 259, 360–369.

Otvos, L., Jr., Bokonyi, K., Varga, I., Otvos, B.I., Hoffmann, R. *et al.* (2000) Insect peptides with improved protease-resistance protect mice against bacterial infection. *Protein Science* 9, 742–749.

Overhage, J., Campisano, A., Bains, M., Torfs, E.C., Rehm, B.H. and Hancock, R.E. (2008) Human host defense peptide LL-37 prevents bacterial biofilm formation. *Infection and Immunity* 76, 4176–4182.

Papo, N. and Shai, Y. (2004) Effect of drastic sequence alteration and D-amino acid incorporation on the membrane binding behavior of lytic peptides. *Biochemistry* 43, 6393–6403.

Papo, N. and Shai, Y. (2005) Host defense peptides as new weapons in cancer treatment. *Cellular and Molecular Life Sciences* 62, 784–790.

Papo, N., Oren, Z., Pag, U., Sahl, H.G. and Shai, Y. (2002) The consequence of sequence alteration of an amphipathic alpha-helical antimicrobial peptide and its diastereomers. *Journal of Biological Chemistry* 277, 33913–33921.

Papo, N., Braunstein, A., Eshhar, Z. and Shai, Y. (2004) Suppression of human prostate tumor growth in mice by a cytolytic D-, L-amino acid peptide: membrane lysis, increased necrosis, and inhibition of prostate-specific antigen secretion. *Cancer Research* 64, 5779–5786.

Papo, N., Seger, D., Makovitzki, A., Kalchenko, V., Eshhar, Z., Degani, H. and Shai, Y. (2006) Inhibition of tumor growth and elimination of multiple metastases in human prostate and breast xenografts by systemic inoculation of a host defense-like lytic peptide. *Cancer Research* 66, 5371–5378.

Park, C.B., Kim, H.S. and Kim, S.C. (1998) Mechanism of action of the antimicrobial peptide buforin II: buforin II kills microorganisms by penetrating the cell membrane and inhibiting cellular functions. *Biochemical and Biophysical Research Communications* 244, 253–257.

Patra, C.R., Rupasinghe, C.N., Dutta, S.K., Bhattacharya, S., Wang, E., *et al.* (2012) Chemically-modified peptides targeting the PDZ domain of GIPC as a therapeutic approach for cancer. *ACS Chemical Biology* 7, 770–779.

Patrzykat, A., Friedrich, C.L., Zhang, L., Mendoza, V. and Hancock, R.E. (2002) Sublethal concentrations of pleurocidin-derived antimicrobial peptides inhibit macromolecular synthesis in *Escherichia coli*. *Antimicrobial Agents and Chemotherapy* 46, 605–614.

Pearson, C.S., Kloos, Z., Murray, B., Tabe, E., Gupta, M., *et al.* (2016) Combined bioinformatic and rational design approach to develop antimicrobial peptides against mycobacterium tuberculosis. *Antimicrobial Agents and Chemotherapy* 60, 2757–2764.

Percy, M.G. and Grundling, A. (2014) Lipoteichoic acid synthesis and function in Gram-positive bacteria. *Annual Review of Microbiology* 68, 81–100.

Pouny, Y. and Shai, Y. (1992) Interaction of D-amino acid incorporated analogues of pardaxin with membranes. *Biochemistry* 31, 9482–9490.

Qi, G., Zhu, F., Du, P., Yang, X., Qiu, D., *et al.* (2010) Lipopeptide induces apoptosis in fungal cells by a mitochondria-dependent pathway. *Peptides* 31, 1978–1986.

Raetz, C.R. and Whitfield, C. (2002). Lipopolysaccharide endotoxins. *Annual Review of Biochemistry* 71, 635–700.

Raj, P.A., Soni, S.D. and Levine, M.J. (1994) Membrane-induced helical conformation of an active candidacidal fragment of salivary histatins. *Journal of Biological Chemistry* 269, 9610–9619.

Rapaport, D. and Shai, Y. (1992) Aggregation and organization of pardaxin in phospholipid membranes: a fluorescence energy transfer study. *Journal of Biological Chemistry* 267, 6502–6509.

Rathinakumar, R., Walkenhorst, W.F. and Wimley, W.C. (2009) Broad-spectrum antimicrobial peptides by rational combinatorial design and high-throughput screening: the importance of interfacial activity. *Journal of the American Chemical Society* 131, 7609–7617.

Reddy, K.V., Yedery, R.D. and Aranha, C. (2004) Antimicrobial peptides: premises and promises. *International Journal of Antimicrobial Agents* 24, 536–547.

Rerole, A.L., Gobbo, J., De Thonel, A., Schmitt, E., Pais De Barros, J.P., *et al.* (2011) Peptides and aptamers targeting HSP70: a novel approach for anticancer chemotherapy. *Cancer Research* 71, 484–495.

Rietschel, E.T., Brade, H., Holst, O., Brade, L., Muller-Loennies, S., *et al.* (1996) Bacterial endotoxin: chemical constitution, biological recognition, host response, and immunological detoxification. *Current Topics in Microbiology and Immunology* 216, 39–81.

Robbel, L. and Marahiel, M.A. (2010) Daptomycin: a bacterial lipopeptide synthesized by a nonribosomal machinery. *Journal of Biological Chemistry* 285, 27501–27508.

Rosca, E.V., Koskimaki, J.E., Rivera, C.G., Pandey, N.B., Tamiz, A.P. and Popel, A.S. (2011) Anti-angiogenic peptides for cancer therapeutics. *Current Pharmaceutical Biotechnology* 12, 1101–1116.

Rosenfeld, Y., Papo, N. and Shai, Y. (2006) Endotoxin (lipopolysaccharide) neutralization by innate immunity host-defense peptides: peptide properties and plausible modes of action. *Journal of Biological Chemistry* 281, 1636–1643.

Rosenfeld, Y., Sahl, H.G. and Shai, Y. (2008) Parameters involved in antimicrobial and endotoxin detoxification activities of antimicrobial peptides. *Biochemistry* 47, 6468–6478.

Rozek, A., Friedrich, C.L. and Hancock, R.E. (2000) Structure of the bovine antimicrobial peptide indolicidin bound to dodecylphosphocholine and sodium dodecyl sulfate micelles. *Biochemistry* 39, 15765–15774.

Sass, V., Schneider, T., Wilmes, M., Korner, C., Tossi, A.. *et al.* (2010) Human beta-defensin 3 inhibits cell wall biosynthesis in Staphylococci. *Infection and Immunity* 78, 2793–2800.

Sato, Y., Goto, Y., Narita, N. and Hoon, D.S. (2009) Cancer cells expressing toll-like receptors and the tumor microenvironment. *Cancer Microenvironment* 2, Suppl. 1, 205–214.

Schweizer, F. (2009). Cationic amphiphilic peptides with cancer-selective toxicity. *European Journal of Pharmacology* 625, 190–194.

Scocchi, M., Tossi, A. and Gennaro, R. (2011) Proline-rich antimicrobial peptides: converging to a non-lytic mechanism of action. *Cellular and Molecular Life Sciences* 68, 2317–2330.

Scott, M.G. and Hancock, R.E. (2000) Cationic antimicrobial peptides and their multifunctional role in the immune system. *Critical Reviews in Immunology* 20, 407–431.

Scott, M.G., Gold, M.R. and Hancock, R.E. (1999) Interaction of cationic peptides with lipoteichoic acid and Gram-positive bacteria. *Infection and Immunity* 67, 6445–6453.

Scott, M.G., Vreugdenhil, A.C., Buurman, W.A., Hancock, R.E. and Gold, M.R. (2000) Cutting edge: cationic antimicrobial peptides block the binding of lipopolysaccharide (LPS) to LPS binding protein. *Journal of Immunology* 164, 549–553.

Scott, M.G., Davidson, D.J., Gold, M.R., Bowdish, D. and Hancock, R.E. (2002) The human antimicrobial peptide LL–37 is a multifunctional modulator of innate immune responses. *Journal of Immunology* 169, 3883–3891.

Segev-Zarko, L., Saar-Dover, R., Brumfeld, V., Mangoni, M.L. and Shai, Y. (2015) Mechanisms of biofilm inhibition and degradation by antimicrobial peptides. *Biochemical Journal* 468, 259–270.

Sengupta, D., Leontiadou, H., Mark, A.E. and Marrink, S.J. (2008) Toroidal pores formed by antimicrobial peptides show significant disorder. *Biochimica et Biophysica Acta* 1778, 2308–2317.

Shai, Y. (1999) Mechanism of the binding, insertion and destabilization of phospholipid bilayer membranes by alpha-helical antimicrobial and cell non-selective membrane-lytic peptides. *Biochimica et Biophysica Acta* 1462, 55–70.

Shai, Y. (2002) Mode of action of membrane active antimicrobial peptides. *Biopolymers* 66, 236–248.

Shai, Y., Bach, D. and Yanovsky, A. (1990) Channel formation properties of synthetic pardaxin and analogues. *Journal of Biological Chemistry* 265, 20202–20209.

Silhavy, T.J., Kahne, D. and Walker, S. (2010) The bacterial cell envelope. *Cold Spring Harbor Perspectives in Biology* 2, a000414.

Sinha, S., Cheshenko, N., Lehrer, R.I. and Herold, B.C. (2003) NP-1, a rabbit alpha-defensin, prevents the entry and intercellular spread of herpes simplex virus type 2. *Antimicrobial Agents and Chemotherapy* 47, 494–500.

Sitaram, N. and Nagaraj, R. (1999) Interaction of antimicrobial peptides with biological and model membranes: structural and charge requirements for activity. *Biochimica et Biophysica Acta* 1462, 29–54.

Song, B.H., Lee, G., Moon, M.S., Cho, Y.H. and Lee, C.H. (2001) Human cytomegalovirus binding to heparan sulfate proteoglycans on the cell surface and/or entry stimulates the expression of human leukocyte antigen class I. *Journal of General Virology* 82, 2405–2413.

Steiner, H., Hultmark, D., Engstrom, A., Bennich, H. and Boman, H.G. (1981) Sequence and specificity of two antibacterial proteins involved in insect immunity. *Nature* 292, 246–248.

Straus, S.K. and Hancock, R.E. (2006) Mode of action of the new antibiotic for Gram-positive pathogens daptomycin: comparison with cationic antimicrobial peptides and lipopeptides. *Biochimica et Biophysica Acta* 1758, 1215–1223.

Tada, R., Latge, J.P. and Aimanianda, V. (2013) Undressing the fungal cell wall/cell membrane: the antifungal drug targets. *Current Pharmaceutical Design* 19, 3738–3747.

Takahashi, D., Shukla, S.K., Prakash, O. and Zhang, G. (2010) Structural determinants of host defense peptides for antimicrobial activity and target cell selectivity. *Biochimie* 92, 1236–1241.

Takeuchi, O., Hoshino, K., Kawai, T., Sanjo, H., Takada, H., *et al.* (1999) Differential roles of TLR2 and TLR4 in recognition of Gram-negative and Gram-positive bacterial cell wall components. *Immunity* 11, 443–451.

Tam, V.H., Schilling, A.N., Vo, G., Kabbara, S., Kwa, A.L., Wiederhold, N.P. and Lewis, R.E. (2005) Pharmacodynamics of polymyxin B against *Pseudomonas aeruginosa*. *Antimicrobial Agents and Chemotherapy* 49, 3624–3630.

Tossi, A., Sandri, L. and Giangaspero, A. (2000) Amphipathic, alpha-helical antimicrobial peptides. *Biopolymers* 55, 4–30.

Uyterhoeven, E.T., Butler, C.H., Ko, D. and Elmore, D.E. (2008) Investigating the nucleic acid interactions and antimicrobial mechanism of buforin II. *FEBS Letters* 582, 1715–1718.

Van Der Weerden, N.L., Bleackley, M.R. and Anderson, M.A. (2013) Properties and mechanisms of action of naturally occurring antifungal peptides. *Cellular and Molecular Life Sciences* 70, 3545–3570.

Van Zoggel, H., Carpentier, G., Dos Santos, C., Hamma-Kourbali, Y., Courty, J., Amiche, M. and Delbe, J. (2012) Antitumor and angiostatic activities of the antimicrobial peptide dermaseptin B2. *PLoS One* 7, e44351.

Vollmer, W. and Bertsche, U. (2008) Murein (peptidoglycan) structure, architecture and biosynthesis in *Escherichia coli*. *Biochimica et Biophysica Acta* 1778, 1714–1734.

Wadhwani, P., Epand, R.F., Heidenreich, N., Burck, J., Ulrich, A.S. and Epand, R.M. (2012) Membrane-active peptides and the clustering of anionic lipids. *Biophysical Journal* 103, 265–274.

Wang, C., Tian, L.L., Li, S., Li, H.B., Zhou, Y., *et al.* (2013) Rapid cytotoxicity of antimicrobial peptide tempoprin-1CEa in breast cancer cells through membrane destruction and intracellular calcium mechanism. *PLoS One* 8, e60462.

Wang, Y.S., Li, D., Shi, H.S., Wen, Y.J., Yang, L., *et al.* (2009) Intratumoral expression of mature human neutrophil peptide-1 mediates antitumor immunity in mice. *Clinical Cancer Research* 15, 6901–6911.

Winder, D., Gunzburg, W.H., Erfle, V. and Salmons, B. (1998) Expression of antimicrobial peptides has an antitumour effect in human cells. *Biochemical and Biophysical Research Communications* 242, 608–612.

Wingender, J., Strathmann, M., Rode, A., Leis, A. and Flemming, H.C. (2001) Isolation and biochemical characterization of extracellular polymeric substances from *Pseudomonas aeruginosa*. *Methods in Enzymology* 336, 302–314.

Xhindoli, D., Pacor, S., Benincasa, M., Scocchi, M., Gennaro, R. and Tossi, A. (2016) The human cathelicidin LL-37: a pore-forming antibacterial peptide and host-cell modulator. *Biochimica et Biophysica Acta* 1858, 546–566.

Xiong, Y.Q., Bayer, A.S. and Yeaman, M.R. (2002) Inhibition of intracellular macromolecular synthesis in *Staphylococcus aureus* by thrombin-induced platelet microbicidal proteins. *Journal of Infectious Diseases* 185, 348–356.

Xu, H., Chen, C.X., Hu, J., Zhou, P., Zeng, P., Cao, C.H. and Lu, J.R. (2013) Dual modes of antitumor action of an amphiphilic peptide A(9)K. *Biomaterials* 34, 2731–2737.

Yao, J., Liu, H., Zhou, T., Chen, H., Miao, Z., Sheng, C. and Zhang, W. (2012) Total synthesis and structure–activity relationships of new echinocandin-like antifungal cyclolipohexapeptides. *European Journal of Medicinal Chemistry* 50, 196–208.

Yasin, B., Wang, W., Pang, M., Cheshenko, N., Hong, T., *et al.* (2004) Theta defensins protect cells from infection by herpes simplex virus by inhibiting viral adhesion and entry. *Journal of Virology* 78, 5147–5156.

Yeaman, M.R. and Yount, N.Y. (2003) Mechanisms of antimicrobial peptide action and resistance. *Pharmacological Reviews* 55, 27–55.

Yount, N.Y. and Yeaman, M.R. (2013). Peptide antimicrobials: cell wall as a bacterial target. *Annals of the New York Academy of Sciences* 1277, 127–138.

Zasloff, M. (1987) Magainins, a class of antimicrobial peptides from Xenopus skin: isolation, characterization of two active forms, and partial cDNA sequence of a precursor. *Proceedings of the National Academy of Sciences of the United States of America* 84, 5449–5453.

Zasloff, M. (2002) Antimicrobial peptides of multicellular organisms. *Nature* 415, 389–395.

Zhang, L., Benz, R. and Hancock, R.E. (1999) Influence of proline residues on the antibacterial and synergistic activities of alpha-helical peptides. *Biochemistry* 38, 8102–8111.

Zhang, L., Dhillon, P., Yan, H., Farmer, S. and Hancock, R.E. (2000) Interactions of bacterial cationic peptide antibiotics with outer and cytoplasmic membranes of *Pseudomonas aeruginosa*. *Antimicrobial Agents and Chemotherapy* 44, 3317–3321.

8 Microbial Membranes and the Action of Antimicrobial Peptides

José Carlos Bozelli, Jr[1,2], Shirley Schreier[2] and Richard M. Epand[1,*]

[1]*Department of Biochemistry and Biomedical Sciences, McMaster University, Health Sciences Centre, Hamilton, Ontario L8S 4K1 Canada;* [2]*Laboratory of Structural Biology, Department of Biochemistry, Institute of Chemistry, University of São Paulo (USP), São Paulo, São Paulo, C.P. 26077, 05513-970, Brazil*

Abstract

Since their discovery, antimicrobial peptides (AMPs) have excited researchers worldwide, mainly due to their wide spectrum of activity and rapid action. As for the latter feature, it is believed to be a consequence of their membrane-targeting properties. In the present chapter we will describe this fine-tuned interaction between peptides and lipids in a biophysical context. We took advantage of the antimicrobial peptide database to identify physicochemical properties of AMPs based on their target microorganisms. In spite of the fact that cell envelopes of microorganisms present different molecular composition, as well as molecular organization, the physicochemical properties of membrane-interacting AMPs have been found to be similar. The interactions of AMPs with different components of the cell envelope and their consequence for the peptide's toxicity are discussed. In addition, membrane–peptide interactions are described with a focus on bacterial membranes, since they vary for different bacterial species and can contribute to the efficacy of some AMPs. Finally, we will outline novel strategies for using the interaction of AMPs with components of the microbial membranes both directly as antimicrobial agents, and by altering membrane properties so as to sensitize microorganisms to different cytotoxic drugs.

8.1 Introduction

In the 1980s, cecropin, magainin and defensin were isolated and purified, leading to increased prominence and expansion of the field of antimicrobial peptides (AMPs) (Steiner *et al.*, 1981; Ganz *et al.*, 1985; Zasloff, 1987; see also Chapter 1). Currently, over 2700 AMPs have been isolated and characterized or had their sequence predicted from the host genome (Wang *et al.*, 2016). Properties such as the wide spectrum of activity and a fast timescale of action compared to conventional drugs against microorganisms render these ubiquitous molecules very attractive. The broad action spectrum of AMPs is exemplified in the Venn diagram of Fig. 8.1, built using data from the antimicrobial peptide database (http://aps.unmc.edu/AP). This diagram clearly shows the activity overlap of AMPs against different organisms. Moreover, the

* Corresponding author e-mail: epand@mcmaster.ca

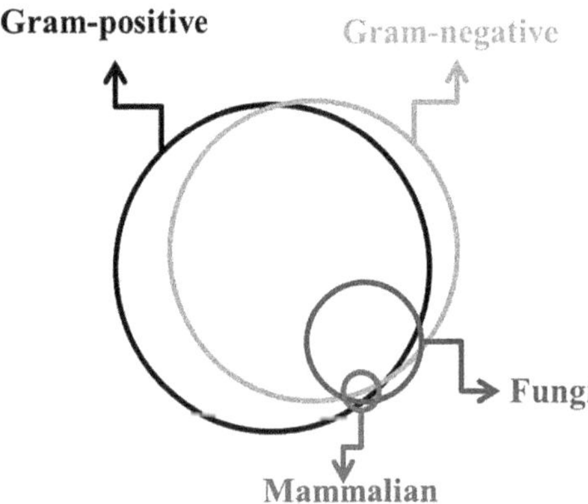

Fig. 8.1. Venn diagram representing the population of AMPs with activity against Gram-positive bacteria, Gram-negative bacteria, fungi and mammalian cells. Data to build the diagram were obtained from the antimicrobial peptide database (Wang *et al.*, 2016).

small number of AMPs with activity against mammalian cells as compared to bacteria or fungi points to their potential use as therapeutic agents. Besides bearing activity against bacteria and fungi, AMPs have also been reported to act against viruses, parasites and cancer cells (Dotiwala *et al.*, 2016; Gaspar and Castanho, 2016; Sousa *et al.*, 2016).

The fast timescale at which AMPs are able to kill microorganisms (minutes to hours) represents an advantage in avoiding development of resistance. This is believed to be due to the action of these peptides at the membrane level. In 1989, studies with human defensin suggested that this peptide's bactericidal activity was related to permeabilization of the plasma membrane (Lehrer *et al.*, 1989). Following this, studies with cecropin A, amidated magainin II and melittin showed that their mechanism of action is due to a direct interaction between peptides and cell membrane lipids, without any stereospecific interaction with receptors and/or enzymes (Wade *et al.*, 1990). Since then, a collection of experimental results have suggested that the mechanism of action of these peptides is related to AMP-induced alteration of membrane properties (Schibli *et al.*, 2002; Shai, 2002; Huang *et al.*, 2004; Salay *et al.*, 2004; Lohner

and Blondelle, 2005; Epand *et al.*, 2008a; Bozelli *et al.*, 2012). Additionally, more recent studies have shown that some of these peptides act by interacting with other cellular targets (for a comprehensive description of these mechanisms of action see Chapter 9). In the present chapter we will present biophysical insights of membrane-targeting AMPs. We will further outline novel strategies for using the interaction of antimicrobial agents with components of the microbial membranes both directly as antimicrobial agents, and by altering membrane properties so as to sensitize microbes to different drugs.

8.2 Physicochemical Properties of AMPs and the Molecular Organization of the Cell Envelope of Different Microorganisms

AMP-induced alteration of membrane properties leading to microorganism death is a fine-tuned interplay between the ability of lipids to modulate the conformation of AMPs (encoded by their amino acid sequence), and the ability of the peptides to affect the molecular arrangement of lipids in the membrane (as a consequence of their conformation, amino acid composition, and dynamics). However, in order for this interaction between lipids and peptides to occur it is necessary for the peptide to circumvent several barriers presented by the microorganism's cell wall (see below).

AMPs do not present high sequence homologies and most of their structures are unknown (70, 60, 57, and 60% of AMPs in the antimicrobial peptide database with activity against Gram-positive bacteria, Gram-negative bacteria, fungi and mammalian cells, respectively, have unknown structures). However, they exhibit similar general physicochemical properties. In Fig. 8.2 we present the distribution of sizes (Fig. 8.2A), net charges (Fig. 8.2B), and percentages of hydrophobic residues (Fig. 8.2C) for those AMPs active against Gram-positive and Gram-negative bacteria, fungi and mammalian cells (data from the antimicrobial peptide database: Wang *et al.*, 2016). It is worth mentioning that regardless of target, their physicochemical properties are similar and in agreement with the overlap in activity (Fig. 8.1). Most AMPs (as judged by the mode of the distribution) are 21–30 residues long, have a net charge at physiological pH between +1 and +5, and bear 40–50% of hydrophobic residues

(interestingly, AMPs presenting activity against mammalian cells bear slightly higher content of hydrophobic residues, between 50–60%). These properties are believed to be requisites for peptide-membrane interaction. The short size contributes to peptide flexibility, while the positive net charge would act as a selective filter towards microbial targets, the

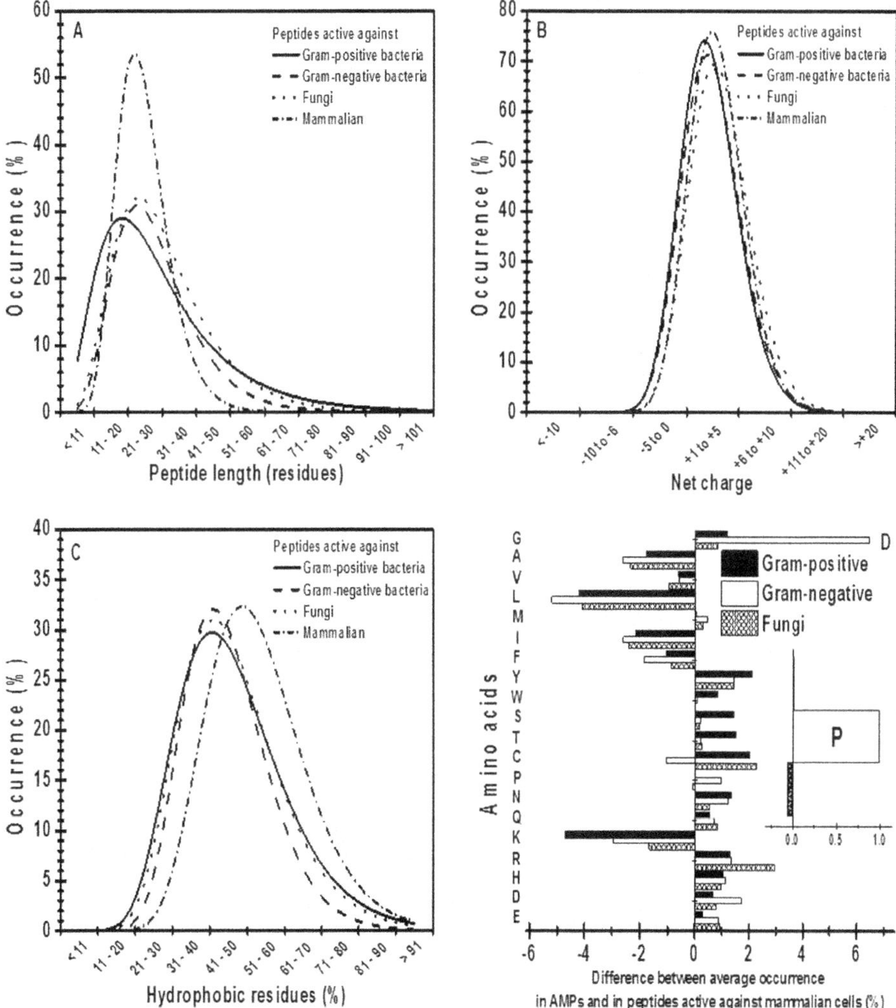

Fig. 8.2. Physical properties of antimicrobial peptides (AMPs) and the cell envelope of different organisms. Distribution of AMPs (A) size, (B) net charge and (C) percentage of hydrophobic residues for AMPs active against different organisms. (D) Difference between the average occurrence of the 20 common amino acids in AMPs active against Gram-positive bacteria, Gram-negative bacteria, and fungi, and the average occurrence of these amino acids in peptides active against mammalian cells. Insert shows an expansion of the difference of average occurrence of P residues.

Continued

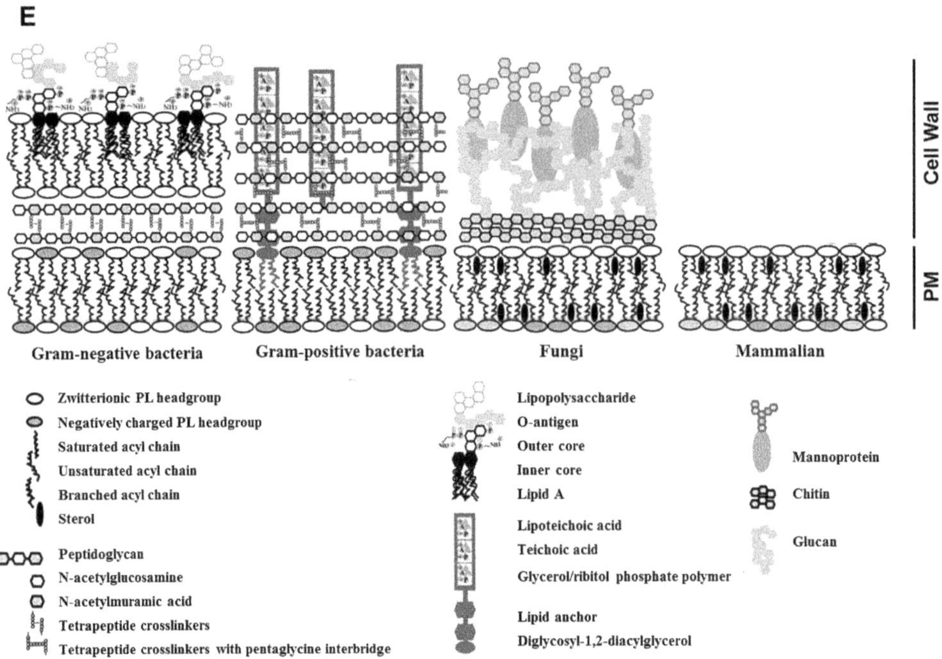

Fig. 8.2. (Continued) (E) Schematic depiction of the cell envelope of some microbes and mammalian cells. AMPs physical properties graphics were build using data from the antimicrobial peptide database (Wang *et al.*, 2016). Cell envelope schemes were adapted and altered from Malanovic and Lohner, 2016.

amphipathic nature of their amino acid sequence is suitable for interaction with membranes (or with other interfaces), and the hydrophobic residues are necessary for insertion and membrane perturbation.

When the average occurrence of each of the 20 usual amino acids in AMPs active against Gram-positive bacteria, Gram-negative bacteria and fungi is compared to that found in peptides active against mammalian cells, some striking differences emerge (Fig.8.2D). The latter present more L residues than do AMPs that are active against microorganisms, which is in agreement with their higher content of hydrophobic residues. In addition, peptides active against mammalian cells present a higher content of K residues, which is surprising, since several studies in the literature with point substitution of R to K residues report a decrease in haemolytic activity (Schibli *et al.*, 2006; Yang *et al.*, 2003; Zhang *et al.*, 2016). This finding suggests that the whole amino acid sequence,

rather than specific residues, encodes the activity of these peptides.

In the case of AMPs active against microorganisms, the most striking observation is the higher content of G residues in those active against Gram-negative bacteria. In contrast to all other common amino acids, G bears a hydrogen atom as side chain, allowing for a higher degree of conformational flexibility. It is proposed that peptides with higher conformational flexibility and/or bearing less ordered secondary structure could translocate across the outer membrane (OM) of Gram-negative bacteria more easily. In this context, it is interesting that AMPs active against Gram-negative bacteria are the only ones that present a higher average occurrence of P residues (although small, there is 1% difference: Fig. 8.2D). Proline has a dual role in modulating peptide conformational flexibility. Locally, on a short length scale, Pro restricts rotation around the nitrogen in the amide bond because of the ring structure. However, because the amide bond geometry of Pro is not compatible with α-helices, this residue breaks up such longer range ordered structures. In model amphipathic α-helical peptides, the presence of a central P residue limits the formation of highly helical aggregates in aqueous environment, while in membrane-mimetic environments it (partially) distorts the stable α-helix (Yang *et al.*, 2006). As a consequence of the structural distortions imposed by the central P residue, peptides were faster in transposing the peptidoglycan layer in Gram-positive bacteria. The statistical analysis presented here suggests that P residues might be more important for AMPs active against Gram-negative bacteria. Since Gram-negative bacteria have an additional barrier (the outer membrane), the presence of P residues might facilitate these peptides transposing the additional barrier as a consequence of the loss of ordered secondary structure.

One of the remarkable differences between the cell envelope of microbes – Gram-negative and Gram-positive bacteria, and fungi – and that of mammalian cells is the presence of a cell wall surrounding the plasma membrane of microbes (Fig. 8.2E). The cell envelope of Gram-negative bacteria has a higher complexity, since it has an additional (outer) membrane. From the cell exterior to the interior this envelope is composed of: (i) OM; (ii) periplasm, containing a layer of peptidoglycan; and (iii) plasma membrane. The OM is unique in its properties and composition (Epand and Epand, 2010). It is an asymmetric bilayer, where phospholipids are the main components of the inner leaflet and lipopolysaccharides (LPS) are the major components of the outer leaflet. In addition, the presence of porins, β-barrel proteins that have an aqueous core, in the OM allows the passage of small molecules with molecular mass up to 700 Da. Between the outer and inner membranes is the periplasm, which contains a single layer of peptidoglycan. Finally, there is the plasma membrane, whose structure is based on a phospholipid bilayer. In order to gain access to the plasma membrane of a Gram negative bacteria, an antimicrobial agent

must first traverse the sugar chains in the O-antigen layer (up to 30 nm thick) and then cross the LPS layer (*c.*8 nm thick), followed by a peptidoglycan layer (a porous sacculus 7–8 nm thick).

Compared to Gram-negative bacteria, Gram-positive bacteria and fungi have simpler cell envelopes. Gram-positive bacteria have a single bilayer membrane, surrounded by a cell wall composed of a thick layer of peptidoglycan (40–80 nm) and lipoteichoic acid (LTA). LTA is anchored to the cell membrane by diacylglycerol. A single plasma membrane is also present in fungi, surrounded by a cell wall consisting of various layers of the polysaccharides chitin, β-glucan and mannan in the form of mannoproteins (whose thickness varies from 50 to 1000 nm depending on cell developmental stage). Given the number of physical barriers and sites for interaction that AMPs are exposed to during their journey towards the plasma membrane, AMPs emerge as truly amazing agents.

8.3 The Role of Cell Wall Components on AMP Toxicity

In addition to the cytoplasmic membrane damage caused by AMPs that may lead to toxicity, one must also consider possible roles for the cell wall components. The cell wall provides structural rigidity and plays a role in cell shape and homeostasis, acting, for instance, in protection against cell damage caused by osmotic stress. Several classical drugs act by affecting the synthesis of cell wall components.

The OM of Gram-negative bacteria can act as a barrier for the passage of antimicrobial agents to the plasma membrane. The interaction of cationic antimicrobial agents with negatively charged LPS can prevent the toxicity of these agents by inhibiting access or decreasing the concentration of AMPs that reach the plasma membrane. An interesting example is the blockage of penetration of the small cationic peptides, the temporins (Mangoni *et al.*, 2008). This study showed the dependence of the OM barrier function on the length of the lipopolysaccharide chain (LPS). In addition, synergistic action between pairs of temporin molecules was demonstrated.

An increase of acidic phospholipids in the OM could also contribute to inhibit AMP access or effective concentration. It has been shown that the *Salmonella* two-component regulatory system, PhoPQ, regulates acidic lipids by increasing the levels of CL and palmitoylated acylphosphatidyl-glycerols within the OM, suggesting that these lipids cooperate with lipid A (the bioactive component of LPS) to form an OM barrier critical for AMP resistance and intracellular survival of *S. typhimurium* (Dalebroux *et al.*, 2014).

Although generally the OM acts as a barrier to protect against AMPs, under certain conditions, some AMPs can block the passage of polar molecules across the OM leading to microbial toxicity, rather than protection. In this manner, the agent can inhibit growth of the organism without accessing or damaging the plasma membrane. Elucidation of this mechanism was facilitated by the availability of a strain of *E. coli*, ML-35p, especially constructed to simultaneously monitor the passage of chromogenic substrates across the inner and the outer membrane (Lehrer *et al.*, 1988). An example of an antimicrobial agent that blocks the flux of small molecules across the OM of *E. coli* is a flexible sequence-random polymer containing cationic and lipophilic subunits that acts as a functional mimic of AMPs (Epand *et al.*, 2008b). At low concentrations, the polymer permeabilizes the outer and inner membranes, but at higher concentrations, permeabilization of the outer membrane is progressively diminished, while the inner membrane remains unaffected. Although, in general, several oligo-acyl-lysine (OAKs) have been shown to have antibacterial action only to bacterial species that can cluster anionic lipids (see Section 8.5), there is also an additional mechanism exhibited by certain miniature OAKs against Gram-negative bacteria (Epand *et al.*, 2009a). These miniature OAKs can inhibit permeabilization across the OM by a non-specific mechanism, which, in turn, leads to cell death.

The role of the peptidoglycan layer on the toxicity of AMPs is less studied and, hence, not well understood. However, the peptidoglycan sacculus is porous and does not represent a permeability barrier for molecules up to 50 kDa (Malanovic and Lohner, 2016). In Gram-negative bacteria, it seems that the interaction of AMPs with the peptidoglycan layer does not affect toxicity. It has recently been shown that an antimicrobial homologue of the peptide melittin does not affect the thickness, nor the mechanical properties of this layer. Furthermore, removal of this layer in bacterial mutants did not increase lysis by the peptide (Mularski *et al.*, 2015). The peptidoglycan layer in Gram-positive bacteria is much thicker than that of Gram-negative bacteria and the presence of anionic teichoic acids in the cell wall of Gram-positive bacteria can actually facilitate AMP entry into Gram-positive bacteria by adding an additional site for interaction with AMPs.

In a study of the activity of human β-defensin 3 towards *S. aureus*, it was shown that the activity depends on the initial interaction with cell wall teichoic acids, since a mutant lacking them (tagO) was highly resistant to the peptide (Koprivnjak *et al.*, 2008). On the other hand, it has also been reported that the interaction of the AMPs PBP 10, LL-37 and melittin with LTA inhibits their activity, probably by inhibiting or decreasing the effective concentration of the peptides on the plasma membrane (Bucki and Janmey, 2006). In addition, it has been demonstrated that D-alanylation of LTA in group B *Streptococcus* confers resistance to LL-37, magainin II, polymyxin B and colistin (Saar-Dover *et al.*, 2012). It was proposed that D-alanylation changes LTA conformation. Hence, peptides become sequestered at the cell wall, decreasing the effective concentration that reaches the plasma membrane. Another example of cell wall components acting to hinder the activity of AMPs is their effect on peptide conformation. It has been reported that the binding of a β-bungarotoxin B chain, an antibacterial cationic polypeptide from snake venom, to LTA promotes a conformational change, which, in turn, leads to a decrease in the peptide's activity (Wen *et al.*, 2013).

The interaction of peptides with fungal cell wall components impairs the cell wall integrity, leading to cell vulnerability and hampering its development (Lohner and Leber, 2016). It has been reported that echinocandins, semi-synthetic lipopeptides, act as non-competitive inhibitors of (1,3)-β-D-glucan synthase, an enzymatic complex that forms the glucan layer, impairing cell wall structural integrity and resulting in cell vulnerability to osmotic lysis (Grover, 2010). Inhibitors of chitin synthase, such as nikkomycins (a group of peptidyl nucleosides), have also been reported to inhibit the growth of filamentous fungi and yeasts (Feng *et al.*, 2014). In addition, it has been shown that hevein-like peptides, cyclothiazomycin B1 and penaeidins impair cell development (Destoumieux *et al.*, 2000; Mizuhara *et al.*, 2011; Rogozhin *et al.*, 2015). The activity of these peptides has been described as a consequence of their ability to bind chitin, which probably induces cell wall fragility.

8.4 Membrane Lipid Composition and AMP Sensitivity

Although less common, the activity of some antimicrobial agents is related to specificity towards microbial membrane lipid components. These lipid components either (i) may not be present in mammalian membranes as is the case of lipid II which is specifically targeted by the antimicrobial peptide nisin (Breukink and de Kruijff, 1999); or (ii) bear structural differences, as is the case of fungi sphingolipids, which display structural differences with respect to those found in mammalian cells, such as the 9-methyl group branching of the sphingoid base, and different degrees of unsaturation (Thevissen *et al.*, 2005). In *S. cerevisiae*, when the biosynthetic pathway for the sphingolipid mannosyl di-(inositol phosphoryl) ceramide is disrupted,

the cells become resistant to plant defensin DmAMP1 and synthetic amphipathic peptide LTX109, suggesting that the sphingolipid is essential for activity (Thevissen *et al.*, 2000; Bojsen *et al.*, 2013). Depletion of the sphingolipid glucosylceramide in *S. cerevisiae* also promotes cell resistance to the plant defensin RSAFP2, suggesting a specific interaction between this sphingolipid and the peptide (Thevissen *et al.*, 2004). Another possibility is for the specific microbial lipid target not to be accessible in mammalian membranes. The zwitterionic phospholipid phosphatidylethanolamine (PE), present on the outer leaflet of bacterial membranes, is a specific target for duramycin and cinnamycin, two antimicrobial peptides of the same lantibiotic class as nisin (Clejan *et al.*, 1989; Fredenhagen *et al.*, 1991; Sahl *et al.*, 1995; Epand *et al.*, 2015; Phoenix *et al.*, 2015). However, this phospholipid is present in the inner leaflet of fungi and mammalian plasma membranes, making the targeting of these antibiotics specific for some bacteria.

The activity of AMPs at the membrane level often involves less specific interactions with membrane lipids, such as electrostatic or H-bonding interactions, which could influence potency and/or mechanism of action of these agents. This can be particularly important because the lipid compositions of bacterial membranes vary widely, resulting in certain bacterial species being more susceptible to some antimicrobial agents. The relationship between PE content and the antimicrobial action of the cationic sterol compound CSA-8 illustrates the importance of membrane phospholipid content for the potency of this antimicrobial agent (Epand *et al.*, 2007). This conclusion was further confirmed using an *E. coli* mutant unable to synthesize PE (Epand *et al.*, 2007). In this context, it has been reported that the activity and mechanism of action of the cecropin-melittin hybrid peptide BP100 depend on the content of the negatively charged phospholipid phosphatidylglycerol (PG) of the target membrane (Manzini *et al.*, 2014). Additionally, the toxicity of certain OAK is higher against bacteria that contain both anionic and either zwitterionic lipids or in their membranes (Epand *et al.*, 2008a). The activity of the antifungal peptide syringomycin E, a small cyclic lipodepsipeptide, depends on the presence of sterols in the plasma membrane (Takemoto *et al.*, 1993). This peptide activity is sensitive to the type of sterol. While its activity decreases in bilayers containing cholesterol, the opposite occurs in bilayers containing ergosterol (the sterol found in fungal membranes) (Feigin *et al.*, 1997; Blasko *et al.*, 1998). Peptides such as Psd1 (a defensin) and human neutrophil peptide 1 (HNP1) also have been reported to preferentially interact with ergosterol-containing bilayers in comparison to cholesterol-containing bilayers *in vitro* (Gonçalves *et al.*, 2012a, b).

8.5 Antimicrobial Agents that Promote Clustering of Anionic Lipids

In general, plasma membranes of Gram-positive and Gram-negative bacteria have a higher fraction of anionic lipids than do eukaryotic membranes. In Gram-negative bacteria the major negatively charged phospholipid is PG, while in Gram-positive bacterial membranes, in addition to PG, there is a high content of cardiolipin (CL) (Epand and Epand, 2009). The major zwitterionic bacterial lipid is PE, but high PE concentrations are generally found only in Gram-negative bacteria and in Gram-positive species of *Bacillus*. Fungi, on the other hand, are eukaryotes, and their plasma membranes present a high content of zwitterionic phospholipids, as well as ergosterol.

AMP-induced lipid clustering usually depends on the presence of anionic lipids in the plasma membrane of the target cell. These lipids are not present in the outer leaflet of mammalian or fungi plasma membranes. The ability of certain antimicrobial agents to cluster anionic lipids could explain the selective toxicity of these agents toward certain bacterial species. Such agents are generally more toxic to Gram-negative bacteria than to Gram-positive

ones. The glycolipids segregation of anionic lipids into domains can result in the arrest of cell growth, or cell death. Although not reported yet, clustering of anionic lipids could also be important for the toxicity of AMPs towards cancer cells and parasites, since their plasma membranes contain negatively charged lipids in the outer leaflet.

Anionic lipids clustering in lipid mixtures corresponding to those found in bacterial membranes has been reported by several methods (Epand and Epand, 2009; Epand *et al.*, 2009b; Epand *et al.*, 2010; Epand and Epand, 2011). The results of these analyses allow the prediction of which bacterial species will be most susceptible to the action of a particular antimicrobial agent based on the lipid composition of their membranes (Epand *et al.*, 2008a). The cecropin-melittin hybrid peptide, BP100, was shown to be selective for Gram-negative bacteria (Badosa *et al.*, 2007). *In vitro* studies showed that at high peptide concentration there is fast leakage of lipid vesicle content as a consequence of large-scale peptide and lipid clustering, typical of a carpet-like mechanism (Manzini *et al.*, 2014). A role for peptide acylation in lipid clustering has also been demonstrated. While a group of acylated and non-acylated cationic peptides all caused anionic lipid clustering, only the acylated peptides were able to promote the formation of PE-rich domains (Zweytick *et al.*, 2014). A recent study of a group of cyclic hexapeptides showed that their ability to promote PG clustering in a PG/PE mixture was related to their antimicrobial activity (Finger *et al.*, 2015). All the peptides had three positively charged groups and three aromatic groups. The charged groups were required for electrostatic binding to lipid, but the position of the aromatic residues in the sequence also contributed to binding and to lipid clustering. The antimicrobial agent 3',6-dinonoyl neamine was shown by a variety of methods to act by clustering anionic lipids, particularly CL (Sautrey *et al.*, 2016). A simple qualitative correlation has been shown between a peptide's net charge and its ability to promote lipid clustering, independently of the peptide's secondary structure (Wadhwani *et al.*, 2012).

8.6 Synergistic Action of AMPs and Other Antimicrobial Agents

Several cellular processes depend on ion or electrical gradients across the plasma membrane. These functions include signal transduction, bioenergetics and active transport (Kaneti *et al.*, 2016; Mor, 2016). The alteration of membrane properties induced by AMPs could disrupt these gradients. The damage to the membrane caused by these perturbations could be below the agent's minimal inhibition concentration, i.e. it would not have to be enough to kill the microorganism. This also prevents dying microorganisms releasing toxic factors that would stimulate an acute immune response. However, the loss of membrane potential would make the cell more sensitive to other drugs by inhibiting drug efflux pumps that depend on proton gradients for their function. This would suggest that certain combinations of antimicrobial agents could be particularly effective in controlling microbial infections.

The above strategy was found to be effective in sensitizing drug-resistant Gram-negative bacteria to the action of intracellular targeting antibiotics (Goldberg *et al.*, 2013). It was shown that a low concentration of an OAK could transiently depolarize a bacterial cell membrane and, thus, inactivate proton gradient-dependent drug efflux pumps. This resulted in resistant bacteria becoming sensitive to a variety of intracellular targeting antibiotics. A similar result was obtained with combinations of OAKs and rifampin. Interestingly, mixtures of certain OAKs and phospholipids form aggregates with cochleate morphology (Livne *et al.*, 2010; Epand *et al.*, 2011; Sarig *et al.*, 2011). Each of these antibiotics was ineffective against a resistant Gram-negative strain of *Klebsiella*, but the combination of the two drugs showed synergistic action that could be explained by the OAK damaging the membrane and dissipating the membrane potential, thus inactivating drug efflux pumps and sensitizing the bacteria to the action of rifampin, both *in vitro* as well as *in vivo* in mice (Jammal *et al.*, 2015).

Synergistic action has also been reported for AMPs and conventional antibiotics or antifungal agents against Gram-positive bacteria and fungi, respectively. In a recent study, the antimicrobial activities based on the synergistic effects of traditional antibiotics (imipenem, cefepime, levofloxacin hydrochloride, and vancomycin) and antimicrobial peptides (PL-5, PL-31, PL-32, PL-18, PL-29 and PL-26) against three Gram-positive bacteria (*Staphylococcus aureus*, *Streptococcus pneumonia*, and *Staphylococcus epidermidis*) were investigated (Feng *et al.*, 2015). Besides showing a synergistic effect *in vitro*, a strong effect was observed with PL-5 and levofloxacin hydrochloride in mice. In a study with *Candida* species, a substantial cooperative effect was reported upon use of the combination of lactoferrin with amphotericin B, fluconazole or 5-fluorocytosine (Kuipers *et al.*, 1999). A synergistic effect was also reported by a combination of amphotericin B with two AMPs, histatin-5 and PGLa against *Aspergillus*, *Candida* and *Cryptococcus* strains (van't Hof *et al.*, 2000). A successful combined antifungal therapy of a difficult-to-treat systemic fungal infection by *Aspergillus flavus* was reported in a clinical trial; the treatment was performed with liposomal amphotericin B and caspofungin, with a deep fungal infection being resolved in 30 days (Krivan *et al.*, 2006). The subinhibitory concentrations of AMPs could avoid cytotoxic effects, while enhancing the activity of conventional drugs, suggesting that the combination therapy might be a promising strategy for the treatment of complex infections.

8.7 Summary and Future Perspective

Antimicrobial peptides have been demonstrated to be extremely versatile molecules presenting activity towards a wide spectrum of infectious bacterial, viral, fungal and parasitic pathogens. Nevertheless, it is surprising that peptides with quite similar physicochemical properties act upon this broad range of pathogenic microorganisms with clearly distinct cell envelopes. At this stage, we are starting to understand the interrelationship between structural determinants and activity of antimicrobial peptides. We know that some biophysical properties are similar (length, net charge, amphipathicity and hydrophobicity); however, information regarding their three-dimensional configuration is lacking (conformation, polar angle and overall stereo geometry). A deeper understanding of structure–activity relationships of AMPs should provide new models and strategies for developing novel antimicrobial agents, which could augment immunity, restore potency, or amplify the mechanisms of action of more conventional drugs.

Among the target microorganisms, bacteria are the most studied with the aim of understanding the mechanism of action of AMPs. It has been shown that clustering anionic lipids is a component of the mechanism of action of many antimicrobial agents, including OAKs, some amphipathic helical peptides, and small arginine- and lysine-rich peptides. This phenomenon is more important for antimicrobial agents that have a high number and density of positive charges, that are conformationally flexible, and that are sufficiently hydrophobic to cross the outer membrane of Gram-negative bacteria. Optimizing the potency and effectiveness of agents that promote this phenomenon will allow the targeting of antimicrobial agents to specific strains of bacteria. In addition, it may provide a mechanism of bactericidal action that does not involve lysis and disruption of bacteria and may, therefore, have fewer toxic side effects when applied to humans, allowing for faster clearance of bacteria by macrophages. Further studies are required to fully elucidate how lipid clustering leads to bacteriostatic effects, as well as to understand the relationship between membrane domains normally present in bacteria and those that are formed as a result of the interaction of antimicrobial agents with bacterial membranes. In addition, there has been interest in cationic antimicrobial agents that can function as anticancer and antiparasitic agents. The role of clustering anionic lipids in cancer cells and parasites by antimicrobial agents should be investigated.

Acknowledgements

SS acknowledges the receipt of a research fellowship from CNPq, JCBJr has a postdoctoral fellowship from CNPq Science without Borders Program (201111/2015-2), and RME acknowledges NSERC.

References

Badosa, E., Ferre, R., Planas, M., Feliu, L., Besalú, E., *et al.* (2007) A library of linear undecapeptides with bactericidal activity against phytophatogenic bacteria. *Peptides* 28, 2276–2285. DOI: 10.1016/j.peptides.2007.09.010

Blasko, K., Schagina, L.V., Agner, G., Kaulin, Y.A. and Takemoto, J.Y. (1998) Membrane sterol composition modulates the pore forming activity of syringomycin E in human red blood cells. *Biochimica et Biophysica Acta (BBA)* 1373, 163–169.

Bojsen, R., Torbensen, R., Larsen, C.E., Folkesson, A. and Regenberg, B. (2013) The synthetic amphipathic peptidomimetic LTX109 is a potent fungicide that disturbs plasma membrane integrity in a sphingolipid dependent manner. *PLoS ONE*, 8, e69483. DOI: 10.1371/journal.pone.0069483

Bozelli, J.C., Jr., Sasahara, E.T., Pinto, M.R., Nakaie, C.R. and Schreier, S. (2012) Effect of head group and curvature on binding of the antimicrobial peptide tritrpticin to lipid membranes. *Chemistry and Physics of Lipids* 165, 365–373. DOI: 10.1016/j.chemphyslip.2011.12.005

Breukink, E. and de Kruijff, B. (1999) The lantibiotic nisin, a special case or not? *Biochimica et Biophysica Acta (BBA)* 1462, 223–234.

Bucki, R. and Janmey, P.A. (2006) Interaction of the gelsolin-derived antibacterial PBP 10 peptide with lipid bilayers and cell membranes. *Antimicrobial Agents and Chemotherapy* 50, 2932–2940. DOI: 10.1128/AAC.00134-06

Clejan, S., Guffanti, A.A., Cohen, M.A. and Krulwich, T.A. (1989) Mutation of *Bacillus firmus* OF4 to duramycin resistance results in substantial replacement of membrane lipid phosphatidylethanolamine by its plasmalogen form. *Journal of Bacteriology* 171, 1744–1746.

Dalebroux, Z.D., Matamouros, S., Whittington, D., Bishop, R.E. and Miller, S.I. (2014) PhoPQ regulates acidic glycerophospholipid content of the *Salmonella typhimurium* outer membrane. *Proceedings of National Academy of Sciences of the United States of America* 111, 1963–1968. DOI: 10.1073/pnas.1316901111

Destoumieux, D., Muñoz, M., Cosseau, C., Rodriguez, J., Bulet, P., Comps, M. and Bachère, E. (2000) Penaeidins, antimicrobial peptides with chitin-binding activity, are produced and stored in shrimp granulocytes and released after microbial challenge. *Journal of Cell Science* 113, 461–469.

Dotiwala, F., Mulik, S., Polidoro, R.B., Ansara, J.A., Burleigh, B.A., *et al.* (2016) Killer lymphocytes use granulysin, perforin and granzymes to kill intracellular parasites. *Nature Medicine* 22, 210–218. DOI: 10.1038/nm.4023

Epand, R.F., Savage, P.B. and Epand, R.M. (2007) Bacterial lipid composition and the antimicrobial efficacy of cationic steroid compounds (Ceragenins). *Biochimica et Biophysica Acta (BBA)* 1768, 2500–2509. DOI: 10.1016/j.bbamem.2007.05.023

Epand, R.M., Rotem, S., Mor, A., Berno, B. and Epand, R.F. (2008a) Bacterial membranes as predictors of antimicrobial potency. *Journal of American Chemical Society* 130, 14346–14352. DOI: 10.1021/ja8062327

Epand, R.F., Mowery, B.P., Lee, S.E., Stahl, S.S., Lehrer, R.I., Gellman, S.H. and Epand, R.M. (2008b) Dual mechanism of bacterial lethality for a cationic sequence-random copolymer that mimics host-defense antimicrobial peptides. *Journal of Molecular Biology* 379, 38–50. DOI: 10.1016/j.jmb.2008.03.047

Epand, R.F., Sarig, H., Mor, A. and Epand, R.M. (2009a) Cell-wall interactions and the selective bacteriostatic activity of a miniature oligo-acyl-lysyl. *Biophysical Journal* 97, 2250–2257. DOI: 10.1016/j.bpj.2009.08.006

Epand, R.F., Wang, G., Berno, B. and Epand, R.M. (2009b) Lipid segregation explains selective toxicity of a series of fragments derived from the human cathelicidin LL-37. *Antimicrobial Agents and Chemotherapy* 53, 3705–3714. DOI: 10.1128/AAC.00321-09

Epand, R.F., Sarig, H., Ohana, D., Papahadjopoulos-Sternberg, B., Mor, A. and Epand, R.M. (2011) Physical properties affecting cochleate formation and morphology using antimicrobial oligo-acyl-lysyl peptide mimetics and mixtures mimicking the composition of bacterial membranes in the absence of divalent cations. *Journal of Physical Chemistry B* 115, 2287–2293. DOI: 10.1021/jp111242q

Epand, R.M. and Epand, R.F. (2009) Domains in bacterial membranes and the action of antimicrobial agents. *Molecular Biosystems* 5, 580–587. DOI: 10.1039/b900278m

Epand, R.M. and Epand, R.F. (2010) Biophysical analysis of membrane-targeting antimicrobial peptides: membrane properties and the design of peptides specifically targeting Gram-negative bacetria. In: Wang, G. (ed.) *Antimicrobial Peptides: Discovery, Design and Novel Therapeutic Strategies.* CABI, Wallingford, UK, pp. 116–127.

Epand, R.M. and Epand, R.F. (2011) Bacterial membrane lipids in the action of antimicrobial agents. *Journal of Peptide Sciences* 17, 298–305. DOI: 10.1002/psc.1319

Epand, R.M., Epand, R.F., Arnusch, C.J., Papahadjopoulos-Sternberg, B., Wang, G. and Shai, Y. (2010) Lipid clustering by three homologous arginine-rich antimicrobial peptides is insensitive to amino acid arrangement and induced secondary structure. *Biochimica et Biophysica Acta (BBA)* 1798, 1272–1280. DOI: 10.1016/j.bbamem.2010.03.012

Epand, R.M., Walker, C., Epand, R.F. and Magarvey, N.A. (2015) Molecular mechanisms of membrane targeting antibiotics. *Biochimica et Biophysica Acta (BBA)* 1858, 980–987. DOI: 10.1016/j.bbamem.2015.10.018

Feigin, A.M., Schagina, L.V., Takemoto, J.Y., Teeter, J.H. and Brand, J.G. (1997) The effect of sterols on the sensitivity of membranes to the channel-forming antifungal antibiotic, syringomycin E. *Biochimica et Biophysica Acta (BBA)* 1324, 102–110.

Feng, C., Ling, H., Du, D., Zhang, J., Niu, G. and Tan, H. (2014) Novel nikkomycin analogues generated by mutasynthesis in *Streptomyces ansochromogenes*. *Microbial Cell Factories* 13, 59. DOI: 10.1186/1475-2859-13-59

Feng, Q., Huang, Y., Chen, M., Li, G. and Chen, Y. (2015) Functional synergy of α-helical antimicrobial peptides and traditional antibiotics against Gram-negative and Gram-positive bacteria in vitro and in vivo. *European Journal of Clinical Microbiology and Infectious Diseases* 34, 197–204. DOI: 10.1007/s10096-014-2219-3

Finger, S., Kerth, A., Dathe, M. and Blume, A. (2015) The efficacy of trivalent cyclic hexapeptides to induce lipid clustering in PG/PE membranes correlates with their antimicrobial activity. *Biochimica et Biophysica Acta (BBA) – Biomembranes* 1848, 2998–3006. DOI: 10.1016/j.bbamem.2015.09.012

Fredenhagen, A., Märki, F., Fendrich, G., Märki, W., Gruner, J., Van, Oostrum, J., Raschdorf, F. and Peter, H.H. (1991) Duramycin B and C, two new lanthionine-containing antibiotics as inhibitors of phospholipase A2, and structural revision of duramycin and cinnamycin. In: Jung, G. and Sahl, H.-G. (eds) *Nisin and Novel Lantibiotics*. ESCOM, Leiden, Netherlands, pp. 131–140.

Ganz, T., Selsted, M.E., Szklarek, D., Harwig, S.S.L., Daher, K., Bainton, D.F. and Lehrer, R.I. (1985) Defensins: natural peptides antibiotics of human neutrophils. *Journal of Clinical Investigation* 76, 1427–1435. DOI: 10.1172/JCI112120

Gaspar, D. and Castanho, M.A.R.B. (2016) Anticancer peptides: prospective innovation in cancer therapy. In: Epand, R.M. (ed.) *Host Defense Peptides and Their Potential as Therapeutic Agents*. Springer, Switzerland, pp. 95–109.

Goldberg, K., Sarig, H., Zaknoon, F., Epand, R.F., Epand, R.M. and Mor, A. (2013) Sensitization of Gram-negative bacteria by targeting the membrane potential. *FASEB Journal* 27 3818–3826. DOI: 10.1096/fj.13-227942

Gonçalves, S., Abade, J., Teixeira, A. and Santos, N.C. (2012a) Lipid composition is a determinant for human defensin HNP1 selectivity. *Biopolymers* 98, 313–321.

Gonçalves, S., Teixeira, A., Abade, J., de Medeiros, L.N., Kurtenbach, E. and Santos, N.C. (2012b) Evaluation of the membrane lipid selectivity of the pea defensin Psd1. *Biochimica et Biophysica Acta (BBA) – Biomembranes* 1818, 1420–1426. DOI: 10.1016/j/bbamen.2012.02.012

Grover, N.D. (2010) Echinocandins: a ray of hope in antifungal drug therapy. *Indian Journal of Pharmacology* 42, 9–11. DOI: 10.4103/0253-7613.62396

Huang, H.W., Chen, F.-Y. and Lee, M.-T. (2004) Molecular mechanism of peptide-induced pores in membranes. *Physical Review Letter* 92, 198304. DOI: 10.1103/PhysRevLett.92.198304

Jammal, J., Zaknoon, F., Kaneti, G., Goldberg, K. and Mor, A. (2015) Sensitization of Gram-negative bacteria to rifampin and OAK combinations. *Scientific Reports* 5, 9216. DOI: 10.1038/srep09216

Kaneti, G., Meir, O. and Mor, A. (2016) Controlling bacterial infections by inhibiting proton-dependent processes. *Biochimica et Biophysica Acta (BBA) – Biomembranes* 1858, 995–1003. DOI: 10.1016/j.bbamem.2015.10.022

Koprivnjak, T., Weidenmaier, C., Peschel, A. and Weiss, J.P. (2008) Wall teichoic acid deficiency in *Staphylococcus aureus* confers selective resistance to mammalian group IIA phospholipase A(2) and human beta-defensin 3. *Infection and Immunity* 76, 2169–2176. DOI: 10.1128/IAI.01705-07

Krivan, G., Sinkó, J., Nagy, I.Z., Goda, V., Reményi, P., *et al.* (2006) Successful combined antifungal salvage therapy with liposomal amphothericin B and caspofungin for invasive *Aspergillus flavus* infection in a child following allogeneic bone marrow transplantation. *Acta Biomedica* 77, 17–21.

Kuipers, M.E., de Vries, H.G., Eikelboom, M.C., Meijer, D.K. and Swart, P.J. (1999) Synergistic fungistatic effects of lactoferrin in combination with antifungal drugs against clinical *Candida* isolates. *Antimicrobial Agents and Chemotherapy* 43, 2635–2641.

Lehrer, R.I., Barton, A. and Ganz, T. (1988) Concurrent assessment of inner and outer membrane permeabilization and bacteriolysis in *E. coli* by multiple-wavelength spectrophotometry. *Journal of Immunological Methods* 108, 153–158. DOI: 10.1016/0022-1759(88)90414-0

Lehrer, R.I., Barton, A., Daher, K.A., Harwig, S.S.L., Ganz, T. and Selsted, M.E. (1989) Interaction of human defensins with *Escherichia coli*: Mechanism of bactericidal activity. *Journal of Clinical Investigation* 84, 553–561. DOI: 10.1172/JCI114198

Livne, L., Epand, R.F., Papahadjopoulos-Sternberg, B., Epand, R.M. and Mor, A. (2010) OAK-based cochleates as a novel approach to overcome multidrug resistance in bacteria. *FASEB Journal* 24, 5092–5101. DOI: 10.1096/fj.10-167809

Lohner, K. and Blondelle, S.E. (2005) Molecular mechanisms of membrane perturbation by antimicrobial peptides and the use of biophysical studies in the design of novel peptide antibiotics. *Combinatorial Chemistry and High Throughput Screening* 8, 241–256.

Lohner, K. and Leber, R. (2016) Antifungal host defense peptides. In: Epand, R.M. (ed.) *Host Defense Peptides and Theeir Potential as Therapeutic Agents*. Springer, Switzerland, pp. 27–56.

Malanovic, N. and Lohner, K. (2016) Gram-positive bacterial cell envelopes: the impact on the activity of antimicrobial peptides. *Biochimica et Biophysica Acta (BBA)* 1858, 936–946. DOI: 10.1016/j.bbamem.2015.11.004

Mangoni, M.L., Epand, R.F., Rosenfeld, Y., Peleg, A., Barra, D., Epand, R.M. and Shai, Y. (2008) Lipopolysaccharide, a key molecule involved in the synergism between temporins in inhibiting bacterial growth and in endotoxin neutralization. *Journal of Biological Chemistry* 283, 22907–22917. DOI: 10.1074/jbc.M800495200

Manzini, M.C., Perez, K.R., Riske, K.A., Bozelli, J.C. Jr., Santos, T.L., *et al.* (2014) Peptide:lipid ratio and membrane surface charge determine the mechanism of action of the antimicrobial peptide BP100. Conformational and functional studies. *Biochimica et Biophysica Acta (BBA) – Biomembranes* 1838, 1985–1999. DOI: 10.1016/j.bbamem.2014.04.004

Mizuhara, N., Kuroda, M., Ogita, A., Tanaka, T., Usuki, Y. and Fujita, K. (2011) Antifungal thipeptidecyclothiazomycin B1 exhibits growth inhibition accompanying morphological changes via binding to fungal cell wall chitin. *Bioorganic and Medical Chemistry* 19, 5300–5310. DOI: 10.1016/j.bmc.2011.08.010

Mor, A. (2016) Enginereed OAKs against antibiotic resistance and for bacterial detection. In: Epand, R.M. (ed.) *Host Defense Peptides and Their Potential as Therapeutic Agents*. Springer, Switzerland, pp. 205–226.

Mularski, A., Wilksch, J.J., Wang, H., Hossain, M.A., Wade, J.D., Separovic, F., Strugnell, R.A. and Gee M.L. (2015) Atomic force microscopy reveals the mechanobiology of lytic peptide action on bacteria. *Langmuir* 31, 6164–6171. DOI: 10.1021/acs.langmuir.5b01011

Phoenix, D.A., Harris, F., Mura, M. and Dennison, S.R. (2015) The increasing role of phosphatidylethanolamine as a lipid receptor in the action of host defence peptides. *Progress in Lipid Research* 59, 26–37. DOI: 10.1016/j.plipres.2015.02.003

Rogozhin, E.A., Slezina, M.P., Slavokhotova, A.A., Istomina, E.A., Korostyleva, T.V., *et al.* (2015) A novel antifungal peptide from leaves of the weed *Stellaria media L. Biochimie* 116, 125–132. DOI: 10.1016/j.biochi.2015.07.014

Saar-Dover, R., Bitler, A., Nezer, R., Shmuel-Galia, L., Firon, A., Shimoni, E., Trieu-Cuot, P. and Shai, Y. (2012) D-alanylation of lipoteichoic acids confers resistance to cationic peptides in group B streptococcus by increasing the cell wall density. *PLoS Pathogens* 8, e1002891. DOI: 10.1371/journal.ppat.1002891

Sahl, H.G., Jack, R.W. and Bierbaum, G. (1995) Biosynthesis and biological activities of lantibiotics with unique post-translational modifications. *European Journal of Biochemistry* 230, 827–853.

Salay, L.C., Procopio, J., Oliveira, E., Nakaie, C.R. and Schreier, S. (2004) Ion channel-like activity of the antimicrobial peptide tritrpticin in planar lipid bilayers. *FEBS Letters* 565, 171–175. DOI: 10.1016/j.febslet.2004.03.093

Sarig, H., Ohana, D., Epand, R.F., Mor, A. and Epand, R.M. (2011) Functional studies of cochleate assemblies of an oligo-acyl-lysyl with lipid mixtures for combating bacterial multidrug resistance. *FASEB Journal* 25, 3336–3343. DOI: 10.1096/fj.11-183764

Sautrey, G., El Khoury, M., dos Santos, A.G., Zimmermann, L., Deleu, M., Lins, L., Decout, J.L. and Mingeot-Leclercq, M.P. (2016) Negatively charged lipids as a potential target for new amphiphilic aminoglycoside antibiotics: a biophysical study. *Journal of Biological Chemistry* 291, 13864–13874. DOI: 10.1074/jbc.M115.665364

Schibli, D.J., Epand, R.F., Vogel, H.J. and Epand, R.M. (2002) Tryptophan-rich antimicrobial peptides: comparative properties and membrane interactions. *Biochemistry and Cell Biology* 80, 667–677.

Schibli, D.J., Nguyen, L.T., Kernaghan, S.D., Rekdal, Ø. and Vogel, H.J. (2006) Structure-function analysis of tritrpticin analogues: potential relationships between antimicrobial activities, model membrane interactions, and their micelle bound NMR structures. *Biophysical Journal* 91, 4413–4426. DOI: 10.1529/biophysj.106.085837

Shai, Y. (2002) Mode of action of membrane active antimicrobial peptides. *Biopolymers* 66, 236–248. DOI: 10.1002/bip.10260

Sousa, F.H., Casanova, V., Stevens, C. and Barlow, P.G. (2016) Antiviral host defense peptides. In: Epand, R.M. (ed.) *Host Defense Peptides and Their Potential as Therapeutic Agents.* Springer, Switzerland, pp. 57–94.

Steiner, H., Hultmark, D., Engstrom, A., Bennich, H. and Boman, H.G. (1981) Sequence and specificity of two antibacterial proteins involved in insect immunity. *Nature* 292, 246–248.

Takemoto, J.Y., Yu, Y., Stock, S.D. and Miyakawa, T. (1993) Yeast genes involved in growth inhibition by *Pseudomonas syringae* pv *syringae* syringomycin family lipodepsipeptides. *FEMS Microbiology Letters* 114, 339–342.

Thevissen, K., Cammue, B.P., Lemaire, K., Winderickx, J., Dickson, R.C., Lester, R.L., Ferket, K.K., van Even, F., Parret, A.H. and Broekaert, W.F. (2000) A gene encoding a sphingolipid biosynthesis enzyme determines the sensitivity of *Saccharomyces cerevisiae* to an antifungal plant defensin from dahlia (*Dahlia merckii*). *Proceedings of National Academy of Sciences of the United States of America* 97, 9531–9536. DOI: 10.1073/pnas.100077797

Thevissen, K., Warnecke, D.C., François, I.E.J.A., Leipelt, M., Heinz, E., *et al.* (2004) Defensins from insects and plants interact with fungal glucosylceramides. *Journal of Biological Chemistry* 279, 3900–3905. DOI: 10.1074/jbc.M311165200

Thevissen, K., François, I.E.J.A., Aerts, A.M. and Cammue, B.P.A. (2005) Fungal sphingolipids as targets for the developments of selective antifungal therapeutics. *Current Drug Targets* 6, 923–928.

van't Hof, W., Reijnders, I.M., Helmerhorst, E.J., Walgreen-Weterings, E., Simoons-Smit, I.M., Veerman, E.C. and Amerongen, A.V. (2000) Synergistic effects of low doses of histatin 5 and its analogues on amphotericin B anti-mycotic activity. *Antonie Van Leeuwenhoek* 78, 163–169.

Wade, D., Boman, A., Wåhlin, B., Drain, C.M., Andreu, D., Boman, H.G. and Merrifield, R.B. (1990) All-D amino acid-containing channel-forming antibiotic peptides. *Proceedings of National Academy of Sciences of the United States of America* 87, 4761–4765. DOI: 10.1073/pnas.87.12.4761

Wadhwani, P., Epand, R.F., Heidenreich, N., Burck, J., Ulrich, A.S. and Epand, R.M. (2012) Membrane-active peptides and the clustering of anionic lipids. *Biophysical Journal* 103, 265–274. DOI: 10.1016/j.bpj.2012.06.004

Wang, G., Li, X. and Wang, Z. (2016) APD3: the antimicrobial peptide database as a tool for research and education. *Nucleic Acids Research* 44, D1087–D1093. DOI: 10.1093/nar/gkv1278

Wen, Y.L., Wu, B.J., Kao, P.H., Fu, Y.S. and Chang, L.S. (2013) Antibacterial and membrane-damaging activities of beta-bungarotoxin B chain. *Journal Peptide Sciences* 19, 1–8. DOI: 10.1002/psc.2463

Yang, S.-T., Shin, S.Y., Lee, C.W., Kim, Y.-C., Hahm, K.-S. and Kim, J.I. (2003) Selective cytotoxicity following Arg-to-Lys substitution in tritrpticin adopting a unique amphipathic turn structure. *FEBS Letters* 540, 229–233.

Yang, S.-T., Lee, J.Y., Kim, H.-J., Eu, Y.-J., Shin, S.Y., Hahm, K.-S. and Kim, J.I. (2006) Contribution of a central proline in model amphipathic α-helical peptides to self-association, interaction with phospholipids, and antimicrobial mode of action. *FEBS Journal* 273, 4040–4054. DOI: 10.1111/j.1742-4658.2006.05407.x

Zasloff, M. (1987) Magainins, a class of antimicrobial peptides from *Xenopus* skin: isolation, characterization of two active forms, and partial cDNA sequence of a precursor. *Proceedings of National Academy of Sciences of the United States of America* 84, 5449–5453.

Zhang, S.-K., Song, J.-W., Gong, F., Li, S.-B., Chang, H.-Y., *et al.* (2016) Design of an α-helical antimicrobial peptide with improved cell-selective and potent anti-biofilm activity. *Scientific Reports* 6, 27394. DOI: 10.1038/srep27394

Zweytick, D., Japelj, B., Mileykovskaya, E., Zorko, M., Dowhan, W., *et al.* (2014) N-acylated peptides derived from human lactoferricin perturb organization of cardiolipin and phosphatidylethanolamine in cell membranes and induce defects in *Escherichia coli* cell division. *PLoS One* 9, e90228. DOI: 10.1371/journal.pone.0090228

9 Non-membranolytic Mechanisms of Action of Antimicrobial Peptides – Novel Therapeutic Opportunities?

Marco Scocchi*, Mario Mardirossian, Giulia Runti and Monica Benincasa

Department of Life Sciences, University of Trieste, via Giorgieri 5, 34127 Trieste, Italy

Abstract

Antimicrobial peptides (AMPs) possess a remarkable capacity to inactivate and kill microorganisms by their well-established lytic activity on target membranes. However, an ever-increasing set of data highlights the importance of non-lytic modes of action for a number of AMPs, which affect target microorganisms acting through their interaction with specific molecular targets. Data indicate that these non-membrane-permeabilizing AMPs inhibit protein synthesis, nucleic acid functions and essential intracellular enzymes, or affect cell wall synthesis. Recent findings on these non-lytic modes of antimicrobial action, which appear to be alternative or complementary to membrane lysis, are reviewed here with specific attention to those for which sufficient data have been collected to support a mode of action with a real contribution of killing without lytic activity. A detailed knowledge of this class of AMPs and of their mechanism of action is very important in the design of novel antibacterial agents against unexploited targets, endowed with the capacity to penetrate into pathogen cells and kill them from within.

9.1 Introduction

Bacterial resistance to antibiotics is on the rise and a return to the 'pre-antibiotic' era has become a frightening possibility (Frère and Rigali, 2016). The problem is so serious that in some cases antibiotic resistance now represents a potential public health disaster, with a real threat that infectious diseases may soon be untreatable in certain circumstances (Whiley *et al.*, 2012). For this reason, the development of new bactericidal agents which target resistant pathogens is a compelling need. Increasing antibiotic-resistance limits the useful lifespan of antibiotics and results in the requirement for a constant introduction of new compounds, possibly with mechanisms of action different from those of known antibiotics, which could raise problems in terms of cross-resistance (Coates *et al.*, 2011).

Antimicrobial peptides (AMPs) represent promising therapeutic agents because of their rapid and broad-spectrum antimicrobial properties (Hadley and Hancock, 2010). AMPs are a vast group of oligopeptides with wide variations in their mass, amino acid residue composition, charge, three-dimensional structure and biological

* Corresponding author e-mail: mscocchi@units.it

characteristics (Brogden and Brogden, 2011). They are widely distributed throughout nature and produced by organisms of all kingdoms of life. In some species AMPs serve as the primary antimicrobial defence mechanism, yet in other species they are multifunctional molecules with a central role in infection and inflammation, and serve as an adjunct to existing innate and adaptive immune systems (Hadley and Hancock, 2010; Brogden and Brogden, 2011). All AMPs show direct antimicrobial activity against bacteria, several of them also demonstrate efficacy against viruses, fungi and parasites (Bahar and Ren, 2013). Moreover, certain AMPs are known to stimulate cytokine release, chemotaxis, antigen presentation, angiogenesis and wound healing (Diamond *et al.*, 2009; Lai and Gallo, 2009) or have been shown to be cytotoxic for certain tumours (Gaspar *et al.*, 2013).

Generally, two physical features are common for AMPs. Firstly they are generally cationic in physiological conditions due to a high content of arginine and lysine residues that promotes selectivity for negatively charged microbial cytoplasmic membranes over zwitterionic mammalian membranes. Secondly, most classes have a high proportion (up to 50%) of hydrophobic residues that allow them to fold or arrange into a variety of amphipathic structures and conformations, and to interact with lipids (Nguyen *et al.*, 2011). Amphipathic residue arrangement and positive charges explain their high propensity for *in vitro* interaction with anionic lipid bilayers (Shai, 2002; Scocchi *et al.*, 2005; Nguyen *et al.*, 2011).

Based on their amino acid composition and secondary structure, all AMPs can be divided into four major classes: α-helical, β-sheet, β-hairpin and peptides with extended conformation (Tossi *et al.*, 2000; Brogden, 2005; see also Chapter 1). Extensive studies carried out on members of all four classes of AMPs indicate that the damage and/or permeabilization of microbial cytoplasmic membranes is the major mechanism for killing cells for most AMPs (Sitaram and Nagaraj, 1999). The membrane-permeation process takes place via two major consecutive steps: (i) peptides initially bind onto the membrane surface until a threshold concentration is reached; and (ii) peptides organize themselves to form a permeation pathway (Shai, 2002; Zasloff, 2002). This process does not involve the binding to specific receptors on the cell membrane but rather a non-specific interaction with membrane phospholipids (Yeaman and Yount, 2003). Details on the modes of action of AMPs based on membrane permeabilization are described in a number of excellent reviews (Shai, 2002; Wimley, 2010; Brogden and Brogden, 2011; Nguyen *et al.*, 2011).

Not all AMPs are believed to exert their killing action solely via bacterial membranes. In the last few years an increasing number of AMPs have been shown to kill microorganisms by a mechanism different from, or in addition to, membrane-permeabilizing/disrupting activity (Brogden, 2005; Hale and Hancock, 2007; Nicolas, 2009; Scocchi *et al.*, 2016; Wang *et al.*, 2015). These peptides, collectively named 'non-lytic AMPs', generally either translocate across bacterial membranes and bind to intracellular targets, or exert their activity at the level of the cell wall. In any case the killing event, determined by their activity, is thought to be different from membranolysis (Otvos, 2005; Scocchi *et al.*, 2016).

It is widely recognized that virtually all AMPs have a high affinity for microbial membranes, leading to a certain degree of perturbation (Melo *et al.*, 2009; Nicolas, 2009; Zasloff, 2002). For non-lytic peptides the membrane-permeabilizing effects become significant only when their concentrations are increased well above their minimum inhibitory concentration (MIC) values. For example, the α-helical pleurocidins from winter flounder do not permeabilize the *E. coli* cytoplasmic membrane when applied at five times its MIC value, but they cause membrane depolarization when applied at ten times the MIC (Patrzykat *et al.*, 2002). The proline-rich peptide Bac7, at near-MIC concentrations, inactivates *E. coli* via a mechanism based on a specific uptake that is followed by its binding to intracellular targets, but it can also kill bacteria through a secondary membranolytic mechanism when applied at concentrations several times its MIC value (Podda *et al.*, 2006).

The temporal dissociation between cell death and changes in membrane permeability are common and important aspects observed in non-lytic AMPs. Lysis of the microbial membrane and cell killing are rapid and concomitant events for lytic antimicrobial peptides, (Yount *et al.*, 2006). Conversely, non-lytic AMPs often show a lag period after cell killing before membrane damage is observed. The lag period is interpreted as a secondary effect due to the decomposition of already non-viable bacteria (Schneider *et al.*, 2010) and it has also been observed with some antibiotics having intracellular targets (Walberg *et al.*, 1997; Wickens *et al.*, 2000). These observations suggest that in a non-membranolytic killing, membrane damage and cell death are independent events that occur at different times and/or concentrations.

9.2 Intracellular Mode of Action

Several non-lytic AMPs act inside the bacterial cells against intracellular targets (Nicolas, 2009; Scocchi *et al.*, 2016). Despite their intracellular localization, the precise mechanism whereby some AMPs enter bacterial cells is not clear. Two major mechanisms have been proposed: (i) translocation mediated by bacterial proteins; and (ii) spontaneous translocation.

Membrane translocation mediated by a bacterial protein has been observed for the proline-rich group of antimicrobial peptides (PR-AMPs) (Mattiuzzo *et al.*, 2007; Scocchi *et al.*, 2011; Berthold and Hoffmann, 2014). Different PR-AMPs expressed in mammals, insects and crustaceans, including PR-39, Bac7, apidaecin 1b, oncocin and arasin 1, exploit the inner membrane protein SbmA to efficiently penetrate into *E. coli* and other Gram-negative bacteria (Mattiuzzo *et al.*, 2007; Runti *et al.*, 2013; Berthold and Hoffmann, 2014; Paulsen *et al.*, 2016). In *E. coli* some PR-AMPs appear to rely exclusively on the SbmA

uptake system (Krizsan *et al.*, 2015a) whereas others, including Bac7(1-35) and oncocin, are quite active also in SbmA-deleted strains probably because of the presence of a second bacterial transport system recently identified as the *yjiL-mdtM* gene cluster (Krizsan *et al.*, 2015a). Spontaneous translocation has been proposed by the Shai-Matsuzaki-Huang model (Huang, 2000; Matsuzaki, 1998; Shai, 2002). According to this model, peptides first bind to the membrane surface and then insert into the membrane as a result of their amphipathic structure, forming transient pores. Upon disintegration of these pores, some peptides become translocated to the inner leaflet of the membrane. Below the critical peptide concentration that can cause a collapse of the membrane itself, peptide passage preserves the integrity of the membrane, which is only transiently breached. Direct translocation has been observed for certain cell-penetrating peptides, sharing some features with AMPs that spontaneously translocate across synthetic lipid bilayer membranes without permeabilizing them (Marks *et al.*, 2011; Di Pisa *et al.*, 2015).

Both single and multiple targets have been proposed for different non-lytic AMPs. The main mechanisms of action include inhibition of protein synthesis, DNA binding affecting transcription/replication, and inactivation of fundamental enzyme activities (Fig 9.1). Different levels of understanding and knowledge have been reached for the different mechanisms. Some examples of the most documented/studied are shown in Table 9.1.

9.2.1 Inhibition of molecular chaperones and protein synthesis

Some non-lytic peptides have been shown to interfere with protein synthesis. Evidence of this mode of action has been reported for a derivative of pleurocidin (Patrzykat *et al.*, 2002), for CP10A, a variant of the indolicidin (Friedrich *et al.*, 2001), and for lactoferricin B (Ulvatne *et al.*, 2004) even if its specificity for inhibition of

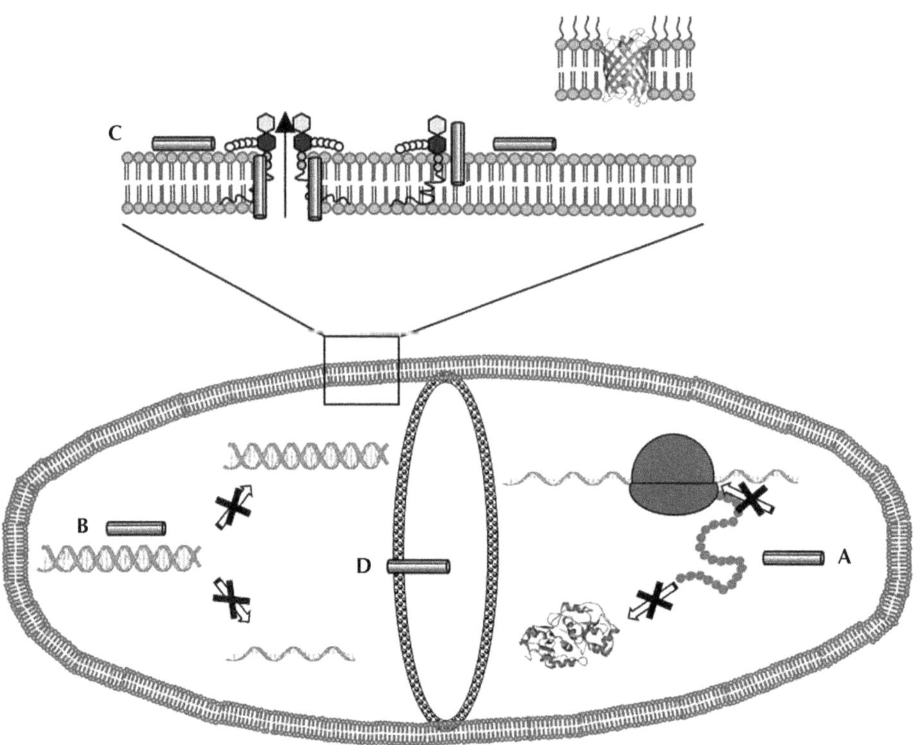

Fig. 9.1. Schematic diagram (unscaled) of the different mechanisms of action of non-lytic AMPs. Iinhibition of protein synthesis and/or chaperones (A), binding to DNA and inhibition of transcription/replication (B), inhibition of cell wall synthesis and outer membrane biogenesis (C), and inhibition of cytokinesis (D). Peptides were schematically represented with cylinders ▬▬.

protein synthesis was unclear. Bacterial protein synthesis and the inhibition of molecular chaperones have been shown to represent a relevant target also for proline-rich antimicrobial peptides (PR-AMPs) isolated from different organisms ranging from mammals (Gennaro *et al.*, 1989; Agerberth *et al.*, 1991) to insects (Casteels *et al.*, 1989; Knappe *et al.*, 2010). First evidence of non-lytic activity was observed for the honeybee AMP apidaecin, for which a hypothesis of inhibition of protein synthesis in living bacteria has been formulated (Castle *et al.*, 1999). The inhibition of protein – but also the macromolecular synthesis in general – has been observed for the native full-length porcine peptide PR-39 and for the bovine Bac7. These peptides, in poor media and near the bacteriostatic concentration, inhibit DNA or DNA and RNA synthesis respectively (Boman *et al.*, 1993; Skerlavaj *et al.*, 1990). Moreover, a sub-lethal concentration of Bac7 induces in *E. coli* the overexpression of many genes involved in the transcription/translation process (Tomasinsig *et al.*, 2004), suggesting that bacteria modulate their gene expression to counteract the interfering activity of the peptide on these processes.

Further evidence has been provided suggesting that PR-AMPs interfere with the biosynthesis of correctly folded proteins. The insect pyrrhocoricin, drosocin and apidaecin have been shown to bind specifically the heat-shock protein DnaK, and in a minor extent also the chaperone GroEL (Morell *et al.*, 2008; Otvos *et al.*, 2000). A link was found between the antimicrobial potency of some pyrrhocoricin fragments and their capability to inhibit DnaK, indicating that this chaperone was at least one of the final intracellular targets.

Table 9.1.   List of representative AMPs with description of their non-lytic modes of action.

Mode of action	Peptide	Additional remarks	References
Inhibition of chaperones and protein synthesis	Pleurocidin	Inhibition of protein synthesis *in vivo*.	(Patrzykat *et al.*, 2002)
	Lactoferricin B	Specificity for protein synthesis not completely clear.	(Ulvatne *et al.*, 2004)
	Apidaecin	Binding to DnaK, GroEL and trigger factor. Binding to specific ribosomal proteins and inhibition of protein synthesis *in vitro* and *in vivo*.	(Otvos *et al.*, 2000; Volke *et al.*, 2015; Krizsan *et al.*, 2014; Mardirossian *et al.*, 2014; Farkas *et al.*, 2014)
	Pyrrhocoricin	Binding to DnaK and GroEL. Inhibition of *in vitro* translation. Resolved crystallographic structure in complex with ribosomes.	(Otvos *et al.*, 2000; Taniguchi *et al.*, 2016; Seefeldt *et al.*, 2016; Gagnon *et al.*, 2016)
	Drosocin	Binding to DnaK and GroEL.	(Otvos *et al.*, 2000)
	Oncocin	Binding to DnaK and specific ribosomal proteins. Inhibition of protein synthesis *in vitro* and *in vivo*. Resolved crystallographic structure in complex with ribosomes.	(Knappe *et al.*, 2011; Volke *et al.*, 2015; Krizsan *et al.*, 2014; Mardirossian *et al.*, 2014; Farkas *et al.*, 2014; Seefeldt *et al.*, 2015; Roy *et al.*, 2015)
	Bac7	Binding to DnaK and specific ribosomal proteins. Inhibition of protein synthesis *in vitro* and *in vivo*. Resolved crystallographic structure in complex with ribosomes.	(Scocchi *et al.*, 2009; Zahn *et al.*, 2014; Krizsan *et al.*, 2014; Mardirossian *et al.*, 2014; Farkas *et al.*, 2014; Seefeldt *et al.*, 2016; Gagnon *et al.*, 2016)
	PR-39	Inhibition of protein synthesis *in vivo*.	(Boman *et al.*, 1993)
Binding to DNA and inhibition of transcription/ replication	Buforin II	Binding *in vitro* to duplex DNA.	(Park *et al.*, 1998; Park *et al.*, 2000; Uyterhoeven *et al.*, 2008; Cho *et al.*, 2009; Lan *et al.*, 2010; Hao *et al.*, 2013; Cutrona *et al.*, 2015)
	Indolicidin	Inhibition of DNA synthesis.	(Subbalakshmi and Sitaram, 1998; Friedrich *et al.*, 2001; Hsu *et al.*, 2005; Shaw *et al.*, 2006; Nan *et al.*, 2009; Ghosh *et al.*, 2014)
	Fallaxin	Inhibition of DNA synthesis and induction of the SOS DNA damage response.	(Gottschalk *et al.*, 2015)
Inhibition of cell-wall synthesis and outer membrane biogenesis	Nisin	Binding and relocation of lipid II in the membrane.	(Wiedemann *et al.*, 2001; Hasper *et al.*, 2004; 't Hart *et al.*, 2016)
	Mutacin 1140	Lipid II segregation observed in GUVs and *in vivo*.	(Hasper *et al.*, 2006)
	Plectasin	Binding to lipid I and lipid II.	(Schneider *et al.*, 2010)
	Copsin	Binding to lipid II.	(Essig *et al.*, 2014)
	L27-11 and POL7001	Binding to LptD and impairment of its function.	(Srinivas *et al.*, 2010)
Inhibition of cytokinesis	CRAMP	Binding to FtsZ and inhibition of septum formation *in vivo*.	(Rosenberger *et al.*, 2004; Ray *et al.*, 2014)
Other membrane-independent mechanisms	Daptomycin	Misregulated recruitment of the cell division protein DivIVC.	(Pogliano *et al.*, 2012; Taylor and Palmer, 2016)
	θ-defensins	Release of autolytic enzymes responsible for cell wall degradation.	(Wilmes *et al.*, 2014)
	Magainin-2	Effects resembling typical apoptosis hallmarks.	(Lee and Lee, 2014)

The inhibition is explained primarily by the steric block of the chaperone and secondly by a competition between the peptide and the proteins for the chaperone's active site (Kragol *et al.*, 2001; Kragol *et al.*, 2002). Interestingly the all-D isomers of some PR-AMPs are inactive, suggesting that the interaction between PR-AMPs and DnaK is stereospecific (Kragol *et al.*, 2001; Scocchi *et al.*, 2009). More recently, the binding to DnaK has also been reported for other PR-AMPs, i.e. different apidaecins (Czihal *et al.*, 2012) and oncocins (Knappe *et al.*, 2011), as well as many fragments and derivatives of pyrrhocoricin, drosocin and A3-APO (Zahn *et al.*, 2013). In addition other chaperones, such as GroEL, and the trigger factor have been identified as *in vivo* interacting partners of the apidaecin derivative Api88 (Volke *et al.*, 2015). The bovine Bac7 also binds DnaK (Scocchi *et al.*, 2009; Zahn *et al.*, 2014) and interferes with the activity of the DnaK/DnaJ/GrpE/ATP complex (Scocchi *et al.*, 2009). The targeting to DnaK has also been exploited to rationally design the artificial PR-AMP A3-APO with enhanced antimicrobial activity (Otvos *et al.*, 2005). However, at least for Bac7 and oncocin, the inhibition of DnaK activity is insufficient to kill bacteria. In fact, *E. coli* cells lacking DnaK at permissive temperature are still susceptible to these molecules, suggesting the existence of other targets (Scocchi *et al.*, 2009; Krizsan *et al.*, 2014).

Recently, ribosomes and protein synthesis have been indicated as a main target for different PR-AMPs. The PR-AMPs derivatives Api88, Onc72 and Bac7(1-35) inhibit protein synthesis *in vitro* (Krizsan *et al.*, 2014; Mardirossian *et al.*, 2014) as well as in living *E. coli* cells (Mardirossian *et al.*, 2014). The *in vitro* inhibition of bacterial translation was also observed for other PR-AMPs including pyrrhocoricin (Seefeldt *et al.*, 2016; Taniguchi *et al.*, 2016) and for metalnikowin1 (Seefeldt *et al.*, 2016). Api88 was shown to bind bacterial ribosomes by specific interactions with ribosomal proteins (Volke *et al.*, 2015) and, more recently, crystallographic studies carried out with *Thermus thermophilus* 70S ribosome have identified the A-site and the exit tunnel of the ribosome as the site of binding of the 19-residue PR-AMP Onc112 (Roy *et al.*, 2015; Seefeldt *et al.*, 2015). This binding site and mechanism of inhibition have been confirmed also for Bac7(1-16) and Bac7(1-35), metalnikowin1, pyrrhocoricin and Onc112 derivatives (Gagnon *et al.*, 2016; Seefeldt *et al.*, 2016). Biochemical evidence indicates that all these peptides prevent bacterial ribosomes from entering the elongation phase of protein synthesis (Gagnon *et al.*, 2016; Seefeldt *et al.*, 2015; Seefeldt *et al.*, 2016), whereas apidaecin-type peptides have a different mechanism, blocking the assembly of the large (50S) subunit of the ribosome (Krizsan *et al.*, 2015b).

Surprisingly, Bac7 fragments also inhibit *in vitro* the eukaryotic translation, even if less efficiently than bacterial translation (Seefeldt *et al.*, 2016). This result seems in contrast to previous data showing that Bac7 fragments, as for most PR-AMPs (Hansen *et al.*, 2012), exhibit very low cytotoxicity (Benincasa *et al.*, 2010; Pelillo *et al.*, 2014; Tomasinsig *et al.*, 2006). Since Bac7(1-35) penetrates eukaryotic cells mainly by macropinocytosis (Tomasinsig *et al.*, 2006) it probably does not freely diffuse into the cytosol and hence it does not interact with ribosomes.

Bacterial protein synthesis is also affected by AMPs other than PR-AMPs. The cysteine-rich antimicrobial peptide NCR247 from the plant *Medicago truncatula* interacts with ribosomal proteins of the bacterial endosymbiont *Synorhizobium meliloti*, hosted in root nodules (Farkas *et al.*, 2014). Two interesting short peptides, GE81112 and GE82832, isolated from metabolites of *Actinomicetes*, block *in vitro* and *in vivo* bacterial protein synthesis in a different manner from that of PR-AMPs. These peptides bind to the small ribosomal subunit and inhibit respectively the starting of the translocation and the EF-G-catalysed translocation (Bulkley *et al.*, 2014; Brandi *et al.*, 2006a; Brandi *et al.*, 2006b; Brandi *et al.*, 2012).

Understanding the mechanisms by which all these non-lytic AMPs inhibit protein synthesis could provide an opportunity for structure-based design of new-generation therapeutics. These peptides are particularly active against Gram-negative strains (Benincasa *et al.*, 2004; Bluhm *et al.*, 2015) but the spectrum of activity has been extended to Gram-positive species by rational design of new apidaecin and oncocin derivatives (Bluhm *et al.*, 2015; Knappe *et al.*, 2016b) or by using them in combination with other AMPs (Knappe *et al.*, 2016a). Oncocins and apidaecins were demonstrated to have *in vivo* antimicrobial activity in murine *E. coli* and *K. pneumoniae* infections (Knappe *et al.*, 2012; Ostorhazi *et al.*, 2014; Knappe *et al.*, 2015; Schmidt *et al.*, 2016), while Bac7(1-35) provided a protective effect on mice infected by *S. typhimurium* (Benincasa *et al.*, 2010) and the artificial A3-APO PR-AMP gave promising results when tested on mice with *E. coli* bacteriaemia (Szabo *et al.*, 2010). The designer A3-APO is also involved in immunostimulation and epithelial tissue repair, eliminating wound infections and promoting wound healing in Gram-positive and Gram-negative mouse skin burns (Otvos and Ostorhazi, 2015). Recent elucidation of the molecular mechanism of action will help us design more potent peptides based on PR-AMPs and to extend the potential therapeutic applications.

9.2.2 Binding to DNA and inhibition of transcription/replication

Several studies highlight the capability of a number of AMPs to interact *in vitro* with nucleic acids (DNA and/or RNA) (Park *et al.*, 1998; Subbalakshmi and Sitaram, 1998; Yonezawa *et al.*, 1992; Haney *et al.*, 2013). This is not surprising given that these molecules are highly positively charged (Scocchi *et al.*, 2016), although it is difficult to infer if this interaction has a relevant biological effect. The most cited example of DNA-binding AMP is represented by buforin II, a H2A-histone derivative from the toad *Bufo bufo gargarizans*. In the original study Park *et al.* (1998) determined that buforin II is able to translocate into *E. coli* without membrane damage and to bind to DNA (Park *et al.* 1998; Park

et al., 2000; Cho *et al.*, 2009; Cutrona *et al.*, 2015), a mode of action also exhibited by the histone-derived AMP DesHDAPs (Pavia *et al.*, 2012). Subsequently it was shown that buforin with increased arginine content exhibited improved antibacterial activity and translocation effects (Cutrona *et al.*, 2015). This peptide adopts an extended conformation when bound to DNA. (Lan *et al.*, 2010). The *in vitro* binding of buforin to duplex DNA was also confirmed by its variants (Lan *et al.*, 2010), which suggests a relationship between DNA affinity and antimicrobial efficacy (Hao *et al.*, 2013; Uyterhoeven *et al.*, 2008). In particular, the reallocation of the central proline residue seems to be crucial for the internalization of buforin variants (Cutrona *et al.*, 2015; Kobayashi *et al.*, 2000).

There are several other examples of AMPs that are thought to bind to and inhibit important DNA functions. However, it is worth noting that most studies do not explain in detail the mechanism by which the AMP is internalized into the cells and/or do not report whether the *in vitro* intracellular activity is measured under non-membrane-permeabilizing conditions. For example, gel-retardation assays and footprinting analysis highlight the DNA binding ability of the 17 amino-acid horseshoe crab peptide tachyplesin I (Imura *et al.*, 2007; Yonezawa *et al.*, 1992). By microscopic techniques, it has also been shown that tachyplesin I at active concentrations forms pores in the cell membrane without flow of cytoplasmic content (Hong *et al.*, 2015), making it uncertain whether DNA interaction has a physiological relevance in the activity of this peptide. Retarded migration of DNA bound by short arginine-, lysine- and tryptophan-containing lipopeptides, such as C10-RIKWWK and C10-RKWWK, in a DNA-binding assay is in agreement with an intracellular mechanism of action. However, these AMPs efficiently disrupt the integrity of bacterial membranes making the contribution of DNA binding to their antimicrobial activity uncertain (Fang *et al.*, 2014).

The study of the modes of action of different Trp-rich peptides such as the 13-mer cathelicidin indolicidin has provided controversial results. This very small peptide inhibits DNA synthesis (Subbalakshmi and Sitaram, 1998; Hsu *et al.*, 2005) but also promotes significant membrane depolarization and lysis (Shaw *et al.*, 2006; Nan *et al.*, 2009). The structural details of its interaction with DNA have been investigated at an atomic resolution in a recent study (Ghosh *et al.*, 2014). Results of microscopy studies in conjunction with spectroscopic data confirmed that the DNA duplex is stabilized by indolicidin, thereby inhibiting DNA replication and transcription (Ghosh *et al.*, 2014).

Replacement of three proline residues of indolicidin with three alanine residues resulted in the peptide CP10A, which retained full antibacterial activity and showed multiple intracellular modes of action (Friedrich *et al.*, 2001). Electron microscopy showed minimal effects of the peptide on the cell wall; however membrane depolarization by CP10A was very efficient. Macromolecular synthesis assays indicated that nucleic acid and protein production were also affected by the peptide (Friedrich *et al.*, 2001).

Biophysical characterization of PuroB, another Trp-rich peptide designed on the sequence of puroindoline proteins, suggests that the principal mechanism of action of this peptide does not involve the disruption of the bacterial membrane, but indicates that the PuroB peptides cross the bacterial cytoplasmic membrane and bind to nucleic acids within the cell, blocking macromolecular synthesis of DNA, RNA and proteins (Haney *et al.*, 2013). However, the exact mechanism of PuroB membrane translocation remains to be elucidated (Haney *et al.*, 2013).

The DNA binding property has been reported with an increasing range of AMPs. Recently, it has been shown that synthetic polymers with a polyamide backbone (SAMPs) are active against *Mycobacterium smegmatis*. They are able to bind to DNA and to inhibit PCR amplifications of DNA extracted from peptide-treated cells (Sharma *et al.*, 2015). In another recent study, an analogue of the amphibian AMP

fallaxin has been found to have a dual mode of action against *S. aureus*. At MIC, it binds to DNA, inhibits DNA synthesis and induces the SOS DNA damage response, whereas at concentrations above the MIC the peptide causes membrane disruption (Gottschalk *et al.*, 2015).

9.3 Cell Surface Modes of Action

Antibacterial activity of a group of AMPs is directed against important superficial structures of the target bacteria, despite evidence suggesting that their action is primarily based on non-lytic interactions. The cell wall is an important cell surface structure and its inhibition represents an important target for AMPs.

9.3.1 Cell wall inhibition

Different AMPs have been found to inhibit the synthesis of peptidoglycan, the main constituent of the bacterial cell wall which is not present in eukaryotic cells and therefore represents an interesting target for therapeutic applications.

Lantibiotics are a class of post-translationally modified bacteriocins produced by Gram-positive bacteria, containing unusual amino acids (Hechard and Sahl, 2002) and classified as type-A (linear peptides) or type-B (globular peptides), on the basis of their structure (Islam *et al.*, 2012). Although most lantibiotics show membrane-disrupting activities, a number of bacteriocins have specific target-mediated activity. The biosynthesis of cell wall components is a multi-step process in which lipid II is a central building block of the peptidoglycan biosynthesis. Lipid II has been identified as a principal target for lantibiotics (Hechard and Sahl, 2002; Willey and van der Donk, 2007) and other AMPs (Ling *et al.*, 2015, Sass *et al.*, 2010; Schneider *et al.*, 2010). The best characterized among type A lantibiotics, nisin, initially forms a complex with the membrane-bound lipid II thereby inhibiting the cell-wall biosynthesis, and then aggregates by incorporating further peptides, leading to a pore in the bacterial membrane ('t Hart *et al.*, 2016). Nisin variants binding to lipid II without disrupting the membrane have also been described (Hasper *et al.*, 2004; Wiedemann *et al.*, 2001), indicating that the binding and relocation of lipid II in the membrane is sufficient *per se* to inhibit cell wall synthesis and cause cell death. An example of this mode of action has been described for the lantibiotic mutacin 1140 (Hasper *et al.*, 2006). It has been shown that the addition of the epidermin-like lantibiotic mutacin 1140 to fluorescently labelled lipid II in giant unilamellar vesicles (GUVs) induces hot spots without causing membrane permeabilization. In fact the impermeable soluble fluorescent marker Texas Red remains extracellular. The lipid II segregation observed in GUVs was then also confirmed *in vivo* in *Bacillus* and *Lactococcus* cells, suggesting that it may be responsible for the inhibition of cell wall synthesis and ultimately cell death (Hasper *et al.*, 2006).

Type B lantibiotics such as mersacidin also use lipid II as a docking molecule, but they can only inhibit cell wall biosynthesis without forming pores (Brotz *et al.*, 1997). On the other hand, even for those lantibiotics (such as plantaricin C, gallidermin and epidermin) that are known to induce pore formation, this effect has been shown to be strain-specific. These results suggest that the *in vivo* activity of lantibiotics cannot be assigned exclusively to the interaction with isolated cell-wall precursors such as lipid II; rather, cell wall synthesis inhibition and membrane disruption may contribute differently to the antimicrobial activity depending on the target strain (Bonelli *et al.*, 2006; Wiedemann *et al.*, 2006).

Lantibiotics are not the only AMPs to target lipid II as part of their activity. Other examples include some defensins, defensin-like peptides and teixobactin. Plectasin (Schneider *et al.*, 2010), and copsin (Essig *et al.*, 2014) are defensins of fungal origin that bind respectively to lipid I and lipid II. Human defensin hBD3 has been found to disrupt cell wall biosynthesis by binding

lipid-II-rich regions of the cell wall (Sass *et al.*, 2010). Teixobactin, an 11-residue depsipeptide recently isolated from previously unculturable bacteria, inhibits cell wall synthesis by binding to a highly conserved motif of lipid II and lipid III, a precursor of cell wall teichoic acid (Ling *et al.*, 2015).

AMPs that impair outer membrane structures and cause biogenesis defects have also been reported. A series of interesting peptidomimetics, derived from the membrane-disrupting peptide protegrin, has been shown to kill specifically *Pseudomonas* spp. in a nanomolar range via a mechanism distinct from that of the parent protegrin (Srinivas *et al.*, 2010). The peptidomimetics L27-11 and POL7001 have been shown to target the ß-barrel protein LptD of *P. aeruginosa*, an essential protein involved in the assembly of LPS in the outer leaflet of the outer membrane. Neither L27-11 nor POL7001 caused membrane permeabilization, as demonstrated by the absence of increased fluorescence when bacterial cells were exposed to SYTOX green in the presence of these peptides (Srinivas *et al.*, 2010). Both peptidomimetic antibiotics bind to LptD and impair the LPS transport to the outer membrane resulting in internal accumulation of membrane-like materials and lipid A alterations (Werneburg *et al.*, 2012).

9.3.2 Inhibition of cytokinesis

Inhibition of cytokinesis has been proposed as a possible mode of action of some AMPs. The mouse orthologue of LL-37, CRAMP, impaired *Salmonella* cell division. The resulting long filamentous structures indicate that peptide-treated cells are unable to undergo cell division (Rosenberger *et al.*, 2004). Interestingly, it has been noted that CRAMP has a sequence similar to a 40-amino acid peptide from *Bacillus subtilis*, that inhibits the tubulin-like protein FtsZ preventing inappropriate Z-ring formation during sporulation (Handler *et al.*, 2008). In a recent study, the fragment 16-33 of CRAMP was found to bind FtsZ and to inhibit its assembly and GTPase activity *in vitro*. Furthermore, the authors showed by fluorescence microscopy that the cells treated with CRAMP 16-33 have an elongated morphology, and that FtsZ is either diffused throughout the cells or localized in correspondence of incomplete septum (Ray *et al.*, 2014). Although it is not clear whether CRAMP is internalized in the cytoplasm or inserted into the inner membrane at direct contact with FtsZ, these results highlight an alternative mechanism of action for this peptide, apart from the already known lytic mechanism related to its amphipathic helical nature (Tomasinsig and Zanetti, 2005). An elongated cell morphology has also been observed with the proline-rich PR-39 and the tryptophan-rich indolicidin, although the molecular mechanism of septum inhibition is unknown and could be related to inhibition of DNA replication (Brogden, 2005).

9.4 Other Membrane-independent Mechanisms of Bacterial Killing

Recently, several studies have reported convincing data on non-membranolytic mechanisms of novel/modified AMPs, although in most cases the specific molecular target has not yet been identified. For example the synthetic hexapeptide RWRWRW-NH2, named MP196, a minimal pharmacophore of positively charged and hydrophobic amino acids, localizes at the membrane of *B. subtilis* cells and inserts into the phospholipid bilayer. However, it does so without permeabilizing effects. Instead it causes the delocalization of peripheral membrane proteins essential for respiration and cell wall biosynthesis (Wenzel *et al.*, 2014). Delocalization of membrane proteins, affecting energy metabolism and cell-wall integrity, is a general mode of action that can also be extended to membrane-targeting peptides of other structural classes and may be responsible for the inhibition of cell wall biosynthesis caused by some AMPs (Sass *et al.*, 2010). The interference with many different processes essential for bacterial

survival has been called the 'sand in a gearbox' (Pag *et al.*, 2008) and has been proposed for many AMPs.

A controversial mode of action has been proposed for daptomycin, another lipopeptide which has an extended and partially circular conformation, pointing to the misregulation of the recruitment of the cell division protein DivIVC. Although the effects of this lipopeptide on the bacterial membrane and cell wall are well-known, bacterial lysis has been proposed to occur as a later consequence of a general cell dysfunction, not as the main mode of action (Pogliano *et al.*, 2012; Taylor and Palmer, 2016).

θ-defensins have recently been shown to trigger cell-wall degradation in the septum area between two daughter cells and the authors suggest that the autolysin Atl may be responsible for this phenomenon. The premature release of autolytic enzymes from their anchoring points on lipoteichoic acids eventually leads to cell wall disruption (Wilmes *et al.*, 2014). A similar mechanism, based on bacterial cell lysis promoted by the release of cell wall hydrolases (autolysins) has also been proposed for the bacteriocin Pep5 (Bierbaum and Sahl, 1987). Finally, another example of a membrane-independent killing mechanism was recently proposed for magainin-2. Here, in addition to the membrane-disrupting activity, the possibility of a bacterial apoptosis-like death in *Escherichia coli* cells has been suggested.

Indeed magainin-2 induces effects resembling typical apoptosis hallmarks, such as phosphatidylserine externalization from the inner to outer membrane surface, DNA fragmentation and chromatin condensation (Lee and Lee, 2014).

9.5 Immune Modulatory Effects

As well as having direct antibacterial properties like many other antimicrobial peptides, some non-lytic AMPs show immunomodulating activities. Among the PR-AMPs, most data have been collected using the porcine PR-39 (Veldhuizen *et al.*,

2014). It induces migrations of porcine neutrophils in a calcium-dependent manner, but not of mononuclear cells (Huang *et al.*, 1997), a feature also shared by the precursors of the bovine Bac5 and Bac7 (Verbanac *et al.*, 1993). In addition, PR-39 and some of its shortened peptides induce the production of interleuchin-8 by porcine alveolar macrophages, while the full-length peptide also induces, although to a lesser extent, the production of TNF-α (Veldhuizen *et al.*, 2014). On the other hand, Bac5 and indolicidin do not induce TNF-α in a mammalian (bovine) cell line (Tomasinsig *et al.*, 2010). Indeed, they actually repress the TNF-α secretion induced by LPS, do not recruit monocytic cells and induce interleuchin 8 production by a bronchial cell line (Bowdish *et al.*, 2005). Recently, it has been described that oncocin and apidaecin, two short PR-AMPs (20 amino acids), also lack immuno-modulatory activity. No chemotactic activity towards dendritic cells, no modification of LPS induced immune responses or direct immune stimulating effects on macrophages have been observed for these PR-AMPs. This is in contrast to the murine cathelicidin CRAMP used in the same study (Fritsche *et al.*, 2012). Some studies reported that PR-39 has a promoting role in angiogenesis (Li *et al.*, 2000) and wound healing (Gallo *et al.*, 1994), and that it can reduce the tissue damage due to inflammation events modulating the superoxide anion production by NADPH oxidase in neutrophils (Shi *et al.*, 1996). Similarly to oncocin and apidaecin, daptomycin was also shown to not modulate IL-1β, IL-6 and TNF-α production after exposition *in vitro* of whole human blood to LPS (Thallinger *et al.*, 2008). Lactoferrin B has LPS binding activity and was also shown to modulate the recruitment of cells of the immune system and the production of cytokines (Siqueiros-Cendon *et al.*, 2014). Nisin enhanced the production of the chemokines Gro-α, IL-8 and MCP-1, and decreased the induction of TNF-α after challenging human peripheral blood cells with LPS (Kindrachuk *et al.*, 2013). Moreover, neutrophils exposed to nisin augmented their levels of superoxide and could be induced in producing

neutrophil extracellular traps (Begde *et al.*, 2011). Pleurocidin was shown to activate human mast cells exploiting a signalling based on the G protein coupled receptor FPRL1 (Pundir *et al.*, 2014).

9.6 Towards Novel Therapeutic Opportunities

A considerable number of the AMPs showing non-lytic mechanism of action, and described above, are currently in clinical trials or in preclinical phase, demonstrating that knowledge of AMPs' mechanisms of action increases their potential for therapeutic development. The daptomycin-related lipopeptide surotomycin (CB-315) is in Phase III of clinical trials as a treatment for *Clostridium difficile* infections (Fox, 2013). The indolicidin-derived MBI-226 (omiganan) has completed two separate Phase III clinical trials demonstrating significant efficacy in topical antiseptic prevention of catheter infection (Midura-Nowaczek and Markowska, 2014). The epitope mimetics of protegrin I, POL7080, completed a Phase II trial for non-cystic fibrosis bronchiectasis in November 2015 (Edwards *et al.*, 2016). The success of lantibiotics as a novel treatment of multidrug-resistant infections is illustrated by the clinical development of MU1140 (mutacin 1140) and NAI-107 (microbisporicin), which are in late pre-clinical trials against Gram-positive bacteria; by NVB302, which has completed Phase I clinical trials for the treatment of *C. difficile* infections; and also by duramycin, which has completed Phase II clinical trials in the treatment of cystic fibrosis (Escano and Smith, 2015).

The mechanism of action of PR-AMPs has been elucidated only recently and thus only early preclinical studies have been carried out on these peptides as antimicrobials (see Li *et al.*, 2014 and Section 9.2.1). Interestingly the PR-AMP A3-APO shows broad-spectrum activity in mouse models of systemic *Acinetobacter baumannii* infection (Ostorhazi *et al.*, 2011a) and in wound and lung infections despite low *in vitro* activity, suggesting a mechanism of inhibition mediated by immunostimulation (Ostorhazi *et al.*, 2011b; Sebe *et al.*, 2016).

As well as having direct antimicrobial activity, mammalian and insect PR-AMPs may also have potential in cell drug delivery thanks to their properties to translocate across the cellular membranes of bacteria (Knappe *et al.*, 2010; Mattiuzzo *et al.*, 2007) or eukaryotic cells (Otvos *et al.*, 2004; Tomasinsig *et al.*, 2006) without membrane damage and cytotoxic effects at active concentrations (Pelillo *et al.*, 2014).

Fluorescently labelled Bac7(1-35) is rapidly detected in the cytoplasm of exposed Gram-negative bacteria (Benincasa *et al.*, 2009). It can efficiently internalize small molecules including fluorophores but also conjugated antibiotics (unpublished result) and even 20 kDa covalently-bound polyethylene glycol tail (Benincasa *et al.*, 2015). Similar results were obtained with eukaryotic cells, in which Bac7 fragments were capable of delivering a non-covalently linked protein (Sadler *et al.*, 2002). Even the small 15–24 fragment of Bac7, conjugated to a derivative of Pt(II) coproporphyrin I, resulted in a functional oxygen-sensitive phosphorescent probe for intracellular use (Dmitriev *et al.*, 2010). Further studies indicated that PR-AMPs could help internalization of RNA/PNA molecules. The mammalian PR-39 peptide has been exploited as a carrier to deliver siRNA into cancer cell cytoplasm in order to knock down target gene expression (Tian *et al.*, 2012). In addition, different short PR-AMPs and buforin 2-A have successfully been used as vehicles for delivery of antibacterial peptide nucleic acid oligomers targeting an essential bacterial gene (Hansen *et al.*, 2016).

Interestingly, a recent report showed that short insect PR-AMPs have significant influx into the brain crossing the blood–brain barrier (Stalmans *et al.*, 2014; Schmidt *et al.*, 2016). This effect suggests a possibility for the PR-AMPs not only as potential therapeutics for cerebral infections but also as carriers for brain drug delivery (Li *et al.*, 2014). Overall, these results indicate that these PR-AMPs represent a potentially new class of cell-penetrating peptides (Bechara and Sagan, 2013) for intracellular delivery of impermeant molecular cargo.

9.7 Concluding Remarks

There is mounting evidence that some classes of AMPs act principally through non-membranolytic mechanisms in which the killing event is not based on the disruption of membrane integrity. Despite this, our understanding of internalization routes into the target cell, as well as the precise molecular mechanisms of action, is largely incomplete for most non-lytic AMPs and only speculative for others. Some peptides such as the PR-AMPs seem to be directed towards a single main target, while others seem to interact on multiple targets in a relatively unspecific manner, in which the membranolytic contribution could be different depending on the peptide sequence and concentration. In particular, simultaneous binding to multiple targets or a mixed lytic and non-lytic mode of action is an important factor in order to minimize the likelihood of resistance development. In any case, a deeper knowledge of the molecular interactions between non-lytic AMPs and their bacterial targets would be an important key to future development of peptides as new drugs.

In the last decade, some AMPs have failed to achieve New Drug Application (NDA) approval, despite clinical efficacy. Nowadays, however, the urgency to develop novel antibiotics has promoted a renewed interest from pharmaceutical companies. In this respect, a better understanding of the molecular mechanisms by which AMPs inhibit their targets would be highly desirable for the rational design of new compounds, increasing their attractiveness and probability of success.

Acknowledgements

We gratefully acknowledge Beneficentia Stiftung for generous financial support.

References

Agerberth, B., Lee, J.Y., Bergman, T., Carlquist, M., Boman, H. G., Mutt, V. and Jornvall, H. (1991) Amino acid sequence of PR-39: isolation from pig intestine of a new member of the family of proline-arginine-rich antibacterial peptides. *European Journal of Biochemistry* 202, 849–854.

Bahar, A.A. and Ren, D. (2013) Antimicrobial peptides. *Pharmaceuticals (Basel)* 6, 1543–1575.

Bechara, C. and Sagan, S. (2013) Cell-penetrating peptides: 20 years later, where do we stand? *FEBS Letters* 587, 1693–1702.

Begde, D., Bundale, S., Mashitha, P., Rudra, J., Nashikkar, N. and Upadhyay, A. (2011) Immunomodulatory efficacy of nisin: a bacterial lantibiotic peptide. *Journal of Peptide Science* 17, 438–444.

Benincasa, M., Scocchi, M., Podda, E., Skerlavaj, B., Dolzani, L. and Gennaro, R. (2004) Antimicrobial activity of Bac7 fragments against drug-resistant clinical isolates. *Peptides* 25, 2055–2061.

Benincasa, M., Pacor, S., Gennaro, R. and Scocchi, M. (2009) Rapid and reliable detection of antimicrobial peptide penetration into Gram-negative bacteria based on fluorescence quenching. *Antimicrobial Agents and Chemotherapy* 53, 3501–3504.

Benincasa, M., Pelillo, C., Zorzet, S., Garrovo, C. and Biffi, S., *et al.* (2010) The proline-rich peptide Bac7(1-35) reduces mortality from *Salmonella typhimurium* in a mouse model of infection. *BMC Microbiology* 10, 178.

Benincasa, M., Zahariev, S., Pelillo, C., Milan, A., Gennaro, R. and Scocchi, M. (2015) PEGylation of the peptide Bac7(1-35) reduces renal clearance while retaining antibacterial activity and bacterial cell penetration capacity. *European Journal of Medicinal Chemistry* 95, 210–219.

Berthold, N. and Hoffmann, R. (2014) Cellular uptake of apidaecin 1b and related analogs in Gram-negative bacteria reveals novel antibacterial mechanism for proline-rich antimicrobial peptides. *Protein and Peptide Letters* 21, 391–398.

Bierbaum, G. and Sahl, H.G. (1987) Autolytic system of *Staphylococcus simulans* 22: influence of cationic peptides on activity of N-acetylmuramoyl-L-alanine amidase. *Journal of Bacteriology* 169, 5452–5458.

Bluhm, M.E., Knappe, D. and Hoffmann, R. (2015) Structure–activity relationship study using peptide arrays to optimize Api137 for an increased antimicrobial activity against *Pseudomonas aeruginosa*. *European Journal of Medicinal Chemistry* 103, 574–582.

Boman, H.G., Agerberth, B. and Boman, A. (1993) Mechanisms of action on *Escherichia coli* of cecropin P1 and PR-39: two antibacterial peptides from pig intestine. *Infection and Immunity* 61, 2978–2984.

Bonelli, R.R., Schneider, T., Sahl, H.G. and Wiedemann, I. (2006) Insights into in vivo activities of lantibiotics from gallidermin and epidermin mode-of-action studies. *Antimicrobial Agents and Chemotherapy* 50, 1449–1457.

Bowdish, D.M., Davidson, D.J., Scott, M.G. and Hancock, R.E. (2005) Immunomodulatory activities of small host defense peptides. *Antimicrobial Agents and Chemotherapy* 49, 1727–1732.

Brandi, L., Fabbretti, A., Di Stefano, M., Lazzarini, A., Abbondi, M. and Gualerzi, C.O. (2006a) Characterization of GE82832: a peptide inhibitor of translocation interacting with bacterial 30S ribosomal subunits. *RNA* 12, 1262–1270.

Brandi, L., Fabbretti, A., La Teana, A., Abbondi, M., Losi, D., Donadio, S. and Gualerzi, C.O. (2006b) Specific, efficient, and selective inhibition of prokaryotic translation initiation by a novel peptide antibiotic. *Proceedings of the National Academy of Sciences of the United States of America* 103, 39–44.

Brandi, L., Maffioli, S., Donadio, S., Quaglia, F., Sette, M., *et al.* (2012) Structural and functional characterization of the bacterial translocation inhibitor GE82832. *FEBS Letters* 586, 3373–3378.

Brogden, K.A. (2005) Antimicrobial peptides: pore formers or metabolic inhibitors in bacteria? *Nature Reviews Microbiology* 3, 238–250.

Brogden, N.K. and Brogden, K.A. (2011) Will new generations of modified antimicrobial peptides improve their potential as pharmaceuticals? *International Journal of Antimicrobial Agents* 38, 217–225.

Brotz, H., Bierbaum, G., Reynolds, P.E. and Sahl, H.G. (1997) The lantibiotic mersacidin inhibits peptidoglycan biosynthesis at the level of transglycosylation. *European Journal of Biochemistry* 246, 193–199.

Bulkley, D., Brandi, L., Polikanov, Y.S., Fabbretti, A., O'Connor, M., Gualerzi, C.O. and Steitz, T.A. (2014) The antibiotics dityromycin and GE82832 bind protein S12 and block EF-G-catalyzed translocation. *Cell Reports* 6, 357–365.

Casteels, P., Ampe, C., Jacobs, F., Vaeck, M. and Tempst, P. (1989) Apidaecins: antibacterial peptides from honeybees. *EMBO J* 8, 2387–2391.

Castle, M., Nazarian, A., Yi, S.S. and Tempst, P. (1999) Lethal effects of apidaecin on *Escherichia coli* involve sequential molecular interactions with diverse targets. *Journal of Biological Chemistry* 274, 32555–32564.

Cho, J.H., Sung, B.H. and Kim, S.C. (2009) Buforins: histone H2A-derived antimicrobial peptides from toad stomach. *Biochimica et Biophysica Acta* 1788, 1564–1569.

Coates, A.R.M., Halls, G. and Hu, Y. (2011) Novel classes of antibiotics or more of the same? *British Journal of Pharmacology* 163, 184–194.

Cutrona, K.J., Kaufman, B.A., Figueroa, D.M. and Elmore, D.E. (2015) Role of arginine and lysine in the antimicrobial mechanism of histone-derived antimicrobial peptides. *FEBS Letters,* 589, 3915–3920.

Czihal, P., Knappe, D., Fritsche, S., Zahn, M., Berthold, N., *et al.* (2012) Api88 is a novel antibacterial designer peptide to treat systemic infections with multidrug-resistant Gram-negative pathogens. *ACS Chemical Biology* 7, 1281–1291.

Di Pisa, M., Chassaing, G. and Swiecicki, J.M. (2015) Translocation mechanism(s) of cell-penetrating peptides: biophysical studies using artificial membrane bilayers. *Biochemistry* 54, 194–207.

Diamond, G., Beckloff, N., Weinberg, A. and Kisich, K.O. (2009) The roles of antimicrobial peptides in innate host defense. *Current Pharmaceutical Design* 15, 2377–2392.

Dmitriev, R.I., Ropiak, H.M., Yashunsky, D.V., Ponomarev, G.V., Zhdanov, A.V. and Papkovsky, D.B. (2010) Bactenecin 7 peptide fragment as a tool for intracellular delivery of a phosphorescent oxygen sensor. *FEBS Journal* 277, 4651–4661.

Edwards, I.A., Elliott, A.G., Kavanagh, A.M., Zuegg, J., Blaskovich, M.A. and Cooper, M.A. (2016) Contribution of amphipathicity and hydrophobicity to the antimicrobial activity and cytotoxicity of beta-hairpin peptides. *ACS Infectious Diseases* 2, 442–450.

Escano, J. and Smith, L. (2015) Multipronged approach for engineering novel peptide analogues of existing lantibiotics. *Expert Opinion on Drug Discovery* 10, 857–870.

Essig, A., Hofmann, D., Munch, D., Gayathri, S., Kunzler, M., *et al.* (2014) Copsin: a novel peptide-based fungal antibiotic interfering with the peptidoglycan synthesis. *Journal of Biological Chemistry* 289, 34953–34964.

Fang, Y., Zhong, W., Wang, Y., Xun, T., Lin, D., *et al.* (2014) Tuning the antimicrobial pharmacophore to enable discovery of short lipopeptides with multiple modes of action. *European Journal of Medicinal Chemistry* 83, 36–44.

Farkas, A., Maroti, G., Durgo, H., Gyorgypal, Z., Lima, R.M., *et al.* (2014) *Medicago truncatula* symbiotic peptide NCR247 contributes to bacteroid differentiation through multiple mechanisms. *Proceedings of the National Academy of Sciences of the United States of America* 111, 5183–5188.

Fox, J.L. (2013) Antimicrobial peptides stage a comeback. *Nature Biotechnology* 31, 379–382.

Frère, J.-M. and Rigali, S. (2016) The alarming increase in antibiotic-resistant bacteria. *Drug Target Review* 3, 26–30.

Friedrich, C.L., Rozek, A., Patrzykat, A. and Hancock, R.E. (2001) Structure and mechanism of action of an indolicidin peptide derivative with improved activity against Gram-positive bacteria. *Journal of Biological Chemistry* 276, 24015–24022.

Fritsche, S., Knappe, D., Berthold, N., von Buttlar, H., Hoffmann, R. and Alber, G. (2012) Absence of in vitro innate immunomodulation by insect-derived short proline-rich antimicrobial peptides points to direct antibacterial action in vivo. *Journal of Peptide Science* 18, 599–608.

Gagnon, M.G., Roy, R.N., Lomakin, I.B., Florin, T., Mankin, A.S. and Steitz, T.A. (2016) Structures of proline-rich peptides bound to the ribosome reveal a common mechanism of protein synthesis inhibition. *Nucleic Acids Research* 44, 2439–2450.

Gallo, R.L., Ono, M., Povsic, T., Page, C., Eriksson, E., Klagsbrun, M. and Bernfield, M. (1994) Syndecans, cell surface heparan sulfate proteoglycans, are induced by a proline-rich antimicrobial peptide from wounds. *Proceedings of the National Academy of Sciences of the United States of America* 91, 11035–11039.

Gaspar, D., Veiga, A.S. and Castanho, M.A. (2013) From antimicrobial to anticancer peptides: a review. *Frontiers in Microbiology* 4, 294.

Gennaro, R., Skerlavaj, B. and Romeo, D. (1989) Purification, composition, and activity of two bactenecins: antibacterial peptides of bovine neutrophils. *Infection and Immunity* 57, 3142–3146.

Ghosh, A., Kar, R.K., Jana, J., Saha, A., Jana, B., *et al.* (2014) Indolicidin targets duplex DNA: structural and mechanistic insight through a combination of spectroscopy and microscopy. *ChemMedChem* 9, 2052–2058.

Gottschalk, S., Gottlieb, C.T., Vestergaard, M., Hansen, P.R., Gram, L., Ingmer, H. and Thomsen, L.E. (2015) Amphibian antimicrobial peptide fallaxin analogue FL9 affects virulence gene expression and DNA replication in *Staphylococcus aureus*. *Journal of Medical Microbiology* 64, 1504–1513.

Hadley, E.B. and Hancock, R.E. (2010) Strategies for the discovery and advancement of novel cationic antimicrobial peptides. *Current Topics in Medicinal Chemistry* 10, 1872–1881.

Hale, J.D. and Hancock, R.E. (2007) Alternative mechanisms of action of cationic antimicrobial peptides on bacteria. *Expert Review of Anti-infective Therapy* 5, 951–959.

Handler, A.A., Lim, J.E. and Losick, R. (2008) Peptide inhibitor of cytokinesis during sporulation in *Bacillus subtilis*. *Molecular Microbiology* 68, 588–599.

Haney, E.F., Petersen, A.P., Lau, C.K., Jing, W., Storey, D.G. and Vogel, H.J. (2013) Mechanism of action of puroindoline derived tryptophan-rich antimicrobial peptides. *Biochimica et Biophysica Acta* 1828, 1802–1813.

Hansen, A., Schafer, I., Knappe, D., Seibel, P. and Hoffmann, R. (2012) Intracellular toxicity of proline-rich antimicrobial peptides shuttled into mammalian cells by the cell-penetrating peptide penetratin. *Antimicrobial Agents and Chemotherapy* 56, 5194–5201.

Hansen, A., Bonke, G., Larsen, C.J., Yavari, N., Nielsen, P.E. and Franzyk, H. (2016) Antibacterial peptide nucleic acid-antimicrobial peptide (PNA-AMP) conjugates: antisense targeting of fatty acid biosynthesis. *Bioconjugate Chemistry* 27, 863–867.

Hao, G., Shi, Y.H., Tang, Y.L. and Le, G.W. (2013) The intracellular mechanism of action on *Escherichia coli* of BF2-A/C: two analogues of the antimicrobial peptide Buforin 2. *Journal of Microbiology* 51, 200–206.

Hasper, H.E., de Kruijff, B. and Breukink, E. (2004) Assembly and stability of nisin-lipid II pores. *Biochemistry* 43, 11567–11575.

Hasper, H.E., Kramer, N.E., Smith, J.L., Hillman, J.D., Zachariah, C., Kuipers, O.P., de Kruijff, B. and Breukink, E. (2006) An alternative bactericidal mechanism of action for lantibiotic peptides that target lipid II. *Science* 313, 1636–1637.

Hechard, Y. and Sahl, H.G. (2002) Mode of action of modified and unmodified bacteriocins from Gram-positive bacteria. *Biochimie* 84, 545–557.

Hong, J., Guan, W., Jin, G., Zhao, H., Jiang, X. and Dai, J. (2015) Mechanism of tachyplesin I injury to bacterial membranes and intracellular enzymes, determined by laser confocal scanning microscopy and flow cytometry. *Microbiological Research* 170, 69–77.

Hsu, C.H., Chen, C., Jou, M.L., Lee, A.Y., Lin, Y.C., *et al.* (2005) Structural and DNA-binding studies on the bovine antimicrobial peptide, indolicidin: evidence for multiple conformations involved in binding to membranes and DNA. *Nucleic Acids Research* 33, 4053–4064.

Huang, H.J., Ross, C.R. and Blecha, F. (1997) Chemoattractant properties of PR-39: a neutrophil antibacterial peptide. *Journal of Leukocyte Biology* 61, 624–629.

Huang, H.W. (2000) Action of antimicrobial peptides: two-state model. *Biochemistry* 39, 8347–8352.

Imura, Y., Nishida, M., Ogawa, Y., Takakura, Y. and Matsuzaki, K. (2007) Action mechanism of tachyplesin I and effects of PEGylation. *Biochimica et Biophysica Acta* 1768, 1160–1169.

Islam, M.R., Nagao, J., Zendo, T. and Sonomoto, K. (2012) Antimicrobial mechanism of lantibiotics. *Biochemical Society Transactions* 40, 1528–1533.

Kindrachuk, J., Jenssen, H., Elliott, M., Nijnik, A., Magrangeas-Janot, L., *et al.* (2013) Manipulation of innate immunity by a bacterial secreted peptide: lantibiotic nisin Z is selectively immunomodulatory. *Innate Immunity* 19, 315–327.

Knappe, D., Piantavigna, S., Hansen, A., Mechler, A., Binas, A., *et al.* (2010) Oncocin (VDKPPYL-PRPRPPRRIYNR-NH2): a novel antibacterial peptide optimized against Gram-negative human pathogens. *Journal of Medicinal Chemistry* 53, 5240–5247.

Knappe, D., Zahn, M., Sauer, U., Schiffer, G., Strater, N. and Hoffmann, R. (2011) Rational design of oncocin derivatives with superior protease stabilities and antibacterial activities based on the high-resolution structure of the oncocin-DnaK complex. *ChemBioChem*, 12, 874–876.

Knappe, D., Fritsche, S., Alber, G., Kohler, G., Hoffmann, R. and Muller, U. (2012) Oncocin derivative Onc72 is highly active against *Escherichia coli* in a systemic septicaemia infection mouse model. *Journal of Antimicrobial Chemotherapy* 67, 2445–2451.

Knappe, D., Adermann, K. and Hoffmann, R. (2015) Oncocin Onc72 is efficacious against antibiotic-susceptible *Klebsiella pneumoniae* ATCC 43816 in a murine thigh infection model. *Biopolymers* 104, 707–711.

Knappe, D., Kabankov, N., Herth, N. and Hoffmann, R. (2016a) Insect-derived short proline-rich and murine cathelicidin-related antimicrobial peptides act synergistically on Gram-negative bacteria *in vitro*. *Future Medicinal Chemistry* 8, 1035–1045.

Knappe, D., Ruden, S., Langanke, S., Tikkoo, T., Ritzer, J., *et al.* (2016b) Optimization of oncocin for antibacterial activity using a SPOT synthesis approach: extending the pathogen spectrum to *Staphylococcus aureus*. *Amino Acids* 48, 269–280.

Kobayashi, S., Takeshima, K., Park, C.B., Kim, S.C. and Matsuzaki, K. (2000) Interactions of the novel antimicrobial peptide buforin 2 with lipid bilayers: proline as a translocation promoting factor. *Biochemistry* 39, 8648–8654.

Kragol, G., Lovas, S., Varadi, G., Condie, B.A., Hoffmann, R. and Otvos, L., Jr (2001) The antibacterial peptide pyrrhocoricin inhibits the ATPase actions of DnaK and prevents chaperone-assisted protein folding. *Biochemistry* 40, 3016–3026.

Kragol, G., Hoffmann, R., Chattergoon, M.A., Lovas, S., Cudic, M., *et al.* (2002) Identification of crucial residues for the antibacterial activity of the proline-rich peptide, pyrrhocoricin. *European Journal of Biochemistry* 269, 4226–4237.

Krizsan, A., Volke, D., Weinert, S., Strater, N., Knappe, D. and Hoffmann, R. (2014) Insect-derived proline-rich antimicrobial peptides kill bacteria by inhibiting bacterial protein translation at the 70S ribosome. *Angewandte Chemie International Edition* 53, 12236–12239.

Krizsan, A., Knappe, D. and Hoffmann, R. (2015a) Influence of the yjiL-mdtM gene cluster on the antibacterial activity of proline-rich antimicrobial peptides overcoming *Escherichia coli* resistance induced by the missing SbmA transporter system. *Antimicrobial Agents and Chemotherapy* 59, 5992–5998.

Krizsan, A., Prahl, C., Goldbach, T., Knappe, D. and Hoffmann, R. (2015b) Short proline-rich antimicrobial peptides inhibit either the bacterial 70S ribosome or the assembly of its large 50S subunit. *ChemBioChem* 16, 2304–2308.

Lai, Y. and Gallo, R.L. (2009) AMPed up immunity: how antimicrobial peptides have multiple roles in immune defense. *Trends in Immunology* 30, 131–141.

Lan, Y., Ye, Y., Kozlowska, J., Lam, J.K., Drake, A.F. and Mason, A.J. (2010) Structural contributions to the intracellular targeting strategies of antimicrobial peptides. *Biochimica et Biophysica Acta* 1798, 1934–1943.

Lee, W. and Lee, D.G. (2014) Magainin 2 induces bacterial cell death showing apoptotic properties. *Current Microbiology* 69, 794–801.

Li, J., Post, M., Volk, R., Gao, Y., Li, M., *et al.* (2000) PR39: a peptide regulator of angiogenesis. *Nature Medicine* 6, 49–55.

Li, W., Tailhades, J., O'Brien-Simpson, N.M., Separovic, F., Otvos, L., Jr, Hossain, M.A. and Wade, J.D. (2014) Proline-rich antimicrobial peptides: potential therapeutics against antibiotic-resistant bacteria. *Amino Acids*, 46, 2287–2294.

Ling, L.L., Schneider, T., Peoples, A.J., Spoering, A.L., Engels, I., *et al.* (2015) A new antibiotic kills pathogens without detectable resistance. *Nature* 517, 455–459.

Mardirossian, M., Grzela, R., Giglione, C., Meinnel, T., Gennaro, R., Mergaert, P. and Scocchi, M. (2014) The host antimicrobial peptide Bac71-35 binds to bacterial ribosomal proteins and inhibits protein synthesis. *Chemical Biology* 21, 1639–1647.

Marks, J.R., Placone, J., Hristova, K. and Wimley, W.C. (2011) Spontaneous membrane-translocating peptides by orthogonal high-throughput screening. *Journal of the American Chemical Society* 133, 8995–9004.

Matsuzaki, K. (1998) Magainins as paradigm for the mode of action of pore forming polypeptides. *Biochimica et Biophysica Acta* 1376, 391–400.

Mattiuzzo, M., Bandiera, A., Gennaro, R., Benincasa, M., Pacor, S., Antcheva, N. and Scocchi, M. (2007) Role of the *Escherichia coli* SbmA in the antimicrobial activity of proline-rich peptides. *Molecular Microbiology* 66, 151–163.

Melo, M.N., Ferre, R. and Castanho, M.A. (2009) Antimicrobial peptides: linking partition, activity and high membrane-bound concentrations. *Nature Reviews Microbiology* 7, 245–250.

Midura-Nowaczek, K. and Markowska, A. (2014) Antimicrobial peptides and their analogs: searching for new potential therapeutics. *Perspectives in Medicinal Chemistry* 6, 73–80.

Morell, M., Czihal, P., Hoffmann, R., Otvos, L., Aviles, F.X. and Ventura, S. (2008) Monitoring the interference of protein-protein interactions *in vivo* by bimolecular fluorescence complementation: the DnaK case. *Proteomics* 8, 3433–3442.

Nan, Y.H., Bang, J.K. and Shin, S.Y. (2009) Design of novel indolicidin-derived antimicrobial peptides with enhanced cell specificity and potent anti-inflammatory activity. *Peptides* 30, 832–838.

Nguyen, L.T., Haney, E.F. and Vogel, H.J. (2011) The expanding scope of antimicrobial peptide structures and their modes of action. *Trends in Biotechnology* 29, 464–472.

Nicolas, P. (2009) Multifunctional host defense peptides: intracellular-targeting antimicrobial peptides. *FEBS Journal* 276, 6483–6496.

Ostorhazi, E., Rozgonyi, F., Szabo, D., Binas, A., Cassone, M., *et al.* (2011a). Intramuscularly administered peptide A3-APO is effective against carbapenem-resistant *Acinetobacter baumannii* in mouse models of systemic infections. *Biopolymers*, 96, 126–129.

Ostorhazi, E., Holub, M.C., Rozgonyi, F., Harmos, F., Cassone, M., Wade, J.D. and Otvos, L., Jr (2011b) Broad-spectrum antimicrobial efficacy of peptide A3-APO in mouse models of multidrug-resistant wound and lung infections cannot be explained by in vitro activity against the pathogens involved. *International Journal of Antimicrobial Agents* 37, 480–484.

Ostorhazi, E., Nemes-Nikodem, E., Knappe, D. and Hoffmann, R. (2014) *In vivo* activity of optimized apidaecin and oncocin peptides against a multiresistant, KPC-producing *Klebsiella pneumoniae* strain. *Protein and Peptide Letters* 21, 368–373.

Otvos, L., Jr (2005) Antibacterial peptides and proteins with multiple cellular targets. *Journal of Peptide Science* 11, 697–706.

Otvos, L., Jr and Ostorhazi, E. (2015) Therapeutic utility of antibacterial peptides in wound healing. *Expert Review of Anti-infective Therapy* 13, 871–881.

Otvos, L., Jr, Rogers, M.E., Consolvo, P.J., Condie, B.A., Lovas, S., Bulet, P. and Blaszczyk-Thurin, M. (2000) Interaction between heat shock proteins and antimicrobial peptides. *Biochemistry* 39, 14150–14159.

Otvos, L., Jr, Cudic, M., Chua, B.Y., Deliyannis, G. and Jackson, D.C. (2004) An insect antibacterial peptide-based drug delivery system. *Molecular Pharmacology* 1, 220–232.

Otvos, L., Jr, Wade, J.D., Lin, F., Condie, B.A., Hanrieder, J. and Hoffmann, R. (2005) Designer antibacterial peptides kill fluoroquinolone-resistant clinical isolates. *Journal of Medicinal Chemistry* 48, 5349–5359.

Pag, U., Oedenkoven, M., Sass, V., Shai, Y., Shamova, O., *et al.* (2008) Analysis of *in vitro* activities and modes of action of synthetic antimicrobial peptides derived from an alpha-helical 'sequence template'. *Journal of Antimicrobial Chemotherapy* 61, 341–352.

Park, C.B., Kim, H.S. and Kim, S.C. (1998) Mechanism of action of the antimicrobial peptide buforin II: buforin II kills microorganisms by penetrating the cell membrane and inhibiting cellular functions. *Biochemical and Biophysical Research Communications* 244, 253–257.

Park, C.B., Yi, K. S., Matsuzaki, K., Kim, M.S. and Kim, S.C. (2000) Structure-activity analysis of buforin II, a histone H2A-derived antimicrobial peptide: the proline hinge is responsible for the cell-penetrating ability of buforin II. *Proceedings of the National Academy of Sciences of the United States of America* 97, 8245–8250.

Patrzykat, A., Friedrich, C.L., Zhang, L., Mendoza, V. and Hancock, R.E. (2002) Sublethal concentrations of pleurocidin-derived antimicrobial peptides inhibit macromolecular synthesis in *Escherichia coli*. *Antimicrobial Agents and Chemotherapy* 46, 605–614.

Paulsen, V.S., Mardirossian, M., Blencke, H.M., Benincasa, M., Runti, G., *et al.* (2016) Inner membrane proteins YgdD and SbmA are required for the complete susceptibility of *E. coli* to the proline-rich antimicrobial peptide arasin 1(1-25). *Microbiology* 162 601–609.

Pavia, K.E., Spinella, S.A. and Elmore, D.E. (2012) Novel histone-derived antimicrobial peptides use different antimicrobial mechanisms. *Biochimica et Biophysica Acta* 1818, 869–876.

Pelillo, C., Benincasa, M., Scocchi, M., Gennaro, R., Tossi, A. and Pacor, S. (2014) Cellular internalization and cytotoxicity of the antimicrobial proline-rich peptide Bac7(1-35) in monocytes/ macrophages, and its activity against phagocytosed *Salmonella typhimurium*. *Protein and Peptide Letters* 21, 382–390.

Podda, E., Benincasa, M., Pacor, S., Micali, F., Mattiuzzo, M., Gennaro, R. and Scocchi, M. (2006) Dual mode of action of Bac7, a proline-rich antibacterial peptide. *Biochimica et Biophysica Acta* 1760, 1732–1740.

Pogliano, J., Pogliano, N. and Silverman, J.A. (2012) Daptomycin-mediated reorganization of membrane architecture causes mislocalization of essential cell division proteins. *Journal of Bacteriology* 194, 4494–4504.

Pundir, P., Catalli, A., Leggiadro, C., Douglas, S.E. and Kulka, M. (2014) Pleurocidin, a novel antimicrobial peptide, induces human mast cell activation through the FPRL1 receptor. *Mucosal Immunology* 7, 177–187.

Ray, S., Dhaked, H.P. and Panda, D. (2014) Antimicrobial peptide CRAMP (16-33) stalls bacterial cytokinesis by inhibiting FtsZ assembly. *Biochemistry* 53, 6426–6429.

Rosenberger, C.M., Gallo, R.L. and Finlay, B.B. (2004) Interplay between antibacterial effectors: a macrophage antimicrobial peptide impairs intracellular *Salmonella* replication. *Proceedings of the National Academy of Sciences of the United States of America* 101, 2422–2427.

Roy, R.N., Lomakin, I.B., Gagnon, M.G. and Steitz, T.A. (2015) The mechanism of inhibition of protein synthesis by the proline-rich peptide oncocin. *Nature Structural and Molecular Biology* 22, 466–469.

Runti, G., Lopez Ruiz Mdel, C., Stoilova, T., Hussain, R., Jennions, M., *et al.* (2013) Functional characterization of SbmA, a bacterial inner membrane transporter required for importing the antimicrobial peptide Bac7(1-35). *Journal of Bacteriology* 195, 5343–5351.

Sadler, K., Eom, K.D., Yang, J.L., Dimitrova, Y. and Tam, J.P. (2002) Translocating proline-rich peptides from the antimicrobial peptide bactenecin 7. *Biochemistry* 41, 14150–14157.

Sass, V., Schneider, T., Wilmes, M., Korner, C., Tossi, A., *et al.* (2010) Human beta-defensin 3 inhibits cell wall biosynthesis in Staphylococci. *Infection and Immunity* 78, 2793–2800.

Schmidt, R., Ostorhazi, E., Wende, E., Knappe, D. and Hoffmann, R. (2016) Pharmacokinetics and *in vivo* efficacy of optimized oncocin derivatives. *Journal of Antimicrobial Chemotherapy* 71, 1003–1011.

Schneider, T., Kruse, T., Wimmer, R., Wiedemann, I., Sass, V., *et al.* (2010) Plectasin, a fungal defensin, targets the bacterial cell wall precursor Lipid II. *Science* 328, 1168–1172.

Scocchi, M., Zelezetsky, I., Benincasa, M., Gennaro, R., Mazzoli, A. and Tossi, A. (2005) Structural aspects and biological properties of the cathelicidin PMAP-36. *FEBS Journal* 272, 4398–4406.

Scocchi, M., Lüthy, C., Decarli, P., Mignogna, G., Christen, P. and Gennaro, R. (2009) The proline-rich antibacterial peptide Bac7 binds to and inhibits *in vitro* the molecular chaperone DnaK. *International Journal of Peptide Research and Therapeutics* 15, 147–155.

Scocchi, M., Tossi, A. and Gennaro, R. (2011) Proline-rich antimicrobial peptides: converging to a non-lytic mechanism of action. *Cellular and Molecular Life Sciences* 68, 2317–2330.

Scocchi, M., Mardirossian, M., Runti, G. and Benincasa, M. (2016) Non-membrane permeabilizing modes of action of antimicrobial peptides on bacteria. *Current Topics in Medicinal Chemistry* 16, 76–88.

Sebe, I., Ostorhazi, E., Fekete, A., Kovacs, K.N., Zelko, R., *et al.* (2016) Polyvinyl alcohol nanofiber formulation of the designer antimicrobial peptide APO sterilizes *Acinetobacter baumannii*-infected skin wounds in mice. *Amino Acids* 48, 203–211.

Seefeldt, A.C., Nguyen, F., Antunes, S., Perebaskine, N., Graf, M., *et al.* (2015) The proline-rich antimicrobial peptide Onc112 inhibits translation by blocking and destabilizing the initiation complex. *Nature Structural and Molecular Biology* 22, 470–475.

Seefeldt, A.C., Graf, M., Perebaskine, N., Nguyen, F., Arenz, S., *et al.* (2016) Structure of the mammalian antimicrobial peptide Bac7(1-16) bound within the exit tunnel of a bacterial ribosome. *Nucleic Acids Research* 44, 2429–2438.

Shai, Y. (2002) Mode of action of membrane active antimicrobial peptides. *Biopolymers* 66, 236–248.

Sharma, A., Pohane, A.A., Bansal, S., Bajaj, A., Jain, V. and Srivastava, A. (2015) Cell penetrating synthetic antimicrobial peptides (SAMPs) exhibiting potent and selective killing of mycobacterium by targeting its DNA. *Chemistry* 21, 3540–3545

Shaw, J.E., Alattia, J.R., Verity, J.E., Prive, G.G. and Yip, C.M. (2006) Mechanisms of antimicrobial peptide action: studies of indolicidin assembly at model membrane interfaces by *in situ* atomic force microscopy. *Journal of Structural Biology* 154, 42–58.

Shi, J., Ross, C.R., Leto, T.L. and Blecha, F. (1996) PR-39: a proline-rich antibacterial peptide that inhibits phagocyte NADPH oxidase activity by binding to Src homology 3 domains of p47 phox. *Proceedings of the National Academy of Sciences of the United States of America* 93, 6014–6018.

Siqueiros-Cendon, T., Arevalo-Gallegos, S., Iglesias-Figueroa, B.F., Garcia-Montoya, I.A., Salazar-Martinez, J. and Rascon-Cruz, Q. (2014) Immunomodulatory effects of lactoferrin. *Acta Pharmacologica Sinica* 35, 557–566.

Sitaram, N. and Nagaraj, R. (1999) Interaction of antimicrobial peptides with biological and model membranes: structural and charge requirements for activity. *Biochimica et Biophysica Acta* 1462, 29–54.

Skerlavaj, B., Romeo, D. and Gennaro, R. (1990) Rapid membrane permeabilization and inhibition of vital functions of Gram-negative bacteria by bactenecins. *Infection and Immunity* 58, 3724–3730.

Srinivas, N., Jetter, P., Ueberbacher, B.J., Werneburg, M., Zerbe, K., *et al.* (2010) Peptidomimetic antibiotics target outer-membrane biogenesis in *Pseudomonas aeruginosa*. *Science* 327, 1010–1013.

Stalmans, S., Wynendaele, E., Bracke, N., Knappe, D., Hoffmann, R., *et al.* (2014) Blood-brain barrier transport of short proline-rich antimicrobial peptides. *Protein and Peptide Letters* 21, 399–406.

Subbalakshmi, C. and Sitaram, N. (1998) Mechanism of antimicrobial action of indolicidin. *FEMS Microbiology Letters* 160, 91–96.

Szabo, D., Ostorhazi, E., Binas, A., Rozgonyi, F., Kocsis, B., *et al.* (2010) The designer proline-rich antibacterial peptide A3-APO is effective against systemic *Escherichia coli* infections in different mouse models. *International Journal of Antimicrobial Agents* 35, 357–361.

't Hart, P., Oppedijk, S.F., Breukink, E. and Martin, N.I. (2016) New insights into nisin's antibacterial mechanism revealed by binding studies with synthetic lipid II analogues. *Biochemistry* 55, 232–237.

Taniguchi, M., Ochiai, A., Kondo, H., Fukuda, S., Ishiyama, Y., *et al.* (2016) Pyrrhocoricin, a proline-rich antimicrobial peptide derived from insect, inhibits the translation process in the cell-free *Escherichia coli* protein synthesis system. *Journal of Bioscience and Bioengineering* 121, 591–598.

Taylor, S. D. and Palmer, M. (2016) The action mechanism of daptomycin. *Bioorganic and Medicinal Chemistry* 24, 6253–6268.

Thallinger, C., Rothenburger, M., Marsik, C., Wuenscher, S., Popovic, M., *et al.* (2008) Daptomycin does not exert immunomodulatory effects in an experimental endotoxin model of human whole blood. *Pharmacology* 81, 57–62.

Tian, W., Li, B., Zhang, X., Dang, W., Wang, X., *et al.* (2012) Suppression of tumor invasion and migration in breast cancer cells following delivery of siRNA against Stat3 with the antimicrobial peptide PR39. *Oncology Reports* 28, 1362–1368.

Tomasinsig, L. and Zanetti, M. (2005) The cathelicidins – structure, function and evolution. *Current Protein and Peptide Science* 6, 23–34.

Tomasinsig, L., Scocchi, M., Mettulio, R. and Zanetti, M. (2004) Genome-wide transcriptional profiling of the *Escherichia coli* response to a proline-rich antimicrobial peptide. *Antimicrobial Agents and Chemotherapy* 48, 3260–3267.

Tomasinsig, L., Skerlavaj, B., Papo, N., Giabbai, B., Shai, Y. and Zanetti, M. (2006) Mechanistic and functional studies of the interaction of a proline-rich antimicrobial peptide with mammalian cells. *Journal of Biological Chemistry* 281, 383–391.

Tomasinsig, L., De Conti, G., Skerlavaj, B., Piccinini, R., Mazzilli, M., D'Este, F., Tossi, A. and Zanetti, M. (2010) Broad-spectrum activity against bacterial mastitis pathogens and activation of mammary epithelial cells support a protective role of neutrophil cathelicidins in bovine mastitis. *Infection and Immunity* 78, 1781–1788.

Tossi, A., Sandri, L. and Giangaspero, A. (2000) Amphipathic, alpha-helical antimicrobial peptides. *Biopolymers*, 55, 4–30.

Ulvatne, H., Samuelsen, O., Haukland, H.H., Kramer, M. and Vorland, L.H. (2004) Lactoferricin B inhibits bacterial macromolecular synthesis in *Escherichia coli* and *Bacillus subtilis*. *FEMS Microbiology Letters* 237, 377–384.

Uyterhoeven, E.T., Butler, C.H., Ko, D. and Elmore, D.E. (2008) Investigating the nucleic acid interactions and antimicrobial mechanism of buforin II. *FEBS Letters* 582, 1715–1718.

Veldhuizen, E.J., Schneider, V.A., Agustiandari, H., van Dijk, A., Tjeersdma-van Bokhoven, J.L., *et al.* (2014) Antimicrobial and immunomodulatory activities of PR-39 derived peptides. *PLoS One* 9, e95939.

Verbanac, D., Zanetti, M. and Romeo, D. (1993) Chemotactic and protease-inhibiting activities of antibiotic peptide precursors. *FEBS Letters* 317, 255–258.

Volke, D., Krizsan, A., Berthold, N., Knappe, D. and Hoffmann, R. (2015) Identification of Api88 binding partners in *Escherichia coli* using a photoaffinity-cross-link strategy and label-free quantification. *Journal of Proteome Research* 14, 3274–3283.

Walberg, M., Gaustad, P. and Steen, H.B. (1997) Rapid assessment of ceftazidime, ciprofloxacin, and gentamicin susceptibility in exponentially-growing *E. coli* cells by means of flow cytometry. *Cytometry* 27, 169–178.

Wang, G., Mishra, B., Lau, K., Lushnikova, T., Golla, R. and Wang, X. (2015) Antimicrobial peptides in 2014. *Pharmaceuticals (Basel)* 8, 123–150.

Wenzel, M., Chiriac, A.I., Otto, A., Zweytick, D., May, C., *et al.* (2014) Small cationic antimicrobial peptides delocalize peripheral membrane proteins. *Proceedings of the National Academy of Sciences of the United States of America* 111, E1409–E1418.

Werneburg, M., Zerbe, K., Juhas, M., Bigler, L., Stalder, U., *et al.* (2012) Inhibition of lipopolysaccharide transport to the outer membrane in *Pseudomonas aeruginosa* by peptidomimetic antibiotics. *ChemBioChem* 13, 1767–1775.

Whiley, D.M., Goire, N., Lahra, M.M., Donovan, B., Limnios, A.E., Nissen, M.D. and Sloots, T.P. (2012) The ticking time bomb: escalating antibiotic resistance in *Neisseria gonorrhoeae* is a public health disaster in waiting. *The Journal of Antimicrobial Chemotherapy* 67, 2059–2061.

Wickens, H.J., Pinney, R.J., Mason, D.J. and Gant, V.A. (2000) Flow cytometric investigation of filamentation, membrane patency, and membrane potential in *Escherichia coli* following ciprofloxacin exposure. *Antimicrobial Agents and Chemotherapy* 44, 682–687.

Wiedemann, I., Bottiger, T., Bonelli, R.R., Schneider, T., Sahl, H.G. and Martinez, B. (2006) Lipid II-based antimicrobial activity of the lantibiotic plantaricin C. *Applied Environmental Microbiology* 72, 2809–2814.

Wiedemann, I., Breukink, E., van Kraaij, C., Kuipers, O.P., Bierbaum, G., de Kruijff, B. and Sahl, H.G. (2001) Specific binding of nisin to the peptidoglycan precursor lipid II combines pore formation and inhibition of cell wall biosynthesis for potent antibiotic activity. *Journal of Biological Chemistry* 276, 1772–1779.

Willey, J.M. and van der Donk, W.A. (2007) Lantibiotics: peptides of diverse structure and function. *Annual Review of Microbiology* 61, 477–501.

Wilmes, M., Stockem, M., Bierbaum, G., Schlag, M., Gotz, F., *et al.* (2014) Killing of staphylococci by theta-defensins involves membrane impairment and activation of autolytic enzymes. *Antibiotics* 3, 617–631.

Wimley, W.C. (2010) Describing the mechanism of antimicrobial peptide action with the interfacial activity model. *ACS Chemical Biology* 5, 905–917.

Yeaman, M.R. and Yount, N.Y. (2003) Mechanisms of antimicrobial peptide action and resistance. *Pharmacological Review* 55, 27–55.

Yonezawa, A., Kuwahara, J., Fujii, N. and Sugiura, Y. (1992) Binding of tachyplesin I to DNA revealed by footprinting analysis: significant contribution of secondary structure to DNA binding and implication for biological action. *Biochemistry* 31, 2998–3004.

Yount, N.Y., Bayer, A.S., Xiong, Y.Q. and Yeaman, M.R. (2006) Advances in antimicrobial peptide immunobiology. *Biopolymers* 84, 435–458.

Zahn, M., Berthold, N., Kieslich, B., Knappe, D., Hoffmann, R. and Strater, N. (2013) Structural studies on the forward and reverse binding modes of peptides to the chaperone DnaK. *Journal of Molecular Biology* 425, 2463–2479.

Zahn, M., Kieslich, B., Berthold, N., Knappe, D., Hoffmann, R. and Strater, N. (2014) Structural identification of DnaK binding sites within bovine and sheep bactenecin Bac7. *Protein and Peptide Letters* 21, 407–412.

Zasloff, M. (2002) Antimicrobial peptides of multicellular organisms. *Nature* 415, 389–395.

10 Structural Insight into the Mechanisms of Action of Antimicrobial Peptides and Structure-based Design

Guangshun Wang*

*Department of Pathology and Microbiology, College of Medicine,
University of Nebraska Medical Center, Omaha, NE 68198-6495, USA*

Abstract

Antimicrobial peptides (AMPs) are important innate immune molecules that mainly target bacterial membranes, but can also inhibit non-membrane targets such as DNA and ribosomes. Structural studies of AMPs can provide valuable insight into the mechanism of action. Nuclear magnetic resonance (NMR) spectroscopy plays a major role in structural determination of AMPs in membrane-mimetic environments, while X-ray crystallography is the dominant technology for solving the structures of large complexes between AMPs and their targets. Various structural scaffolds have been found and can be classified into four families: α-helices, β-sheets, a mixture of αβ-structures and non-αβ structures (Wang, 2010). This chapter highlights important three-dimensional (3D) structures from each class. The helical family can damage membranes via the carpet or barrel-stave pore model, whereas the Pro-rich members of the non-αβ family inhibit protein synthesis by binding to intracellular ribosomes. The β-sheet containing AMPs can work by different mechanisms such as inhibition of the cell wall synthesis and binding to

specific lipid components in membranes. Finally, high-quality structures of AMPs bound to membrane or non-membrane targets are also useful for more precisely engineering novel medicine.

Antimicrobial peptides (AMPs) are innate immune molecules the host uses to fend off invading pathogens. In multicellular organisms, these peptides are not limited to antimicrobial functions and can have other roles such as immune regulation, apoptosis and wound healing (Zasloff, 2002; Boman, 2003; Hancock *et al*, 2016). AMPs are usually cationic with less than 50 amino acids. They can take a variety of molecular forms, ranging from linear to cyclic. The frequently occurring amino acids appear to determine the molecular scaffolds of AMPs (Chapter 1). While the preceding two chapters have discussed membrane and non-membrane targeting AMPs, this chapter highlights selected three-dimensional (3D) structures of these peptides that shed light on the mechanisms of action. As of November 2016, there were 376 unique structures (328 determined by NMR and 48 by X-ray crystallography) in the Antimicrobial Peptide Database (Wang *et al.*, 2016). These structures can be grouped

---

* Corresponding author e-mail: gwang@unmc.edu

into four classes: α, β, αβ, and non-αβ (Wang, 2010). This chapter also provides examples for structure-based design of novel therapeutic peptides for treatment of infectious diseases and cancer.

10.1 Introduction to Structural Methods and Membrane Models

Most AMPs are cationic (on average +3) and have a hydrophobic content of ~50% (Wang et al., 2016). Such an amphipathic nature enables AMPs to recognize anionic bacterial membranes. As a consequence, structural determination of these peptides in the membrane-bound state should reveal the molecular basis and atomic details of how they might associate with bacterial membranes. According to the statistics in the APD database, such structures are mainly determined by NMR spectroscopy. The wide use of NMR is due to the small size of AMPs and the fact that membrane-targeting peptides are resistant to crystallization. NMR became a structural tool in the 1980s (Wüthrich, 1986; Ernst et al., 1987). It was at a perfect time for AMP research, which also thrived in the same timeframe (Chapter 1). Table 10.1 summarizes the major technologies and membrane models used for structural studies by NMR. Initially, two-dimensional (2D) NMR methods were applied to the studies of gramicidin bound

to the micelles of sodium dodecylsulfate (SDS) (Arseniev et al., 1985), magainin 2 in an aqueous solution of trifluoroethanol (TFE) (Marion et al., 1988), and cecropins in 15% (v/v) hexafluoroisopropyl alcohol (Holak et al., 1988). Since then, micelles of SDS and dodecylphosphocholine (DPC) have been widely accepted and utilized as bacterial membrane-mimetic models (Arseniev et al., 1985; Wüthrich, 1986; Nguyen et al., 2011). During 2003–2004, short-chain phosphatidylglycerols (PGs) were also introduced (Wang et al., 2004; Wang, 2006), enabling a structural determination in complex with short-chain PGs, as well as a direct detection of intermolecular nuclear Overhauser effects (NOE) between cationic peptides and anionic PGs (Wang, 2007). Meanwhile, Wang et al. (2005) measured heteronuclear ^{13}C or ^{15}N chemical shifts of peptides without isotope labelling for validation of ^1H chemical shift assignments and structural refinement. This improved 2D NMR method that includes natural abundance ^{15}N and ^{13}C information led to higher quality 3D structures as demonstrated by different laboratories (Wang et al., 2005; Conibear et al., 2012; Wang, 2013). To gain additional spectral resolution, ^{13}C or ^{15}N-separated 3D NMR spectroscopy can be applied. The use of 3D and 4D triple-resonance (^1H, ^{15}N and ^{13}C) NMR spectroscopy (Kay et al., 1990) makes it possible for NMR studies of more complex antimicrobial peptides and proteins. These NMR

Table 10.1. Methods and models for NMR studies of antimicrobial peptides.

Peptide	NMR method	Model/condition	References
Defensin NP-5	2D NMR	Water	Bach et al., 1987
Magainin 2; Cecropin	2D NMR	Organic solvents (e.g., TFE)	Marion et al., 1988; Holak et al., 1988
Gramicidin A	2D NMR	SDS	Arseniev et al., 1985
Gramicidin A	Solid-state NMR	Lipid bilayers	Ketchem et al., 1993
Nisin	2D NMR	DPC	van den Hooven et al., 1993
Aurein 1.2	Improved 2D NMR	SDS	Wang et al., 2005
KR-12	Improved 2D NMR	D8PG	Wang, 2008
Temporins	Transfer-NOE	LPS	Bhunia et al., 2011
LL-23	3D ^{15}N-separated NMR	SDS, DPC, D8PG	Wang et al., 2012a
LL-37	3D triple-resonance NMR	SDS, LPS, D8PG	Wang, 2008

experiments require isotope labelling of AMPs (Wang, 2008). A detailed description of structural determination of AMPs by multidimensional NMR can be found in the first version of this book (Wang, 2010), including peptide expression and purification, sample preparations, different membrane models, NMR methodology, data collection, sequential signal assignments, structure calculations, validation and deposition. It is important to determine the structure to high resolution under appropriate conditions (Wang, 2013; Wang *et al.*, 2014b).

Not all AMPs, however, target bacterial membranes. Lysozyme is a classic example. Known to cleave polysaccharides in the bacteria cell wall, this small globular protein has been a model for structural studies by X-ray crystallography (Cheetham *et al.*, 1992). Proline-rich antimicrobial peptides (PrAMPs) are now known to bind to ribosomes to shut down the protein synthesis machinery. Such complexes are too large for NMR, but have been determined by X-ray crystallography (Roy *et al.*, 2015; Seefeldt *et al.*, 2015). There are also cases where both NMR spectroscopy and X-ray crystallography were applied. Structural studies of disulfide-stabilized defensins by the two techniques reveal a similar structural fold (Bach *et al.*, 1987; Hill *et al.*, 1991). In addition, these two techniques provide complementary information (Section 10.2.3). In particular, NMR can depict a motional picture for the polypeptide chain as to which part is rigid and which part is mobile. In the following, selected structures from each class are described.

10.2 Three-dimensional Structures of Antimicrobial Peptides

10.2.1 α-helical AMPs

In the APD, 168 AMPs are established to have α-helical structures based on NMR and crystallographic analysis (Wang *et al.*, 2016). These are unique structures that do not include those determined at low resolution, under different conditions, or after a single residue change.

Helical structures in aqueous solution

Due to disulfide bond stabilization, a few AMPs can have a helical structure in aqueous solution. Saposin-like proteins (SAPLIP) occur widely in nature, ranging from protozoan parasites (e.g. *Entamoeba histolytica*) and worms (e.g. *Caenorhabditis elegans*), through to mammals (e.g. *Sus scrofa*), including humans (*Homo sapiens*). The helix-bundle structures of these antimicrobial proteins are stabilized by three disulfide bonds. In the structure of caenopore-5 from *C. elegans* (Pro81 cis conformer in Fig. 10.1A), the five helices are located between residues 6-16, 24-36, 45-50, 58-66, and 70-78 (Mysliwy *et al.*, 2010). In addition, there are two S-S bonds (Cys6-Cys80 and Cys9-Cys74) between helices I and V at the N- and C-termini of the protein, a third S-S bond (Cys35-Cys49) is formed between helices II and III. This AMP plays an essential role for the survival of the worm by eliminating *E. coli* ingested. Upon association with bacterial membranes, the helix-bundle structure may open at a site with multiple exposed hydrophobic side chains (arrow in Fig. 10.1A). Despite a similar protein fold, the antibacterial activity of tick microplusin is attributed to Cu^{2+} binding (Silva *et al.*, 2009). Bacterial enterocin AS-48, a circular peptide, also uses the saposin fold. The connection of the N- and C-termini of this bacteriocin by a peptide bond makes the peptide stable to exoproteases (Sánchez-Hidalgo *et al.*, 2011). The inactive dimeric structure of cyclic AS-48 is proposed to dissociate into active monomers to exert effects on bacterial membranes (Cebrián *et al.*, 2015). Another unique AMP that forms a helix-bundle structure in water is distinctin. This amphibian peptide comprises two chains linked by only one S-S bond, which is critical for structure stability to proteases rather than antimicrobial activity (Dalla Serra *et al.*, 2008). Solid-state NMR studies support that both helices are located on the membrane surface of lipid bilayers, excluding the possibility of pore

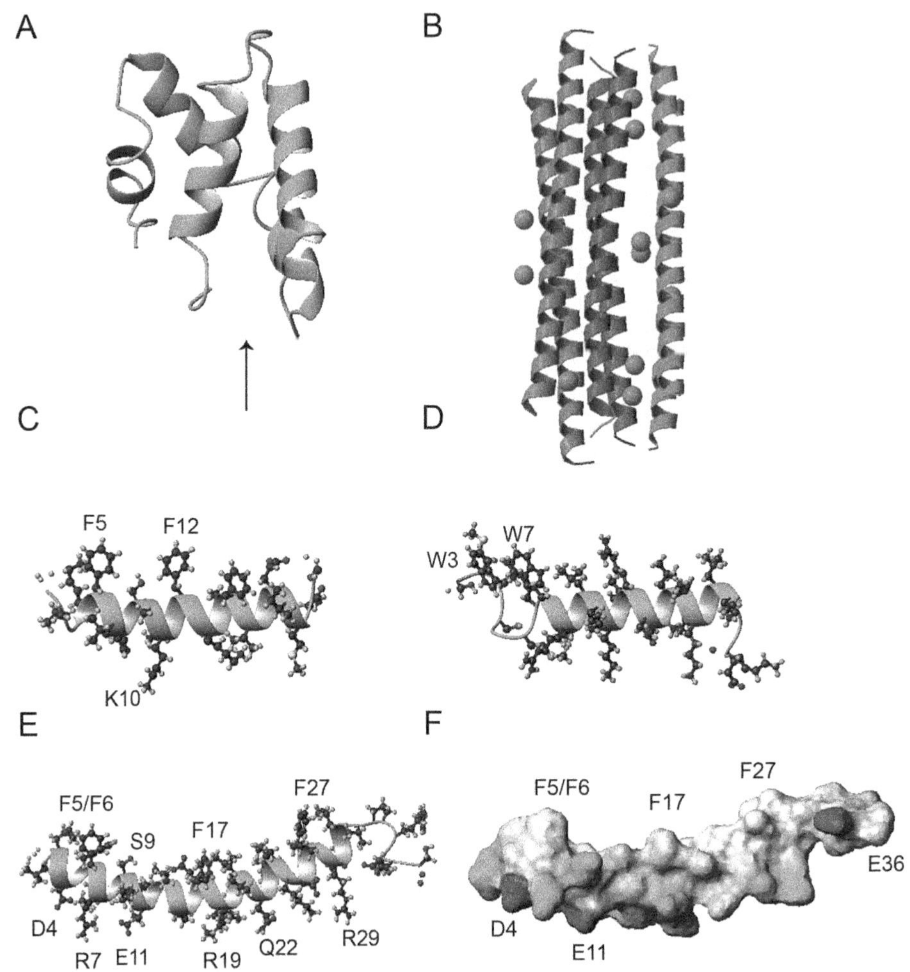

Fig. 10.1. 3D structures of antimicrobial peptides from the α-helix family. Depicted are (A) caenopore-5 from *Caenorhabditis elegans* (PDB ID: 2JS9); (B) human dermcidin (PDB ID: 2YMK); (C) amphibian magainin 2 (PDB ID: 2MAG); (D) spider latarcin 1 (PDB ID: 2PCO); (E) and (F) human cathelicidin LL-37 (PDB ID: 2K6O). In short peptides, aromatic residues (labelled) are common and important for anchoring these AMPs into bacterial membrane. To clearly view the polypeptide fold, the disulfide bonds in panel A are omitted.

formation (Resende *et al.*, 2009). However, there is a proposal that the helix-bundle structure of human dermcidin (Fig. 10.1B) serves as a channel (Song *et al.*, 2013).

Membrane-bound helical structures

Most of the linear AMPs are disordered in water, and can only adopt a helical structure after binding to membranes. Amphibian magainin 2 (Gesell *et al.*, 1997), dermadistinctin K (Verly *et al.*, 2009), fish

pleurocidin (Syvitski *et al.*, 2005), and insect spinigerin (Landon *et al.*, 2006) are such examples. The structure of magainin 2 is determined in the presence of TFE, SDS, or DPC (Gesell *et al.*, 1997). In this case, similar helical structures are found, indicating that these membrane-mimetic models are equally useful. This model peptide possesses a typical amphipathic helical structure for membrane targeting (Fig. 10.1C). It is also likely that magainin 2 works synergistically with another frog peptide PGLa.

Based on solid-state NMR studies, there is no correlation between the observed activity synergy and the topological state of the two peptides in the membrane. Hence, lipid-mediated interactions, rather than the association of the two amphibian peptides, may be responsible for the synergistic activity of the mixture (Marquette *et al.*, 2016).

Some AMPs possess two helical domains. Examples are insect cecropin A (Holak *et al.*, 1988), amphibian gaegurin-4 (Chi *et al.*, 2007), and dermaceptin B2 (Galanth *et al.*, 2009). The linker regions of these peptides are important for antimicrobial activity, allowing optimal binding of both helices to bacterial membranes (Park *et al.*, 2007; Galanth *et al.*, 2009). There are also other molecular defence constructs where the N-terminal portion is not a helix (Wang and Wang, 2016). In the case of latarcin 1, the aromatic rings of W3 and W7 (Fig. 10.1D) might also help anchor the entire peptide onto membranes (Dubovskii *et al.*, 2008). These AMPs could induce a positive membrane curvature, leading to toroidal pore formation or micellization of membranes (Haney *et al.*, 2010; Shai, 2002).

To provide direct evidence for peptide-membrane interactions, NMR studies of human cathelicidin LL-37 have been conducted in complex with either lipopolysaccharides (LPS) or phophatidylglycerols (PGs), which are the key components of the outer and inner membranes of Gram-negative bacteria, respectively. In complex with SDS micelles, LL-37 adopts a long helix between residues 2 and 31 followed by a disordered tail at the C-terminus (Wang, 2008). Such an ordered–disordered structure (Fig. 10.1E) agrees entirely with the backbone dynamics at the ps–ns timescale. Since this LL-37 structure is applicable to the LPS- or PG-bound case (Wang, 2010), it can be used to explain the basis of membrane interactions. First, a unique hydrophilic serine (Ser9) on the hydrophobic surface (Fig. 10.1E) splits the long helix of LL-37 into two domains. Such a two-domain structure is responsible for the synergistic binding of LL-37 to LPS (Turner *et al.*, 1998). Note that the LPS neutralization synergy can also occur between two peptides from the same frog (Mangoni *et al.*, 2008). Temporin L can cause the dissociation of the aggregated form of temporin B, thereby maximizing LPS neutralization by these two amphibian peptides (Bhunia *et al.*, 2011). Second, membrane binding involves the entire long helix of LL-37 since there are direct NOE contacts between the aromatic rings (Phe5, Phe6, Phe17 and Phe27) of the peptide and dioctanoyl phosphatidylglycerol (D8PG). Such favourable contacts are in line with the protruding aromatic rings of the four phenylalanines on the hydrophobic surface (Fig. 10.1F; also see book cover), allowing for membrane anchoring. Third, the central helix (residue 10-31) is found to be critical for antibacterial, antibiofilm and antiviral activities (Wang *et al.*, 2014b). In addition, not all cationic side chains are equal. Based on NMR spectroscopy, only the interfacial basic arginine (R23) of the central helix directly interacts with acidic PGs (Wang, 2007). This electrostatic interaction may constitute the driving force for initial recognition, lipid domain formation (Epand *et al.*, 2009; Chapter 8), or phase changes in lipid bilayers, leading to a toroidal pore formation (Henzler *et al.*, 2003) and even lysis of bacteria (Mishra and Wang, unpublished).

The arginine-PG electrostatic interactions between LL-37 and membranes detected by NMR spectroscopy (Wang, 2008) can also be utilized to understand a counteracting resistance strategy of superbugs. It has been observed that bacteria can make their surfaces less negative via chemical modification (e.g. lysylating PGs). This modification decreases such electrostatic interactions, thereby diminishing the impact of cationic AMPs on bacteria. Modification like this constitutes a resistance mechanism for a pathogen to infect the host (Peschel, 2012), and a survival strategy for commensal bacteria that work in harmony with the host (Wang *et al.*, 2015).

Few AMPs are known to form a barrel-stave pore. Alamethicin is probably the only example of this where multiple copies of the amphipathic helices can be packed into a pore with the hydrophilic side-chains facing inward (to bind ions) and hydrophobic side-chains facing outward (to contact membranes). This voltage-gated ion channel can allow both anionic and cationic ions to go through (Fox and Richards, 1982). In contrast, gramicidin A generates an ion pore by a different molecular assembly. Two molecules stack together via the N-terminus. Each molecule adopts a β-helix in lipid bilayers determined by solid-state NMR (Ketchem *et al.*, 1993) or in SDS micelles determined by liquid-state NMR (Arseniev *et al.*, 1985; Jordan *et al.*, 2005). This head-to-head dimer can then traverse the lipid bilayer with the C-terminal Trp-rich region exposed to the membrane interface. Such an orientation of Trp side-chains, with the five-membered ring more exposed, contributes to the ion channel property. If validated, dermcidin may be another example of ion channel formation in the membranes (Song *et al.*, 2013).

Beyond membranes

Our knowledge of helical AMPs has grown considerably. In particular, AMPs can have multiple functions other than membrane targeting. The pH-dependent oligomerization of LL-37 was observed soon after its discovery. Such a structural transition from random coils at an acidic pH to a helix at pH 7 is supported by both CD (circular dichroism) and NMR studies. Size exclusion chromatography reveals a tetramer of LL-37 at pH 7 (Johansson *et al.*, 1998; Li *et al.*, 2007). The aromatic–aromatic packing between F5 and F6 at the N-terminal region of LL-37 (Fig. 10.1, E, F) may play a role in peptide aggregation (Wang *et al.*, 2014b). Such an aggregated helix bundle could dissociate into monomers when bound to anionic membranes or under acidic conditions (Oren *et al.*, 1999). The physiological role of this pH dependent LL-37 oligomerization has been elucidated recently. At pH 7, DNA can associate with LL-37; this complex, however, is then dissociated in the endosomes at an acidic pH (Singh *et al.*, 2014). In addition, human LL-37 can also stabilize the neutrophil extracellular traps (NETs) structure by binding to DNA (Neumann *et al.*, 2014). Exactly how LL-37 stabilizes these

nucleic acids remains to be determined. The chemotactic property of LL-37 can be attributed to a specific interaction with its receptors. There is no 3D structure available to date. A model is proposed for human LL-37 in complex with formyl peptide receptor 2 (Tripathi *et al.*, 2015). Further characterization of these LL-37 involved complexes will shed light on the basis of specificity.

10.2.2 β-sheet AMPs

Two-stranded β-sheets

A minimal β-sheet peptide contains two β-strands. Several linear AMPs adopt a β-hairpin structure. These include thanatin (Mandard *et al.*, 1998), protegrin-1 (PG-1) (Aumelas *et al.*, 1996), tachyplesins (Laederach *et al.*, 2002), polyphemusin I (Powers *et al.*, 2004), and gomesin (Mandard *et al.*, 2002). Thanatin (Fig. 10.2A) consists of only one S-S bond between C11 and C18. This bridge is essential for specific interaction of the peptide with *E. coli*, but unimportant for non-specific binding to membranes of the Gram-positive bacterium *Micrococcus luteus* (Imamura *et al.*, 2008). Other AMPs listed above contain two S-S bonds. The S-S bond distant to the β-turn region is more important than the one close to the turn, indicative of the importance of the folded structure. The different cationic and hydrophobic side-chains present on the same antiparallel β-sheet structure determine their antimicrobial activity spectrum (Rodziewicz-Motowidło *et al.*, 2010).

θ-Defensins. Different from the open-ended two-stranded β-sheet structures above, the N- and C-termini are closed by a peptide bond in the case of θ-defensins. Like other defensins, they also have three pairs of disulfide bonds to further stabilize the scaffold (Chapter 3). The original structure of RTD-1 has been refined by using the improved 2D NMR method (Table 10.1), thereby identifying the flexible loop regions (Conibear *et al.*, 2012). An accurate mapping of such flexible loops (non-stranded regions in Fig. 10.2B) forms the basis for peptide grafting.

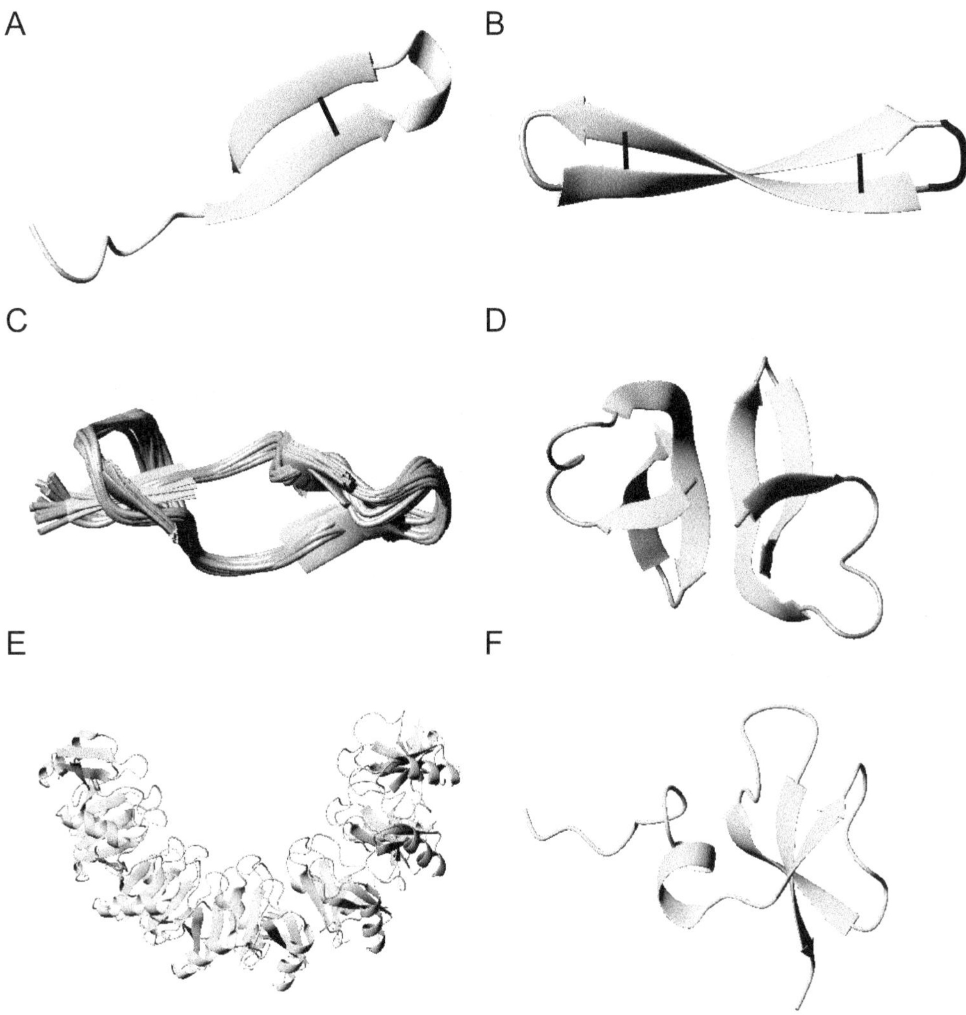

Fig. 10.2. 3D structures of antimicrobial peptides from the β-sheet containing families. Depicted are (A) insect thanatin (PDB ID: 8TFV); (B) monkey RTD-1 (PDB ID: 2LYF); (C) bacterial MccJ25 (PDB ID: 1Q71); (D) human HNP-2 (PDB ID: 1ZMI); (E) plant NaD1 (PDB ID: 4CQK); (F) human hBD-3 (PDB ID: 1KJ6). Structures in panels A, B, C and F are determined by X-ray crystallography and structures in panels D and E are determined by NMR spectroscopy.

Lassos

β-strands have also been observed in lasso peptides. A typical example is bacterial microcin J25 (structural ensemble in Fig. 10.2C). To date, about 40 ribosome synthesized lasso peptides are known (Hegemann *et al.*, 2015). Table 10.2 shows 12 AMPs with a lasso fold. There is a characteristic chemical bond between the amide of residue 1 and the carboxylic side-chain of residue 8 (usually Glu) or 9 (usually Asp). Interestingly, the tail of the peptide can enter the macrolactam ring (Fig. 10.2C, left). Lassos are classified based on disulfide bonds. Type 1 contains disulfide bonds, whereas type 2 does not (Hegemann *et al.*, 2015). The four members in type 1 lassos share a similar length, net charge and hydrophobic content (Pho% in Table 10.2). Type 2 antibacterial lassos appear to vary slightly.

Table 10.2. Select lasso peptides from the APD.[a]

APD ID	Name	Bond type	S-S bond	Length	Net charge	Pho%	Activity
Type I							
28	RP 71955	C1-D9	C1-C13, C7-C19	21	−1	61	V
1137	Siamycin I	C1-D9	C1-C13, C7-C19	21	−1	61	V
590	Siamycin II	C1-D9	C1-C13, C7-C19	21	−1	61	V
2728	Sviceucin	C1-D9	C1-C13, C7-C19	20	−2	60	G+
Type II							
480	MccJ25	G1-E8	None	21	−1	33	G−
1724	Capistruin	G1-E8	None	19	1	31	G−
1728	Lariatin A	G1-E8	None	18	1	33	G+
1729	Lariatin B	G1-E8	None	20	1	30	G+
2053	Astexin-1	G1-E7	None	23	−4	21	G-
2376	Lassomycin	G1-D8	None	16	3	43	G+
2719	Chaxapeptin	G1-D8	None	15	0	40	G+, C
2720	Sunsanpin	G1-D8	None	15	0	40	C

[a]Obtained from the APD at http://aps.unmc.edu/AP. C, anticancer; G-, inhibiting Gram-negative bacteria; G+, inhibiting Gram-positive bacteria; V, antiviral.

For example, the ring is usually formed between amide of G1 and the side-chain of E8 (e.g. MccJ25). However, it can be E7 or D8 as well. Except for lassomycin and astexin-1, lassos have a low net charge (Table 10.2).

Human α-defensins

Human defensins have a folded structure in water, enabling crystallization and structural determination by X-ray crystallography (Hill *et al.*, 1991; Xie *et al.*, 2005). Human α-defensins share a three antiparallel β-strand fold stabilized by three S-S bonds. The disulfide bonds, as well as salt bridges, are critical to maintaining the defensin fold. Using HNP-2 as a model (Fig. 10.2D, dimer in the crystal), the structural basis for the Gly-Xaa-Cys motif has been elucidated. The conserved Gly in the classic β-bulge has the backbone dihedral angles of a D-amino acid. Indeed, the protein fold is retained when Gly16 is changed to a D-amino acid (Ala, Glu, Phe, Arg, Thr, Val or Tyr), but the fold is disrupted when Gly16 is changed to L-Ala (Xie *et al.*, 2005).

Different from HNP-1 to HNP-4 found in neutrophils, HD-5 and HD-6 exist in the human small intestine. How HD-6 works has puzzled researchers, however, progress made recently with HD-6 studies reveals two mechanisms of action. Firstly, HD-6 kills bacteria under a reduced condition, uncovering a mechanism of how nature deploys defence molecules in oxygen-limited cases (Schroeder *et al.*, 2015). Secondly, HD-6 can form nanonets to surround bacteria. Structural analysis supports the essential role of His27 in HD-6 self-association (Chu *et al.*, 2012).

10.2.3 αβ-AMPs

AMPs in the αβ family consist of both α-helices and β-sheets (Fig. 10.2, E, F). In the APD, 103 such AMPs have been found from bacteria, fungi, plants and animals. They have a variety of functions and a few membrane-targeting defensins are highlighted here.

Plant and insect defensins recognize sphingolipids in fungal membranes (Vriens *et al.*, 2014). In the case of plant Psd1 with a βαββ fold, De Medeiros *et al.* (2010) identified the binding sites for glucosylceramide by NMR. The binding involves hydrophobic interactions via residues Val13, Phe15,

Ala18 and Trp38, as well as hydrogen bonding through Thr16 and Asn17. The recognition of unique fungal sphingolipids is essential for plant and insect defensins to induce subsequent events: release of reactive oxygen species (ROS) or cell cycle inhibition that leads to cell death (Aerts *et al.*, 2007; Lobo *et al.*, 2007). Another plant defensin NaD1 can also induce ROS. Its initial action, however, is to bind the plasma membrane phosphatidylinositol 4,5-bisphosphate (PI(4,5)P$_2$) (Lay *et al.*, 2012). In the complex, seven dimers of NaD1 (14 molecules) oligomerize into an arch configuration (Fig. 10.2E) to cooperatively bind the anionic headgroups of 14 phosphatidylinositol PIP(4,5)$_2$ molecules (Poon *et al.*, 2014). This leads to membrane permeation and peptide entry into the cell to produce ROS (Hayes *et al.*, 2013).

Structures of hBD-1, hBD-2 and hBD-3 have been determined by X-ray diffraction and NMR (Hoover *et al.*, 2000; 2001; Bauer *et al.*, 2001; Sawai *et al.*, 2001; Schibli *et al.*, 2002). Human β-defensins, with an αβββ fold, contain one N-terminal helix followed by a three-stranded β-sheet (Fig. 10.2F). X-ray crystallography and NMR provide complementary information under different conditions. While the structural coordinates determined in crystals are normally more accurate, NMR can be applied to the study of peptide dynamics in solution (Skalicky *et al.*, 1994), as well as its interaction with bacterial membranes (Wang, 2006). In addition, NMR also provides insight into the oligomerization of defensins in solution. While a dimer for hBD-1 and octamer for hBD-2 were found under crystal conditions, they are monomers in solution. However, hBD-3 is a dimer in solution, although a monomer is shown in Fig. 10.2F. The dimeric structure of hBD-3 could be more important for its higher antimicrobial activity than hBD-1 or hBD-2 (Schibli *et al.*, 2002). Like plant defensin NaD1 above, hBD-3 can kill cancer cells by targeting PI(4,5)P2. Although the structure of the complex is yet to be determined, the dimeric structure of hBD-3 in solution can be critical for the recognition and subsequent lysis of cancer cells (Phan *et al.*, 2016).

It appears that the structural basis of antimicrobial and chemotactic effects differs. Using hBD-1 as a model, Pazgier *et al.* (2007) determined the structure of 10 mutants by X-ray diffraction. These mutants have a protein fold identical to the wild type. It is proposed that the charged residues Arg29, Lys31, Lys33 and Lys36 are critical for antibacterial activity, whereas the N-terminal helical region (residues 1-8), including adjacent residues such as Lys22, Arg29 and Lys33, form the surface for chemotaxis to CCR6-transfected HEK-293 cells. The Cys residues are not required for antibacterial activity (Hoover *et al.*, 2003). However, the fifth Cys residue is critical for chemotaxis activity. Therefore, the Cys residues are essential for stabilizing the defensin fold required for a specific interaction with chiral molecular targets such as proteins. Indeed, disruption of the S-S bonds of HNP1 and HD5 is detrimental to their binding to Zn^{2+}-dependent metalloprotease (bacterial lethal factor) or HIV gp-120 (Wei *et al.*, 2009).

10.2.4 Non-αβ AMPs

Trp-rich peptides

Several Trp-rich peptides are known to adopt non-αβ amphipathic structures. These structures shine light on the spatial relationships of the Trp rings with adjacent amino acids. In the structure of indolicidin bound to DPC micelles, the aromatic rings of Trp6 and Trp9 pack against Pro7 and Pro10, respectively (Fig. 10.3A). This region is important for anchoring the peptide into the micelle (Rozek *et al.*, 2000). Likewise, the three Trp residues (Fig. 10.3B) are clustered in the amphipathic turn structure of tritrpticin in SDS micelles (Schibli *et al.*, 1999). There is a WW+ motif in the micelle-bound PW2 (Fig. 10.3C), an AMP (sequence: HPLKQYWWRPSI) obtained from phage display libraries (Tinoco *et al.*, 2002). Note that the side-chain of Arg9 packs against the aromatic ring of Trp8, providing an example for the cation-π interaction. The aromatic ring has π electron clouds on the surface, whereas the

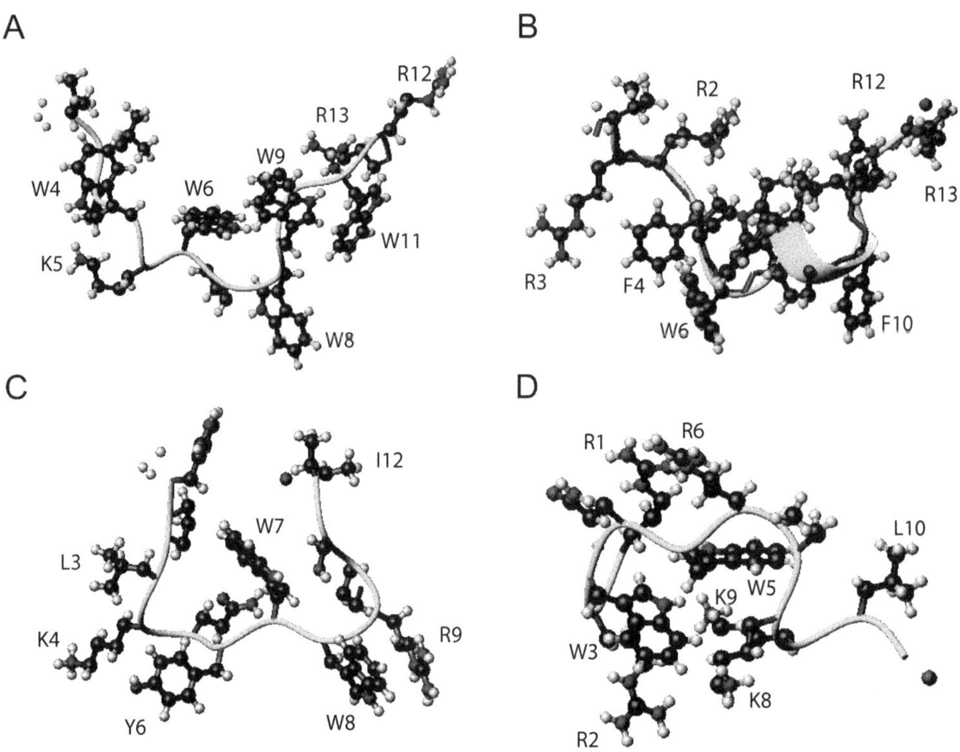

Fig. 10.3. NMR structures of antimicrobial peptides from the non-αβ family. Presented are (A) bovine indolicidin in DPC micelles (PDB ID: 1G89); (B) tritrpticin in SDS micelles (PDB ID: 1D6X); (C) PW2 in SDS micelles (PDB ID: 1M02); (D) lactoferrin B4-14 in SDS micelles (PDB ID: 1Y5C). Key residues are labelled.

arginine side-chain donates positive charge (Burghardt *et al.*, 2002). In SDS micelles, a Trp-rich region of lactoferrin B2 also adopts a non-αβ structure (Fig. 10.3D) with a distorted backbone (Nguyen *et al.*, 2005). In these structures, the six-membered aromatic rings of the Trp residues tend to point towards the membrane (Wang *et al.*, 1996; Yau *et al.*, 1998; Schibli *et al.*, 1999). In contrast, arginine residues may provide positive charges for recognition of negatively charged bacterial membranes in a manner similar to the LL-37 peptides (Wang, 2007). The combination of Trp with Arg may offer two advantages: antimicrobial potency and cell selectivity (Mishra *et al.*, 2017). In addition, a Trp-rich model peptide (sequence RWRWRW-NH$_2$) can exert multiple hits on the membranes, ranging from the classic membrane depolarization to the delocalization of native surface-attached membrane proteins (Wenzel *et al.*, 2014). As part of multiple hits, Trp-rich peptides may also associate with DNA (Arias *et al.*, 2015). (Note that one should not generalize that all Trp-rich peptides adopt non-αβ structures.)

Pro-rich peptides

Unlike the amphipathic helical class, which usually targets bacterial membranes, Pro-rich peptides (PrAMPs) interact with intracellular targets. Recently, ribosomes have been identified as a new target for PrAMPs (Krizsan *et al.*, 2014; Mardirossian *et al.*, 2014). Structural analysis reveals the binding of insect and mammalian PrAMPs to the ribosome tunnel in a non-αβ structure, thereby blocking the entry of the aminoacyl-tRNA to the A-site (Roy *et al.*, 2015; Seefeldt *et al.*, 2015). Such a structure should be useful for rational design of novel peptide antibiotics. It is important to note, however, that the Bac7(1-35) can also enter mammalian cells (Tomasinsig *et al.*, 2006). Therefore, a thorough evaluation of the potential cytotoxicity of AMPs is necessary. In addition, the exact role of the previously identified PrAMP-binding heat shock protein remains to be elucidated. One possibility is that it serves as a vehicle for PrAMPs to reach the ribosome (Knappe *et al.*, 2016).

Nisins–lipid II interactions

Multiple lantibiotics are known to inhibit cell wall synthesis. The interactions of nisin Z with cell wall precursor lipid II have been investigated by NMR (Hsu *et al.*, 2002). There is selective chemical shift perturbation at the N-terminal region of this ^{15}N-labelled lantibiotic, indicating that the N-terminal region, including rings A, B and C, is responsible for nisin recognition. The backbone amides of the N-terminal region actually form hydrogen bonds with the pyrophosphate moiety of lipid II. This cage structure explains the conservation of lanthinone rings of lipid-II binding lantibiotics (Hsu *et al.*, 2004).

10.3 Structure-based Peptide Design

10.3.1 Structural basis for the improvement of peptide druggability

The ultimate goal of peptide engineering is to improve peptide selectivity, efficacy, stability, formulation and delivery. Structure-based design deals with one or more aspects of these properties with a goal to improve peptide druggability. Due to cytotoxicity to human cells, many AMPs cannot be utilized directly. Selected strategies for improving peptide selectivity (or therapeutic index) are discussed in the previous edition (Wang, 2010). These strategies can be grouped into two types based on whether there is a conformational change in the peptide backbone. Firstly, longer peptides, such as human cathelicidin LL-37, can be partially truncated or mutated to reduce hydrophobicity without changing the backbone structure. A successful example is the identification of selective antibacterial peptide template KR-12 from human LL-37 (Wang, 2008). Secondly, peptide hydrophobicity can also be diminished by altering the peptide backbone structure. Compared to the in-phase side-chain packing in a regular amphipathic helix of GF-17 (Wang *et al.*, 2012b), the out-of-phase packing of the hydrophobic side-chains in the non-classic amphipathic structure of GF-17d3 (Li *et al.*, 2006) provides a structural basis for a decrease in peptide hydrophobicity.

Usually, linear peptides are not sufficiently stable to proteases, thereby lacking the needed resilience *in vivo*. A generally useful method to enhance peptide stability is to incorporate D-amino acids, either fully or partially (Wade *et al.*, 1990; Papo and Shai, 2004). This may result from a configuration change in the polypeptide chain, leading to poor association with the active site of proteases. To identify a peptide with stability to chymotrypsin, we screened a peptide library by conducting antimicrobial and stability assays simultaneously. GF-17d3 with 3 D-amino acids, but not peptide analogues with 0, 1 and 2 D-amino acids, is able to inhibit *E. coli* growth in the presence of chymotrypsin. The resultant GF-17d3 template forms the basis for the design of antimicrobial and antibiofilm peptide 17BIPHE2 against a panel of antibiotic-resistant bacteria (superbugs), including methicillin-resistant *Staphylococcus aureus* (Wang *et al.*, 2014a; Mishra *et al.*, 2016). One can also improve peptide stability based on the 3D structure. Introducing a disulfide bond between the termini of the U-shaped structure of CP-11 increases the stability of an indolicidin analogue to trypsin (Rozek *et al.*, 2003). The length of the basic side-chains of bactenecin analogues also influences stability to trypsin (Bagheri *et al.*, 2016).

Blood also influences the activity of AMPs. Serum albumin is an abundant vehicle in human blood. Both neutral and acidic drugs can bind to albumin, and so can basic AMPs. Structural determination reveals basic AMPs binding to drug site II of albumin via hydrophobic interactions (Sivertsen *et al.*, 2014). While reversible binding may help deliver the drug to the needed sites in blood, irreversible binding can cause a loss in activity. However, not all AMPs bind to serum albumin and lose their activity. The D-form of a model peptide remains active, while the L-form is inactive in a mouse model (Braunstein *et al.*, 2004). It is likely that the D-form does not bind to albumin well. Of note is that small lipopeptides also remain active in the presence of serum albumin (Mishra *et al.*, 2015).

10.3.2 Stable scaffold-based grafting

Cyclic peptides, discovered in bacteria, plants and mammals, are usually more stable to proteases. In the case of plant cyclotides, there are three pairs of disulfide bonds that further stabilize the peptide. This scaffold can be utilized to deliver known therapeutic peptides via grafting to the loop regions. Such a grafting can enhance the stability of the peptide motif, thereby improving druggability. In the case of kalata B1, the success of grafting depends on the composition, rather than the length, of the inserted sequence as long as the insert does not disrupt the scaffold (C.K. Wang *et al.*, 2014). Through this approach, anti-HIV or anticancer molecules have been generated (Aboye *et al.*, 2012; Conibear *et al.*, 2016), indicative of the existence of a proper peptide configuration for binding to the molecular target. A similar sequence motif RGDS has been grafted to θ-defensins (Conibear *et al.*, 2016) and the lasso fold on peptides such as MccJ25 (Hegemann *et al.*, 2014). It appears that larger epitopes can be grafted onto cyclotides. However, class II lassos do not have disulfide bonds (Table 10.2), allowing a delivery of the designer molecule under reducing conditions. Therefore, different scaffolds will satisfy the need for delivering different types of therapeutic peptides that modulate protein–protein interactions.

10.4 Concluding Remarks

It is now established that antimicrobial peptides can interact with cell surface components, membranes and intracellular molecular targets. While bacterial lantibiotics can bind to lipid II to block the synthesis of the cell wall of Gram-positive bacteria, human lysozyme is well characterized to cleave saccharides in bacterial cell walls. Recent NMR studies provide insight into the molecular basis of the neutralization of the outer membrane endotoxin LPS of Gram-negative bacteria. While LL-37 can neutralize LPS synergistically via the two-domain helices (Wang *et al.*, 2014b), temporins L and B can work synergistically to achieve optimal LPS neutralization (Mangoni *et al.*, 2008; Bhattacharjya, 2016).

For membrane-targeting peptides, it is believed that damaging the inner membranes is the key event in bacterial killing. To date, only alamethicin is known to form a defined barrel-stave pore in the membrane, whereas some cationic AMPs appear to work via the carpet model (Shai, 2002). We have observed direct interactions of both hydrophobic and cationic moieties of the LL-37 peptides with PGs, providing a structural basis for membrane binding of cationic AMPs. We propose that the two-domain amphipathic structure of LL-37 (Wang, 2008) is important to interact with bacterial membranes, ranging from initial membrane binding, an intermediate toroidal pore formation, to final membrane disruption. Note that bacteriostatic AMPs are unable to disrupt membranes, but can cause a change in membrane phases by forming lipid domains (Chapter 8). A cationic peptide could have multiple actions on the membranes (Wenzel *et al.*, 2014). In addition, insect and plant defensins specifically recognize unique fungal sphingolipids. Some lantibiotics and cyclotides share similar amino acid profiles (Wang, 2010), allowing them to recognize bacterial phosphatidylethanolamines (Iwamoto *et al.*, 2007; Troeira Henriques *et al.*, 2012). The same binding of cyclotides is also responsible for anticancer and cytotoxic effects (Troeira Henriques *et al.*, 2014), making them less useful as potential antibacterial agents. However, the stable scaffolds of cyclotides and lassos can be utilized to deliver peptide epitopes for protein targets related to other diseases such as HIV-1 infection and cancer.

AMPs can also interact with intracellular targets. While bacterial microcin J25 inhibits RNA polymerase (Mukhopadhyay *et al.*, 2004), microcin B, with post-translational modification to generate multiple heterocycles, binds to bacterial DNA gyrase complex (Shkundina *et al.*, 2014). Insect Pro-rich peptides target ribosomes to inhibit protein synthesis. However, a non-specific interaction with eukaryotic cell ribosomes may limit their application as a new antibiotic.

In conclusion, the AMP field is moving forward rapidly in response to the urgent need for novel antibiotics. The combined beneficial effects of AMPs such as bacterial killing, antibiofilm, endotoxin (LPS) neutralization, and immunomodulation are remarkable. Our studies will consolidate new peptides as potential drug candidates. Once a peptide is established as a useful candidate, peptide library screening and structure-based design should play an important role in optimizing and refining the molecules into drug-like candidates (Wang, 2016). Clinically, antibiotics have already been used in combination. As a consequence, a possible synergistic use of newly developed drugs with existing antibiotics can be a realistic avenue (see Chapter 11). This practice can reduce costs by cutting the amount of peptide needed; it can also help to prolong the usefulness of traditional antibiotics by potentiating their antimicrobial effects.

Acknowledgements

GW acknowledges the grant support from the National Institutes of Health, United States (R01 AI105147 and R03 AI128230).
Chapter editor: Michael Zasloff.

References

Aboye, T.L., Ha, H., Majumder, S., Christ, F., Debyser, Z., *et al.* (2012) Design of a novel cyclotide-based CXCR4 antagonist with anti-human immunodeficiency virus (HIV)-1 activity. *Journal of Medicinal Chemistry* 55, 10729–10734.

Aerts, A.M., François, I.E., Meert, E.M., Li, Q.T., Cammue, B.P. and Thevissen, K. (2007) The antifungal activity of RsAFP2, a plant defensin from *Raphanus sativus*, involves the induction of reactive oxygen species in *Candida albicans*. *Journal of Molecular Microbiology and Biotechnology* 13, 243–247.

Arias, M., Jensen, K.V., Nguyen, L.T., Storey, D.G. and Vogel, H.J. (2015) Hydroxy-tryptophan containing derivatives of tritrpticin: modification of antimicrobial activity and membrane interactions. *Biochimica et Biophysica Acta* 1848, 277–288.

Arseniev, A.S., Barsukov, I.L., Bystrov, V.F., Lomize, A.L. and Ovchinnikov, Yu. A. (1985) ^{1}H-NMR study of gramicidin A transmembrane ion channel: head-to-head right-handed, single-stranded helices. *FEBS Letters* 186, 168–174.

Aumelas, A., Mangoni, M., Roumestand, C., Chiche, L., Despaux, E., *et al.* (1996) Synthesis and solution structure of the antimicrobial peptide protegrin-1. *European Journal of Biochemistry* 237, 575–583.

Bach, A.C., II, Selsted, M.E. and Pardi, A. (1987) Two-dimensional NMR studies of the antimicrobial peptide NP-5. *Biochemistry* 26, 4389–4397.

Bagheri, M., Arasteh, S., Haney, E.F. and Hancock, R.E. (2016) Tryptic stability of synthetic bactenecin derivatives is determined by the side chain length of cationic residues and the peptide conformation. *Journal of Medicinal Chemistry* 59, 3079–3086.

Bauer, F., Schweimer, K., Klüver, E., Conejo-Garcia, J.R., Forssmann, W.G., *et al.* (2001) Structure determination of human and murine beta-defensins reveals structural conservation in the absence of significant sequence similarity. *Protein Science* 10, 2470–2479.

Bhattacharjya, S. (2016) NMR structures and interactions of antimicrobial peptides with lipopolysaccharide: connecting structures to functions. *Current Topics in Medicinal Chemistry* 16, 4–15.

Bhunia, A., Saravanan, R., Mohanram, H., Mangoni, M.L. and Bhattacharjya, S. (2011) NMR structures and interactions of temporin-1Tl and temporin-1Tb with lipopolysaccharide micelles: mechanistic insights into outer membrane permeabilization and synergistic activity. *Journal of Biological Chemistry* 286, 24394–24406.

Böhling, A., Hagge, S.O., Roes, S., Podschun, R., Sahly, H., *et al.* (2006) Lipid-specific membrane activity of human beta-defensin-3. *Biochemistry* 45, 5663–5670.

Boman, H.G. (2003) Antibacterial peptides: basic facts and emerging concepts. *Journal of Internal Medicine* 254, 197–215.

Braunstein, A., Papo, N. and Shai, Y. (2004) *In vitro* activity and potency of an intravenously injected antimicrobial peptide and its DL amino acid analog in mice infected with bacteria. *Antimicrobial Agents and Chemotherapy* 48, 3127–3129.

Burghardt, T.P., Juranic, N., Macura, S. and Ajtai, K. (2002) Cation-π interaction in a folded polypeptide. *Biopolymers* 63, 261–272.

Cebrián, R., Martínez-Bueno, M., Valdivia, E., Albert, A., Maqueda, M. and Sánchez-Barrena, M.J. (2015) The bacteriocin AS-48 requires dimer dissociation followed by hydrophobic interactions with the membrane for antibacterial activity. *Journal of Structural Biology* 190, 162–172.

Cheetham, J.C., Artymiuk, P.J. and Phillips, D.C. (1992) Refinement of an enzyme complex with inhibitor bound at partial occupancy. Hen egg-white lysozyme and tri-N-acetylchitotriose at 1.75 Å resolution. *Journal of Molecular Biology* 224, 613–628.

Chi, S.W., Kim, J.S., Kim, D.H., Lee, S.H., Park, Y.H. and Han, K.H. (2007) Solution structure and membrane interaction mode of an antimicrobial peptide gaegurin 4. *Biochemical and Biophysical Research Communications* 352, 592–597.

Chu, H., Pazgier, M., Jung, G., Nuccio, S.P., Castillo, P.A., *et al.* (2012) Human α-defensin 6 promotes mucosal innate immunity through self-assembled peptide nanonets. *Science* 337, 477–481.

Conibear, A.C., Rosengren, K.J., Harvey, P.J. and Craik, D.J. (2012) Structural characterization of the cyclic cystine ladder motif of θ-defensins. *Biochemistry* 51, 9718–9726.

Conibear, A.C., Chaousis, S., Durek, T., Rosengren, K.J., Craik, D.J. and Schroeder, C.I. (2016) Approaches to the stabilization of bioactive epitopes by grafting and peptide cyclization. Biopolymers 106, 89–100.

Dalla Serra, M., Cirioni, O., Vitale, R.M., Renzone, G., Coraiola, M., *et al.* (2008) Structural features of distinctin affecting peptide biological and biochemical properties. *Biochemistry* 47, 7888–7899.

De Medeiros, L.N., Angeli, R., Sarzedas, C.G., Barreto-Bergter, E., Valente, A.P., Kurtenbach, E. and Almeida, F.C. (2010) Backbone dynamics of the antifungal Psd1 pea defensin and its correlation with membrane interaction by NMR spectroscopy. *Biochimica et Biophysica Acta* 1798, 105–113.

Dubovskii, P.V., Volynsky, P.E., Polyansky, A.A., Karpunin, D.V., Chupin, V.V., Efremov, R.G. and Arseniev, A.S. (2008) Three-dimensional structure/hydrophobicity of latarcins specifies their mode of membrane activity. *Biochemistry* 47, 3525–3533.

Epand, R.F., Wang, G., Berno, B. and Epand, R.M. (2009) Lipid segregation explains selective toxicity of a series of fragments derived from the human cathelicidin LL-37. *Antimicrobial Agents and Chemotherapy* 53, 3705–3714.

Ernst, R.R., Bodenhausen, G. and Wokaun, A. (1987) *Principles of Nuclear Magnetic Resonance in One and Two Dimensions.* Clarendon Press, Oxford, UK.

Fox, R.O., Jr and Richards, F.M. (1982) A voltage-gated ion channel model inferred from the crystal structure of alamethicin at 1.5-Å resolution. *Nature* 300, 325–330.

Galanth, C., Abbassi, F., Lequin, O., Ayala-Sanmartin, J., Ladram, A., Nicolas, P. and Amiche, M. (2009) Mechanism of antibacterial action of dermaseptin B2: interplay between helix-hinge-helix structure and membrane curvature strain. *Biochemistry* 48, 313–327.

Gesell, J., Zasloff, M. and Opella, S.J. (1997) Two-dimensional ^{1}H NMR experiments show that the 23-residue magainin antibiotic peptide is an alpha-helix in dodecylphosphocholine micelles, sodium dodecylsulfate micelles, and trifluoroethanol/water solution. *Journal of Biomolecular NMR* 9, 127–135.

Hancock, R.E., Haney, E.F. and Gill, E.E. (2016) The immunology of host defence peptides: beyond antimicrobial activity. *Nature Reviews Immunology* 16, 321–34.

Haney, E.F., Nathoo, S., Vogel, H.J. and Prenner, E.J. (2010) Induction of non-lamellar lipid phases by antimicrobial peptides: a potential link to mode of action. *Chemistry and Physics of Lipids* 163, 82–93.

Hayes, B.M., Bleackley, M.R., Wiltshire, J.L., Anderson, M.A., Traven, A. and van der Weerden, N.L. (2013) Identification and mechanism of action of the plant defensin NaD1 as a new member of the antifungal drug arsenal against *Candida albicans*. *Antimicrobial Agents and Chemotherapy* 57, 3667–3675.

Hegemann, J.D., De Simone, M., Zimmermann, M., Knappe, T.A., Xie, X., *et al.* (2014) Rational improvement of the affinity and selectivity of integrin binding of grafted lasso peptides. *Journal of Medicinal Chemistry* 57, 5829–5834.

Hegemann, J.D., Zimmermann, M., Xie, X. and Marahiel, M.A. (2015) Lasso peptides: an intriguing class of bacterial natural products. *Accounts of Chemical Research* 48, 1909–1919.

Henzler Wildman, K.A., Lee, D.K. and Ramamoorthy, A. (2003) Mechanism of lipid bilayer disruption by the human antimicrobial peptide, LL-37. *Biochemistry* 42, 6545–6558.

Hill, C.P., Yee, J., Selsted, M.E. and Eisenberg, D. (1991) Crystal structure of defensin HNP-3, an amphiphilic dimer: mechanisms of membrane permeabilization. *Science* 251, 1481–1485.

Holak, T.A., Engström, A., Kraulis, P.J., Lindeberg, G., Bennich, H., Jones, T.A., Gronenborn, A.M. and Clore, G.M. (1988) The solution conformation of the antibacterial peptide cecropin A: a nuclear magnetic resonance and dynamical simulated annealing study. *Biochemistry* 27, 7620–7629.

Hoover, D.M., Rajashankar, K.R., Blumenthal, R., Puri, A., Oppenheim, J.J., Chertov, O. and Lubkowski, J. (2000) The structure of human beta-defensin-2 shows evidence of higher order oligomerization. *Journal of Biological Chemistry* 275, 32911–32918.

Hoover, D.M., Chertov, O. and Lubkowski, J. (2001) The structure of human beta-defensin-1: new insights into structural properties of beta-defensins. *Journal of Biological Chemistry* 276, 39021–39026.

Hoover, D.M., Wu, Z., Tucker, K., Lu, W. and Lubkowski, J. (2003) Antimicrobial characterization of human beta-defensin 3 derivatives. *Antimicrobial Agents and Chemotherapy* 47, 2804–2809.

Hsu, S.T., Breukink, E., de Kruijff, B., Kaptein, R., Bonvin, A.M. and van Nuland, N.A. (2002) Mapping the targeted membrane pore formation mechanism by solution NMR: thenisin Z and lipid II interaction in SDS micelles. *Biochemistry* 41, 7670–7676.

Hsu, S.T., Breukink, E., Tischenko, E., Lutters, M.A., de Kruijff, B., *et al.* (2004) The nisin-lipid II complex reveals a pyrophosphate cage that provides a blueprint for novel antibiotics. *Nature Structural and Molecular Biology* 11, 963–967.

Imamura, T., Yamamoto, N., Tamura, A., Murabayashi, S., Hashimoto, S., Shimada, H. and Taguchi, S. (2008) NMR based structure-activity relationship analysis of an antimicrobial peptide, thanatin, engineered by site-specific chemical modification: activity improvement and spectrum alteration. *Biochemical and Biophysical Research Communications* 369, 609–615.

Iwamoto, K., Hayakawa, T., Murate, M., Makino, A., Ito, K., Fujisawa, T., and Kobayashi, T. (2007) Curvature-dependent recognition of ethanolamine phospholipids by duramycin and cinnamycin. *Biophysics Journal* 93, 1608–1619.

Johansson, J., Gudmundsson, G.H., Rottenberg, M.E., Berndt, K.D. and Agerberth, B. (1998) Conformation-dependent antibacterial activity of the naturally occurring human peptide LL-37. *Journal of Biological Chemistry* 273, 3718–3724.

Johnson, L.N. and Phillips, D.C. (1965) Structure of some crystalline lysozyme-inhibitor complexes determined by X-ray analysis at 6 Angstrom resolution. *Nature* 206, 761–3.

Jordan, J.B., Easton, P.L. and Hinton, J.F. (2005) Effects of phenylalanine substitutions in gramicidin A on the kinetics of channel formation in vesicles and channel structure in SDS micelles. *Biophysics Journal* 88, 224–234.

Kay, L.E., Clore, G.M., Bax, A. and Gronenborn, A.M. (1990) Four-dimensional heteronuclear triple-resonance NMR spectroscopy of interleukin-1 beta in solution. *Science* 249, 411–414.

Ketchem, R.R., Hu, W. and Cross, T.A. (1993) High-resolution conformation of gramicidin A in a lipid bilayer by solid-state NMR. *Science* 261, 1457–1460.

Klüver, E., Adermann, K. and Schulz, A. (2006) Synthesis and structure-activity relationship of beta-defensins, multi-functional peptides of the immune system. *Journal of Peptide Science* 12, 243–257.

Knappe, D., Goldbach, T., Hatfield, M.P., Palermo, N.Y., Weinert, S., *et al.* (2016) Proline-rich antimicrobial peptides optimized for binding to *Escherichia coli* chaperone DnaK. *Protein Peptide Letters* 23, 1061–1071.

Krizsan, A., Volke, D., Weinert, S., Strater, N., Knappe, D. and Hoffmann, R. (2014) Insect-derived proline-rich antimicrobial peptides kill bacteria by inhibiting bacterial protein translation at the 70S ribosome. *Angewandte Chemie International Edition in English* 53, 12236–12239.

Laederach, A., Andreotti, A.H. and Fulton, D.B. (2002) Solution and micelle-bound structures of tachyplesin I and its active aromatic linear derivatives. *Biochemistry* 41, 12359–12368.

Landon, C., Meudal, H., Boulanger, N., Bulet, P. and Vovelle, F. (2006) Solution structures of stomoxyn and spinigerin: two insect antimicrobial peptides with an alpha-helical conformation. *Biopolymers* 81, 92–103.

Lay, F.T., Mills, G.D., Poon, I.K., Cowieson, N.P., Kirby, N., *et al.* (2012) Dimerization of plant defensin NaD1 enhances its antifungal activity. *Journal of Biological Chemistry* 287, 19961–19972.

Lee, I.H., Cho, Y., and Lehrer, R.I. (1997) Effects of pH and salinity on the antimicrobial properties of clavanins. *Infection and Immunity* 65, 2898–2903.

Lee, P.H., Ohtake, T., Zaiou, M., Murakami, M., Rudisill, J.A., Lin, K.H. and Gallo, R.L. (2005) Expression of an additional cathelicidin antimicrobial peptide protects against bacterial skin infection. *Proceedings of the National Academy of Sciences of the United States of America* 102, 3750–3755.

Lehrer, R.I., Jung, G., Ruchala, P., Wang, W., Micewicz, E.D., *et al.* (2009) Human alpha-defensins inhibit hemolysis mediated by cholesterol-dependent cytolysins. *Infection and Immunity* 77, 4028–4040.

Li, X., Li, Y., Han, H., Miller, D.W. and Wang, G. (2006) Solution structures of human LL-37 fragments and NMR-based identification of a minimal membrane-targeting antimicrobial and anticancer region. *Journal of the American Chemical Society* 128, 5776–5785.

Li, Y., Li, X., Li, H., Lockridge, O. and Wang, G. (2007) A novel method for purifying recombinant human host defense cathelicidin LL-37 by utilizing its inherent property of aggregation. *Protein Expression and Purification* 54, 157–165.

Lobo, D.S., Pereira, I.B., Fragel-Madeira, L., Medeiros, L.N., Cabral, L.M., *et al.* (2007) Antifungal *Pisum sativum* defensin 1 interacts with *Neurospora crassa* cyclin F related to the cell cycle. *Biochemistry* 46, 987–996.

Mandard, N., Sodano, P., Labbe, H., Bonmatin, J.M., Bulet, P., *et al.* (1998) Solution structure of thanatin, a potent bactericidal and fungicidal insect peptide, determined from proton two-dimensional nuclear magnetic resonance data. *European Journal of Biochemistry* 256, 404–410.

Mandard, N., Bulet, P., Caille, A., Daffre, S. and Vovelle, F. (2002) The solution structure of gomesin: an antimicrobial cysteine-rich peptide from the spider. *European Journal of Biochemistry* 269, 1190–1198.

Mangoni, M.L., Epand, R.F., Rosenfeld, Y., Peleg, A., Barra, D., Epand, R.M. and Shai, Y. (2008) Lipopolysaccharide, a key molecule involved in the synergism between temporins in inhibiting bacterial growth and in endotoxin neutralization. *Journal of Biological Chemistry* 283, 22907–22917.

Mardirossian, M., Grzela, R., Giglione, C., Meinnel, T., Gennaro, R., Mergaert, P. and Scocchi, M. (2014) The host antimicrobial peptide Bac7(1-35) binds to bacterial ribosomal proteins and inhibits protein synthesis. *Chemical Biology* 21, 1639–1647.

Marion, D., Zasloff, M., and Bax, A. (1988) A two-dimensional NMR study of the antimicrobial peptide magainin 2. *FEBS Letters* 227, 21–26.

Marquette, A., Salnikov, E.S., Glattard, E., Aisenbrey, C., and Bechinger, B. (2016) Magainin 2-PGLa interactions in membranes: two peptides that exhibit synergistic enhancement of antimicrobial activity. *Current Topics in Medicinal Chemistry* 16, 65–75.

Mishra, B., Lushnikova, T. and Wang, G. (2015) Small lipopeptides possess anti-biofilm capability comparable to daptomycin and vancomycin. *RSC Advances* 5, 59758–59769.

Mishra, B., Golla, R., Lau, K., Lushnikova, T. and Wang, G. (2016) Anti-staphylococcal biofilm effects of human cathelicidin peptides. *ACS Medicinal Chemistry Letters* 7, 117–121.

Mishra, B., Lushnikova, T., Golla, R.M., Wang, X., and Wang, G. (2017) Design and surface immobilization of short anti-biofilm peptides. *Acta Biomaterialia* 49, 316–328 DOI: 10.1016/j.actbio.2016.11.061

Mukhopadhyay, J., Sineva, E., Knight, J., Levy, R.M. and Ebright, R.H. (2004) Antibacterial peptide microcin J25 inhibits transcription by binding within and obstructing the RNA polymerase secondary channel. *Molecular Cell* 14, 739–751.

Mysliwy. J., Dingley, A.J., Stanisak, M., Jung, S., Lorenzen, I., *et al.* (2010) Caenopore-5: the three-dimensional structure of an antimicrobial protein from *Caenorhabditis elegans*. *Developmental and Comparative Immunology* 34, 323–330.

Neumann, A., Berends, E.T., Nerlich, A., Molhoek, E.M., Gallo, R.L., *et al.* (2014) The antimicrobial peptide LL-37 facilitates the formation of neutrophil extracellular traps. *Biochemical Journal* 464, 3–11.

Nguyen, L.T., Schibli, D.J. and Vogel, H.J. (2005) Structural studies and model membrane interactions of two peptides derived from bovine lactoferricin. *Journal of Peptide Science* 11, 379–389.

Nguyen, L.T., Haney, E.F. and Vogel, H.J. (2011) The expanding scope of antimicrobial peptide structures and their modes of action. *Trends in Biotechnology* 29, 464–472.

Oren, Z., Lerman, J.C., Gudmundsson, G.H., Agerberth, B. and Shai, Y. (1999) Structure and organization of the human antimicrobial peptide LL-37 in phospholipid membranes: relevance to the molecular basis for its non-cell-selective activity. *Biochemical Journal* 341, 501–513.

Papo, N. and Shai, Y. (2004) Effect of drastic sequence alteration and D-amino acid incorporation on the membrane binding behavior of lytic peptides. *Biochemistry* 43, 6393–6403.

Park, S., Son, W.S., Kim, Y.J., Kwon, A.R. and Lee, B.J. (2007) NMR spectroscopic assessment of the structure and dynamic properties of an amphibian antimicrobial peptide (Gaegurin 4) bound to SDS micelles. *Journal of Biochemistry and Molecular Biology* 40, 261–269.

Pazgier, M., Prahl, A., Hoover, D.M. and Lubkowski, J. (2007) Studies of the biological properties of human beta-defensin 1. *Journal of Biological Chemistry* 282, 1819–1829.

Peschel, A. (2012) How do bacteria resist human antimicrobial peptides? *Trends in Microbiol*ogy 10, 179–186.

Phan, T.K., Lay, F.T., Poon, I.K., Hinds, M.G., Kvansakul, M. and Hulett, M.D. (2016) Human β-defensin 3 contains an oncolytic motif that binds PI(4,5)P2 to mediate tumour cell permeabilisation. *Oncotarget* 7, 2054–2069.

Poon, I.Kh., Baxter, A.A., Lay, F.T., Mills, G.D., Adda, C.G., *et al.* (2014) Phosphoinositide-mediated oligomerization of a defensin induces cell lysis. Elife 3:e01808.

Powers, J.P., Rozek, A. and Hancock, R.E. (2004) Structure–activity relationships for the beta-hairpin cationic antimicrobial peptide polyphemusin I. *Biochimica et Biophysica Acta* 1698, 239–250.

Resende, J.M., Moraes, C.M., Munhoz, V.H., Aisenbrey, C., Verly, R.M., *et al.* (2009) Membrane structure and conformational changes of the antibiotic heterodimeric peptide distinctin by solid-state NMR spectroscopy. *Proceedings of the National Academy of Sciences of the United States of America* 106, 16639–16644.

Rodziewicz-Motowidło, S., Mickiewicz, B., Greber, K., Sikorska, E., Szultka, L., Kamysz, E. and Kamysz, W. (2010) Antimicrobial and conformational studies of the active and inactive analogues of the protegrin-1 peptide. *FEBS Journal* 277, 1010–1022.

Roy, R.N., Lomakin, I.B., Gagnon, M.G. and Steitz, T.A. (2015) The mechanism of inhibition of protein synthesis by the proline-rich peptide oncocin. *Nature Structural and Molecular Biology* 22, 466–469.

Rozek, A., Friedrich, C.L. and Hancock, R.E. (2000) Structure of the bovine antimicrobial peptide indolicidin bound to dodecylphosphocholine and sodium dodecyl sulfate micelles. *Biochemistry* 39, 15765–15774.

Rozek, A., Powers, J.P., Friedrich, C.L. and Hancock, R.E. (2003) Structure-based design of an indolicidin peptide analogue with increased protease stability. *Biochemistry* 42, 14310–14318.

Sánchez-Hidalgo, M., Montalbán-López, M., Cebrián, R., Valdivia, E., Martínez-Bueno, M. and Maqueda, M. (2011) AS-48 bacteriocin: close to perfection. *Cellular and Molecular Life Sciences* 68, 2845–2857.

Sawai, M.V., Jia, H.P., Liu, L., Aseyev, V., Wiencek, J.M., *et al.* (2001) The NMR structure of human beta-defensin-2 reveals a novel alpha-helical segment. *Biochemistry* 40, 3810–3816.

Schibli, D.J., Hwang, P.M. and Vogel, H.J. (1999) Structures of the antimicrobial peptide tritrpticin bound to micelles: a distinct membrane-bound peptide fold. *Biochemistry* 38, 16749–16755.

Schibli, D.J., Hunter, H.N., Aseyev, V., Starner, T.D., Wiencek, J.M., *et al.* (2002) The solution structures of the human beta-defensins lead to a better understanding of the potent bactericidal activity of HBD3 against *Staphylococcus aureus*. *Journal of Biological Chemistry* 277, 8279–8289.

Schroeder, B.O., Ehmann, D., Precht, J.C., Castillo, P.A., Küchler, R., *et al.* (2015) Paneth cell α-defensin 6 (HD-6) is an antimicrobial peptide. *Mucosal Immunology* 8, 661–671.

Seefeldt, A.C., Nguyen, F., Antunes, S., Pérébaskine, N., Graf, M., *et al.* (2015) The proline-rich antimicrobial peptide Onc112 inhibits translation by blocking and destabilizing the initiation complex. *Nature Structural and Molecular Biology* 22, 470–475.

Shai, Y. (2002) Mode of action of membrane active antimicrobial peptides. *Biopolymers* 66, 234–248.

Shkundina, I., Serebryakova, M. and Severinov, K. (2014) The C-terminal part of microcin B is crucial for DNA gyrase inhibition and antibiotic uptake by sensitive cells. *Journal of Bacteriology* 196, 1759–1767.

Silva, F.D., Rezende, C.A., Rossi, D.C., Esteves, E., Dyszy, F.H., *et al.* (2009) Structure and mode of action of microplusin: a copper II chelating antimicrobial peptide from the cattle tick *Rhipicephalus (Boophilus) microplus. Journal of Biological Chemistry* 284, 34735–34746.

Singh, D., Vaughan, R., and Kao, C.C. (2014) LL-37 peptide enhancement of signal transduction by toll-like receptor 3 is regulated by pH: identification of a peptide antagonist of LL-37. *Journal of Biological Chemistry* 289, 27614–27624.

Sivertsen, A., Isaksson, J., Leiros, H.S., Svenson, J., Svendsen, J. and Brandsdal, B.O. (2014) Synthetic cationic antimicrobial peptides bind with their hydrophobic parts to drug site II of human serum albumin. *BMC Structural Biology* 14, 4 (PDB: 4BKE).

Skalicky, J.J., Selsted, M.E. and Pardi, A. (1994) Structure and dynamics of the neutrophil defensins NP-2, NP-5, and HNP-1: NMR studies of amide hydrogen exchange kinetics. *Proteins* 20, 52–67.

Song, C., Weichbrodt, C., Salnikov, E.S., Dynowski, M., Forsberg, B.O., *et al.* (2013) Crystal structure and functional mechanism of a human antimicrobial membrane channel. *Proceedings of the National Academy of Sciences of the United States of America* 110, 4586–4591.

Syvitski, R.T., Burton, I., Mattatall, N.R., Douglas, S.E. and Jakeman, D.L. (2005) Structural characterization of the antimicrobial peptide pleurocidin from winter flounder. *Biochemistry* 44, 7282–7293.

Tinoco, L.W., Da Silva, A. Jr, Leite, A., Valente, A.P. and Almeida, F.C. (2002) NMR structure of PW2 bound to SDS micelles: a tryptophan-rich anticoccidial peptide selected from phage display libraries. *Journal of Biological Chemistry* 277, 36351–36356.

Tomasinsig, L., Skerlavaj, B., Papo, N., Giabbai, B., Shai, Y. and Zanetti, M. (2006) Mechanistic and functional studies of the interaction of a proline-rich antimicrobial peptide with mammalian cells. *Journal of Biological Chemistry* 281, 383–391.

Tripathi, S., Wang, G., White, M., Rynkiewicz, M., Seaton, B. and Hartshorn, K. (2015) Identifying the critical domain of LL-37 involved in mediating neutrophil activation in the presence of influenza virus: functional and structural analysis. *PLoS One* 10, e0133454.

Troeira Henriques, S., Huang, Y.H., Castanho, M.A., Bagatolli, L.A., Sonza, S., *et al.* (2012) Phosphatidylethanolamine binding is a conserved feature of cyclotide membrane interactions. *Journal of Biological Chemistry* 287, 33629–33643.

Troeira Henriques, S., Huang, Y.H., Chaousis, S., Wang, C.K., and Craik, D.J. (2014) Anticancer and toxic properties of cyclotides are dependent on phosphatidylethanolamine phospholipid targeting. *ChemBioChem* 15, 1956–1965.

Turner, J., Cho, Y., Dinh, N.-N., Waring, A.J. and Lehrer, R.I. (1998) Activities of LL-37, a cathelin-associated antimicrobial peptide of human neutrophils. *Antimicrobial Agents and Chemotherapy* 42, 2206–2214.

van den Hooven, H.W., Fogolari, F., Rollema, H.S., Konings, R.N., Hilbers, C.W. and van de Ven, F.J. (1993) NMR and circular dichroism studies of the lantibiotic nisin in non-aqueous environments. *FEBS Letters* 319, 189–194.

Verly, R.M., de Moraes, C.M., Resende, J.M., Aisenbrey, C., Bemquerer, M.P., *et al.* (2009) Structure and membrane interactions of the antibiotic peptide dermadistinctin K by multidimensional solution and oriented ^{15}N and ^{31}P solid-state NMR spectroscopy. *Biophysics Journal* 96, 2194–2203.

Vriens, K., Cammue, B.P. and Thevissen, K. (2014) Antifungal plant defensins: mechanisms of action and production. *Molecules* 19, 12280–12303.

Wade, D., Boman, A., Wåhlin, B., Drain, C.M., Andreu, D., Boman, H.G. and Merrifield, R.B. (1990) All-D amino acid-containing channel-forming antibiotic peptides. *Proceedings of the National Academy of Sciences of the United States of America* 87, 4761–4765.

Wang, C.K., Gruber, C.W., Cemazar, M., Siatskas, C., Tagore, P., *et al.* (2014) Molecular grafting onto a stable framework yields novel cyclic peptides for the treatment of multiple sclerosis. *ACS Chemical Biology* 9, 156–163.

Wang, G. (2006) Structural biology of antimicrobial peptides by NMR spectroscopy. *Current Organic Chemistry* 10, 569–581.

Wang, G. (2007) Determination of solution structure and lipid micelle location of an engineered membrane peptide by using one NMR experiment and one sample. *Biochimica et Biophysica Acta* 1768, 3271–3281.

Wang, G. (2008) Structures of human host defense cathelicidin LL-37 and its smallest antimicrobial peptide KR-12 in lipid micelles. *Journal of Biological Chemistry* 283, 32637–32643.

Wang, G. (ed.) (2010) *Antimicrobial Peptides: Discovery, Design and Novel Therapeutic Strategies*, CABI, Wallingford, UK.

Wang, G. (2013) Database-guided discovery of potent peptides to combat HIV-1 or Superbugs. *Pharmaceuticals* 6, 728–758.

Wang, G. (2014) Human antimicrobial peptides and proteins. *Pharmaceuticals* 7, 545–594.

Wang, G. (2016) Structural analysis of amphibian, insect and plant host defense peptides inspires the design of novel therapeutic molecules. In: Epand, R.M. (ed.) *Host Defense Peptides and Their Potential as Therapeutic Agents*. Spinger, Heidelberg, Germany, pp. 229–252.

Wang, G., Pierens, G.K., Treleaven, W.D., Sparrow, J.T. and Cushley, R.J. (1996) Conformations of human apolipoprotein E(263-286) and E(267-289) in aqueous solutions of sodiun dodecyl sulfate by CD and ^{1}H-NMR. *Biochemistry* 35, 10358–10366.

Wang, G., Keifer, P.A. and Peterkofsky, A. (2004) Short-chain diacyl phosphatidylglycerols: Which one to choose for NMR structural determination of a membrane-associated peptide from *Escherichia coli? Spectroscopy* 18, 257–264.

Wang, G., Li, Y. and Li, X. (2005) Correlation of three-dimensional structures with the antibacterial activity of a group of peptides designed based on a non-toxic bacterial membrane anchor. *Journal of Biological Chemistry* 280, 5803–5811.

Wang, G., Elliott, M., Cogen, A.L., Ezell, E.L., Gallo, R.L. and Hancock, R.E. (2012a) Structure, dynamics, antimicrobial and immune modulatory activities of human LL-23 and its single residue variants mutated based on homologous primate cathelicidins. *Biochemistry* 51, 653–664.

Wang, G., Epand, R.F., Mishra, B., Lushnikova, T., Thomas, V.C., Bayles, K.W. and Epand, R. (2012b) Decoding the functional roles of cationic side chains of the major antimicrobial region of human cathelicidin LL-37. *Antimicrobial Agents and Chemotherapy* 56, 845–856.

Wang, G., Hanke, M.L., Mishra, B., Lushnikova, T., Heim, C.E., *et al.* (2014a) Transformation of human cathelicidin LL-37 into selective, stable, and potent antimicrobial compounds. *ACS Chemical Biology* 9, 1997–2002.

Wang, G., Mishra, B., Epand, R.F. and Epand, R.M. (2014b) High-quality 3D structures shine light on antibacterial, anti-biofilm and antiviral activities of human cathelicidin LL-37 and its fragments. *Biochimica et Biophysica Acta* 1838, 2160–2172.

Wang, G., Mishra, B., Lau, K., Lushnikova, T., Golla, R. and Wang, X. (2015) Antimicrobial peptides in 2014. *Pharmaceuticals* 8, 123–150.

Wang, G., Li, X. and Wang, Z. (2016) APD3: the antimicrobial peptide database as a tool for research and education. *Nucleic Acids Research* 44, D1087–D1093.

Wang, X. and Wang, G. (2016) Insights into antimicrobial peptides from spiders and scorpions. *Protein Peptide Letters* 23, 707–721.

Wei, G., de Leeuw, E., Pazgier, M., Yuan, W., Zou, G., *et al.* (2009) Through the looking glass: mechanistic insights from enantiomeria human defensins. *Journal of Biological Chemistry* 284, 29180–29192.

Wenzel, M., Chiriac, A.I., Otto, A., Zweytick, D., May, C., *et al.* (2014) Small cationic antimicrobial peptides delocalize peripheral membrane proteins. *Proceedings of the National Academy of Sciences of the United States of America* 111, E1409–E1418.

Wüthrich, K. (1986) *NMR of Proteins and Nucleic Acids*, Wiley, New York.

Xie, C., Prahl, A., Ericksen, B., Wu, Z., Zeng, P., Li, X., Lu, W.Y., Lubkowski, J. and Lu, W. (2005) Reconstruction of the conserved beta-bulge in mammalian defensins using D-amino acids. *Journal of Biological Chemistry* 280, 32921–32929.

Yau, W.M., Wimley, W.C., Gawrisch, K. and White, S.H. (1998) The preference of tryptophan for membrane interfaces. *Biochemistry* 37, 14713–14718.

Zasloff, M. (2002) Antimicrobial peptides of multicellular organisms. *Nature* 415, 389–395.

11   Synergy of Antimicrobial Peptides

Mobaswar H. Chowdhury, Gill Diamond* and Lisa Kathleen Ryan
University of Florida Colleges of Dentistry and Medicine, Gainesville, Florida, USA

Abstract

Emerging multidrug-resistant organisms challenge the medical community to search for new, effective antimicrobial agents to combat infection. Antimicrobial peptides (AMPs) offer a solution for this challenge and could play a major role in the search for new therapeutic regimens against MDR organisms. These peptides can be utilized in their natural or in synthetic forms, or modulated by agents increasing their natural production *in vivo* via altered gene regulation. Combinations of AMPs with conventional antibiotics and duplicate and triplicate combinations of AMPs are effective in combating Gram-positive and Gram-negative bacteria, as well as parasites and fungi. AMPs of different classes as well as a common class can be combined to induce synergy, enhancing the antimicrobial activity of each peptide or antibiotic compared with its activity alone. Although some specific triple AMP combinations are more effective than specific double AMP combinations, enhancement is generally not a simple stoichiometric relationship. The synergy between AMPs is complex and depends on the concentration and the combination of specific AMPs. Mechanisms include combining membrane-permeabilizing activities as well as modulating the innate immune system to combat inflammatory activity induced by the microorganisms. Mechanisms of AMP-enhanced antibiotic activity are not well studied, although it is postulated that the membrane altering effects allow for increased permeabilization of the membrane to the antibiotic, enhancing antimicrobial activity. Combinations of AMPs with conventional antibiotics serve the advantage of overcoming microbial resistance to the antibiotic as well as decreasing some of the toxicity of certain antibiotics in the patient. Creation of chemical compounds, termed AMP mimetics, that could replace AMPs known to combine with antibiotics to enhance activity would be advantageous in solving the problem of economically feasible AMP production. The examination of synergy with this new class of antibiotics is needed, for the pharmacodynamics of synergy and antagonism between combinations of these agents is complex and varies with the specific combination of agents. So far, research results demonstrate that synergy between AMPs or their mimetics, between themselves or with existing antibiotics offers a solution to the antibiotic resistance problem.

11.1 Introduction

The emergence of multidrug-resistant (MDR) organisms with immunity to many conventional antibiotics is a serious threat

---

* Corresponding author e-mail: GDiamond@dental.ufl.edu

to clinical practice. As a result, research has refocused towards the development of novel antimicrobial drugs (Ventola, 2015). Since their discovery, it has been clear that antimicrobial peptides (AMPs) have the potential to play a major role in the new arsenal of therapeutic antibiotics. Indeed, a number of AMPs have reached the clinical trial phase of development (Brogden and Brogden, 2011; Kang *et al.*, 2014). AMPs have high dose-related toxicity. To overcome this problem, synergistic combinations of AMPs with established antibiotics could be a novel approach for the treatment of infectious diseases. (Cassone and Otvos, 2010; Chongsiriwatana *et al.*, 2011). Since AMPs do not develop microbial resistance easily, combinations of AMPs may also help to overcome the emergence of bacterial resistance and increase the lifespan of existing antibiotics.

Antimicrobial peptides (AMPs) are defined as naturally occurring host defence peptides, which are usually cationic and amphipathic in nature (Bahar and Ren, 2013). The size of these natural peptides ranges from 6 to 40 amino acid residues (Diamond *et al.*, 2009; Bahar and Ren, 2013). Structurally, there are four categories of AMPs: β-sheet, α-helical, loop and extended peptides, all of which display potential activity against different bacteria, viruses, fungi and protozoa (Rahnamaeian, 2011).

AMPs are a key component of the innate immune response, which is the vital defence system for most living organisms, and are present from prokaryotes to humans (Aoki and Ueda, 2003). A wide range of organisms produce AMPs in their immune cells. Examples are natural killer (NK) cells, neutrophils, T-lymphocytes, monocyte/ macrophages, dendritic cells and coelomocytes that occur in organisms such as *C. elegans*, in addition to the exposed surface of skin, gut and lungs, where they provide defence against pathogens (Ryan *et al.*, 1998; Ryan *et al.*, 2011; Choi *et al.*, 2012). Thus, these peptides can be utilized therapeutically both in their purified (or synthetic) forms, as well as *in situ*, where their natural expression can be enhanced through the modification of gene regulation (Liu and Imlay, 2015).

Most importantly, the peptides usually (but not always) act directly on microbial membranes, often forming multimeric pores (Wilmes *et al.*, 2011; Lohner, 2016). This increased understanding of the molecular events that occur between the peptide and the target cell membrane has allowed the examination of the effect of combination therapy, both employing two different peptides, and employing a peptide and a conventional antibiotic.

In addition to naturally occurring AMPs, much research has focused on the enhancement of AMP activity by a number of different types of modifications (reviewed in Scott and Tew, 2016). These include modifying the natural primary amino acid structure, which can change the charge or other structural aspects, or modifying the amino acids themselves. This could include, for example, substitution with the D-form of the amino acid, or by lipidation to enhance the hydrophobicity. In addition, analogues such as β-peptides or peptoids, and small molecule peptide mimics that imitate the amphipathic structure of the natural peptides, have been examined. In addition to their enhanced activity, these new molecules are capable of synergy with each other and with conventional antibiotics.

11.2 Principles of Synergy of Antimicrobial Peptides

In general, drug interaction is defined as the interaction between two or more therapeutic agents resulting in synergistic, additive and antagonistic effects on the target cell or organism. Synergy between drugs, including AMPs, occurs when the effect of combination therapy is greater than the additive effect of each drug alone (Yeh *et al.*, 2009). These interactions may sometimes cause potentiation (one AMP enhances the effect of another AMP or an established antibiotic) and functional diversification, i.e. combinatorial activity increasing the spectrum of responses (Dobson *et al.*, 2013). The synergistic effects of combination therapy can result in increased activity against resistant strains and delay the development of drug resistance, reducing the required dose of an individual drug. By reducing the concentration of the conventional antibiotic, the dose-related toxicity and treatment duration may also be reduced. Synergy in combination therapy enables the direct targeting of specific pathogens, enhances the therapeutic efficacy and robustness of antimicrobial responses, and eventually increases the antimicrobial effect of AMPs at low concentrations (Casteels *et al.*, 1994; Haine *et al.*, 2008; Rahnamaeian *et al.*, 2015).

Quantification of synergy between antimicrobials is a complex matter (extensively reviewed in Greco *et al.*, 1995). Consideration must be paid to whether, for example, both drugs are effective individually, only one is effective individually, or neither is effective on its own. Two basic models that take these factors into consideration are Bliss independence and Loewe additivity, both of which can make different predictions of interactions. Bliss independence supposes that the two drugs being measured have equal probability of inhibiting the growth of the microorganism, including self-interaction. Loewe additivity assumes that the drug cannot affect its own activity. Numerous equations to accurately quantify synergy have thus been developed. Most publications that attempt to quantify synergy or antagonism with AMPs, however, use a simple checkerboard assay, which compares the minimal inhibitory concentrations (MIC) between the two agents, to arrive at a fractional inhibitory concentration (FIC) index. An FIC index of 1.0 indicates simple additive activity, below 1.0 indicates synergy, and above 1.0 indicates antagonism (Hall *et al.*, 1983). While this model is not optimal for all comparisons, it is the one that is most often used to determine whether AMPs exhibit synergy. Baeder *et al.* (2015) proposed a mechanistic based quantification, where for AMPs, the model used ought to depend on the mechanism of action of the peptide. They suggest that Bliss independence should be used for those peptides that form pores in the microbial membrane, while Loewe additivity should be used for peptides that introduce positive charge to the membrane.

Quantification of synergy *in vivo* is more complicated, and is often based on examining statistically significant differences in infectivity using sub-therapeutic concentrations of combinations of the agents compared with therapeutic doses of the agents alone. Thus, synergy with AMPs can be examined as combinations between two different AMPs delivered as drugs (for example, (Westerhoff *et al.*, 1995; Yan and Hancock, 2001; Rahnamaeian *et al.*, 2015), between an AMP and a conventional antimicrobial agent (Cirioni *et al.*, 2008; Yenugu and Narmadha, 2010; Seo *et al.*, 2012), or between an exogenously administered AMP and the patient's endogenous AMPs (Yu *et al.*, 2016). Finally, it is crucial to recognize that the simple administration of a conventional antibiotic can exhibit synergy with endogenous AMPs, which would not be noticed when quantifying *in vitro* activity of the antibiotic using standard MIC assays (Kumaraswamy *et al.*, 2016). Quantification of the MIC of azithromycin, for example, in standard bacterial broth yields a high MIC against the Gram-negative pathogen, *Stenotrophomonas maltophilia*, which would suggest against its use clinically against this pathogen. However, when its activity was measured under conditions that more closely resemble those found *in vivo*, it was discovered that there was synergy with endogenous AMPs and other components of the innate immune system. This has been found with other antibiotics and AMPs (Buyck *et al.*, 2012; Lin *et al.*, 2015) suggesting that this interaction between conventional antibiotics and endogenous AMPs is an important mechanism.

11.3 How Antimicrobial Peptides Synergize to Kill Microorganisms

AMPs kill pathogens through different mechanisms: forming pores on the cell membrane, degrading the membrane lipids, binding with new intracellular targets, promoting the production of reactive oxygen species (ROS) that cause cell death, and modulating the immune system

(Guilhelmelli *et al.*, 2013; Rahnamaeian *et al.*, 2016).

As AMPs often act on different targets, they are very effective in combination with each other (Bahar and Ren, 2013). Examples of the *in vitro* actions of AMP–AMP combinations are summarized in Table 11.1. For example, PGLa and magainin-2 (co-expressed AMPs in *Xenopus laevis* skin) exhibited synergistic effects against *Escherichia coli* and tumour cells (Westerhoff *et al.*, 1995). It was found that the MIC in combination therapy was decreased by twentyfold as compared to the MIC of either peptide alone (Westerhoff *et al.*, 1995). This mechanism of AMP–AMP synergy takes advantage of the strengths of the two different peptides: the pores formed by magainin are very stable, although their formation rate is slow. In contrast, the pores formed by PGLa, while shorter-lived, are fast in formation. Together the two peptides are proposed to form mixed peptide–lipid supramolecular complex pores on the cell membrane (Matsuzaki *et al.*, 1998). Pino-Angeles *et al.* (2016) further reported that synergy occurs between these two peptides via stronger pairwise interactions in the heterodimer rather than in the two homodimers.

AMP–AMP synergy can be observed with numerous peptides from different organisms. Platelet factor-4 and connective tissue activating peptide-3, AMPs from human platelets, synergistically inhibit *E. coli* growth (Tang *et al.*, 2002). AMPs from other mammals (Yan and Hancock, 2001) and insects (Pöppel *et al.*, 2015; Rahnamaeian *et al.*, 2015) are also reported to exert synergistic effects within their respective classes.

Milk-derived antimicrobial peptides LFcin-B and αs2-casein f (183-207) synergistically enhanced the antimicrobial activity of lactoferrin (LF) and the bacterial AMP nisin against the Gram-positive microorganisms *Staphylococcus epidermidis* and *Listeria monocytogenes* (Otvos *et al.*, 2006), and *E. coli* O157:H7 (Murdock *et al.*, 2007), demonstrating synergy between peptides of different classes.

Rahnamaeian *et al.* (2015) demonstrated that combinations of AMPs are therapeutically active against antibiotic resistant Gram-negative bacterial pathogens. They studied functional interaction of co-occurring insect AMPs (the bumblebee linear peptides hymenoptaecin and abaecin), which exhibit synergism in low concentrations against *E. coli* bacteria. Abaecin did not show any activity against *E. coli* when used as an isolated compound at a 200 µM concentration. In combination with hymenoptaecin, abacein enhanced the bactericidal activity of hymenoptaecin even at a 1.25 µM concentration. Abaecin was found

Table 11.1. Synergy among AMPs against various pathogens.

AMP	AMP	Application	References
PGLa	Magainin-2	*Escherichia coli*	(Westerhoff *et al.*, 1995)
LFcin-B	αs2-casein f (183-207)	*Staphylococcus epidermidis*, *Listeria monocytogenes*	(López-Expositó *et al.*, 2008).
Hymenoptaecin	Abaecin	*Escherichia coli*	(Rahnamaeian *et al.*, 2015)
LL 17-29	Cecropin A, melittin, pexiganan, indolicidin and apidaecin	*Escherichia coli*	(Yu *et al.*, 2016)
Defensin	Abaecin, hymenoptaecin	*Crithidia bombi*	(Marxer *et al.*, 2016)
Lysostaphin	Ranalexin	Wound infection and systemic infection	(Graham and Coote, 2007; Clark *et al.*, 1994)
Lactoferrin	Lysostaphin	Various bacterial strains	(Desbois and Coote, 2011)
Lactoferin	Nisin	*Listeria monocytogenes* Scott A ATCC 19111, *Escherichia coli* O157: H7 ATCC 43895	(Murdock *et al.*, 2007)
Polymyxin B	Gramicidin S	*Pseudomonas aeruginosa*	(Berditsch *et al.*, 2015)

to decrease the MIC of hymenoptaecin. Hymenoptaecin forms pores on bacterial cell membranes and hastens the entry of abaecin inside the cell, which binds the bacterial chaperone DnaK (more likely ribosome, see Chapter 9), resulting in the combined AMPs exhibiting greater antimicrobial activity (Rahnamaeian *et al.*, 2015). This has been proposed to be a common mechanism for some synergistic activities of AMPs (Rahnamaeian *et al.*, 2016).

Combinations of AMPs also were shown to inhibit the growth of parasites. Recently, Marxer *et al.* (2016) tested the efficacy of various combinations of AMPs such as proline-rich abaecin, cysteine-rich defensin and glycine-rich hymenoptaecin on the growth rate of *Crithidia bombi*, a trypanosome. These AMPs are expressed in bumblebees, *Bombus terrestris* when infected with *C. bombi*. They found that AMPs inhibit the growth of eight different strains of *C. bombi*, and combinations of AMPs were more potent as compared to AMP when used with a single compound.

AMPs can also combine to act on the innate immune system and exhibit anti-inflammatory activity. For example, Bedran *et al.* (2014) reported that combinations of human β-defensin-3 (hBD-3) and cathelicidin (LL-37) showed synergistic anti-inflammatory activity against a three-dimensional co-culture model of gingival epithelial cells and fibroblasts stimulated with *Aggregatibacter actinomycetemcomitans* lipopolysaccharide.

The pharmacology of AMP–AMP combinations is complex. Yu *et al.* (2016) demonstrated a pharmacodynamics study for the combination therapy among two and three AMPs. They used six different AMPs from different classes of organisms that are commercially available: cecropin A (Cec) (insect), LL 17-29 (LL) (mammal), melittin (Mel) (insect), pexiganan (Pex) (synthesized AMP, an analogue of magainin II), indolicidin (Ind) (mammal), and apidaecin (Api) (insect). They carried out an *in vitro* study of single AMPs, two-AMP and three-AMP combinations on *E. coli* and observed a broad-spectrum synergy for all the two- and three-combined peptides. They showed that

human AMP derivative LL 17-29 synergized in almost all combined therapies with AMP compounds. Further, they illustrated that three-AMP combination therapies have much greater activity than two-AMP combinations.

However, the Yu *et al.* (2016) study showed that enhancement is not a simple stoichiometric relationship. The synergy between AMPs is complex and depends on tho concentration and the combination of specific AMPs. Dual combinations of Pex-Api and Ind-Api were antagonistic in low-concentrations, but synergistic in high-concentrations. In contrast, different dual combinations of AMPs showed the opposite effect: Cec-Api and Mel-Api were synergistic in lower concentration combinations and antagonistic in higher concentration combinations.

Triple AMP combinations also showed similar complex effects. LL-Ind-Api showed synergistic effects in lower-concentration combinations and antagonistic effects in higher-concentration combinations, but Mel-Ind-Api had the opposite effect, with antagonistic effects in lower concentration combinations and synergistic effects at higher concentration combinations (Yu *et al.*, 2016).

The mechanism of antagonism in these AMP combinations is still not clear. However, synergy of combination therapy with increasing numbers of combined AMPs correlates with a decrease of minimum inhibiting concentration (MIC) and an increase of k-values (k-values depict the steepness of the pharmacodynamic curve. If k is high, the range of concentrations from 'no effect' to 'killing' is very small; if k is low, this range is much larger) (Matsuzak *et al.*, 1998; Yan and Hancock, 2001; Rahnamaeian *et al.*, 2015).

11.4 Synergism of Antimicrobial Peptides with Conventional Antibiotics

Combined use of various AMPs and antibiotics to enhance the therapeutic efficacy can occur through a number of different mechanisms. Examples of this type of synergy are shown in Table 11.2.

One mechanism of AMP–antibiotic synergy is through the combination of a standard antibiotic with the immunomodulatory activity of some AMPs (Bowdish *et al.*, 2005). Cationic AMPs derived from porcine leukocytes called protegrins consist of 16–18 amino acids and are highly active against pathogens due to the presence of multiple arginine residues (Cho *et al.*, 1998; Giacometti *et al.*, 2003). Combination of a synthetic protegrin peptide IB-367 with antibiotics daptomycin and teicoplanin synergistically enhanced the antimicrobial activity against methicillin-resistant *Staphylococcus aureus* (MRSA) in *in vivo* studies (Cirioni *et al.*, 2016). This study demonstrated that IB-367 along with daptomycin or teicoplanin showed a four-log decrease of bacterial infection whereas antibiotics alone caused only a one-log decrease of infection. This synergistic effect of combination therapy is due to the modulation by AMPs of both overall and CD11b spleen-specific NK cells, in addition to increasing the Gr-1 leukocyte number, resulting in potentiation of the antibacterial activity of the antibiotics.

Another mechanism of AMP–antibiotic synergy is through the alteration of the bacterial cell wall. In this case, the antibiotic enhances the antimicrobial killing of the AMP. It is reported that the β-lactam antibiotic cefepime potentiates the antibacterial activity of magainin 2 both *in vitro* and *in vivo* against a variety of strains (Darveau *et al.*, 1991). The possible mechanism of AMP–antibiotic synergy may be due to the antibiotic-induced alteration of the bacterial outer membrane structure, which allows for faster entry of the peptides into the inner membrane (Matsuzaki *et al.*, 1998).

In some cases, AMPs retain the activity of the complementary drug by degrading the antimicrobial-inactivating enzymes. For example, a proline-rich antimicrobial peptide, pyrrhocoricin, re-established the antimicrobial activity of amoxicillin against bacteria that expressed the amoxicillin-inactivating β-lactamase enzyme, TEM-1 (Otvos *et al.*, 2006).

Choi and Lee (2012) investigated the combination effect of arenicin-1, a 21-mer AMP, with the conventional antibiotics erythromycin and chloramphenicol. This combination produced synergistic inhibition of bacterial strains. The mechanism of synergy is possibly due to the production of hydroxyl radicals by arenicin-1, which causes oxidative damage to the cell membrane and eventually facilitates chloramphenicol and erythromycin to permeate through the lipid membrane to inhibit the synthesis of protein (Choi and Lee, 2012). This idea is based on the hypothesis of Kohanski *et al.* (2007) that all classes of antibiotics have a common bactericidal mechanism, through which they all lead to the formation of the toxic hydroxyl radical. However, the hydroxyl radical mechanism has been contested by others (Liu and Imlay, 2013; Keren *et al.*, 2013) and thus the actual mechanism may be different.

Most demonstrations of AMP synergy with conventional antibiotics do not examine the mechanism, although it has often been proposed that it involves the increased permeabilization of the membrane to the antibiotic that is induced by the AMP (Lohner, 2016). Naghmouchi *et al.* (2012) studied the antimicrobial activity of bacterial AMPs (nisin Z, pediocin PA-1/AcH and colistin) alone or combined with antibiotics against variants developed from a colistin-sensitive isolate of *Pseudomonas fluorescens* LRC-R73, which were resistant to penicillin G (RvP), streptomycin (RvS), lincomycin (RvL) and rifampicin (RvR). It has been noted that neither nisin Z (a class I bacteriocin) nor pediocin AcH, are effective against Gram-positive bacteria when used alone. However, resistant variants treated with peptide/antibiotic combinations exhibited a synergistic effect with a fractional inhibitory concentration index (FICI) ≤0.5.

Human male reproductive tract antimicrobial peptides HE2a and HE2b cause a synergistic effect when used along with conventional antibiotics to inhibit *Escherichia coli* growth *in vitro* (Yenugu and Narmadha, 2010). Combinations between α-helical AMPs from amphibians or insects

Table 11.2. Synergy between AMPs and conventional antibiotics against various pathogens.

AMP(s)	Conventional antibiotic(s)	Application	References
Pyrrhocoricin	Amoxicillin	Bacteria that secretes drug-inactivated β-lactamase enzyme TEM-1	(Otvos *et al.*, 2006)
Synthetic protegrin peptide IB-367	Daptomycin and teicoplanin	Methicillin-resistant *Staphylococcus aureus* (MRSA)	(Cirioni *et al.*, 2016)
Magainin 2	Cefepime	Various bacterial species	(Darveau *et al.*, 1991)
Nisin Z, pediocin PA-1/ AcH and colistin	Penicillin G, streptomycin, lincomycin and lifampicin	*Pseudomonas fluorescens* LRC-R73	(Naghmouchi *et al.*, 2012)
HE2a and HE2b	Rifampicin	Various bacterial species	(Yenugu and Narmadha, 2010)
Arenicin-1	Erythromycin and chloramphenicol	Various bacterial species	(Kohanski *et al.*, 2007; Choi and Lee, 2012)
PA-KKkK	Rifampicin, colistin, ceftazidime and aztreonam	Antibiotic-resistant *Escherichia coli*	(Hu *et al.*, 2015)
DM1–DM5	Penicillin	*Streptococcus pneumoniae*	(Le *et al.*, 2015)
Lysin Cpl-1	Penicillin G, gentamicin, cefotaxime, daptomycin	*Streptococcus pneumoniae*	(Djurkovic *et al.*, 2005, Vouillamoz *et al.*, 2013)
Lysin ClyS	Vancomycin or Oxacillin	*Staphylococcus aureus*	(Daniel *et al.*, 2010)
Lysostaphin	β-lactum antibiotic	*Staphylococcus aureus*	(Polak *et al.*, 1993, Kokai-Kun *et al.*, 2007, Hertlein *et al.*, 2014)
Antimicrobial cell wall hydrolases (ACWH)	Antibiotics	Various pathogens	(Wittekind and Schuch, 2016)
Cathelicidin AMP LL-37	Azithromycin	*Pseudomonas aeruginosa, Klebsiella pneumoniae* and *Acinetobacter baumannii*	(Lin *et al.*, 2015)
Novicidin	Rifampin, ceftriaxone and ceftazidime	Antibiotic-resistant enterobacteriaceae	(Soren *et al.*, 2015)
Magainin 2, ranalexin, cyclic peptide 6752, cyclic peptide GS14K4, gomesin113 and dermaseptin S3	Echinocandins, caspofungin or anidulafungin	*Candida albicans* and *C. glabrata*	(Harris *et al.*, 2010)
Alamethicin, globomycin, gramicidin S and surfactin	Enrofloxacin	*Mycoplasma pulmonis*	(Fehri *et al.*, 2007)
Human β-defensin 3 (hBD-3)	Lysozyme, metronidazole, amoxicillin and chlorhexidine	*Streptococcus mutans, S. sanguinis, S. sobrinus, Lactobacillus acidophilus, Aggregatibacter actinomycetemcomitans* and *Porphyromonas gingivalis*	(Maisetta *et al.*, 2003)
Aurein 1.2	Clarithromycin, minocycline	*S. aureus, E. faecalis* and *S. pyogenes*	(Giacometti *et al.*, 2007)
Hepicidin 20	Amphotericin B, fluconazol, caspofungin	Clinical isolates of *Candida glabrata*	(Tavanti *et al.*, 2011)

and rifampicin caused inhibition of bacterial growth in rat models of *P. aeruginosa* infection (Cirioni *et al.*, 2008). An AMP from fish skin, pleurocidin, exhibits potent synergy against *Mycobacterium smegmatis* when used together with D-cycloserine (Cole *et al.*, 2000). Aurein 1.2, an AMP derived from granular dorsal glands of frogs, along with clarithromycin and minocycline causes a synergistic effect against *S. aureus*, *Enterococcus faecalis* and *S. pyogenes* (Giacometti *et al.*, 2007).

Synergies between lysins and antibiotics are also reported in several studies. Lysin Cpl-1 exhibited synergy *in vitro* with penicillin G, gentamicin and cefotaxime against *S. pneumoniae*. This compound did not show synergism against quinolones and macrolides (Djurkovic *et al.*, 2005; Rodriguez-Cerrato *et al.*, 2007). In a further study, Cpl-1 showed synergistic activity in combination with daptomycin in the mouse model of peritonitis against *S. pneumoniae* infections (Vouillamoz *et al.*, 2013). It is also reported that the anti-staphylococcal chimeric lysin ClyS exhibited *in vitro* synergy in combination with either vancomycin or oxacillin and the ClyS–oxacillin combination showed potential activity in a mouse model as compared to either single agent when studied *in vivo* (Daniel *et al.*, 2010).

Lysostaphin-β-lactam antibiotics combination therapy showed *in vitro* and *in vivo* synergies against *S. epidermidis* infections as compared to either single agent (Polak *et al.*, 1993; Kokai-Kun *et al.*, 2007; Hertlein *et al.*, 2014). The advantage of this combination therapy is that β-lactam antibiotics can inhibit the development of resistance to lysostaphin (Climo *et al.*, 2001).

Bacterial AMPs that are antimicrobial cell wall hydrolases (ACWH) act through membrane permeabilization of pathogens. ACWHs destroy the integrity of the peptidoglycan in the cell wall at a sub-MIC level, allowing the fast entry of AMP into the cell membrane. This allows for the potent synergistic activity with conventional antibiotics both *in vitro* and *in vivo* (Wittekind and Schuch, 2016).

The bullfrog skin-derived AMP ranalexin (Clark *et al.*, 1994) showed *in vitro* synergy with lysostaphin (Graham and Coote, 2007), and in animal models of wound infection and systemic infection (Desbois *et al.*, 2010). Another report demonstrated that 16 AMPs and bovine lactoferrin each showed synergy with lysostaphin *in vitro* (Desbois and Coote, 2011). Furthermore, short salt-resistant synthetic peptides exhibit synergy with lysostaphin (Mohamed *et al.*, 2014).

It is also reported that azithromycin (AZM) showed multi-log-fold synergies with the antibiotic colistin, or the host cathelicidin AMP, LL-37 (Lin *et al.*, 2015). LL-37 is a host defence peptide, endogenously expressed in humans, and confers defence against microorganisms for the innate immune system. On its own, AZM exhibited bactericidal action against MDR carbapenem-resistant isolates of *Pseudomonas aeruginosa*, *Klebsiella pneumoniae* and *Acinetobacter baumannii*. The AZM–colistin combination showed great results against MDR Gram-negative rod (GNR) infection in murine models and could potentially render beneficial effect in patients with MDR GNR infection. Synergy occurs due to the permeabilization of Gram-negative outer membranes by LL-37 or colistin, which facilitates entry of the large AZM molecules inside the membrane (Lin *et al.*, 2015). The AZM–colistin regimen may allow a lower therapuetic dose while reducing the adverse effects. Recently it was reported that the AMP, novicidin, synergizes with the antibiotics rifampin, ceftriaxone and ceftazidime against antibiotic-resistant *Enterobacteriaceae in vitro*; this combination therapy may have major clinical implications to combat against antibiotic-resistant bacterial infections (Soren *et al.*, 2015).

Berditsch *et al.* (2015) studied the synergy between two cyclic-structured AMPs (polymyxin B and gramicidin S) against 28 different *P. aeruginosa* isolates using a checkerboard assay. In 20 out of 28 strains, combination therapy showed prominent synergism with a fractional inhibitory concentration index (FICI) of <0.5.

Maisetta *et al.* (2003) demonstrated that human β-defensin 3 (hBD-3) in combination with lysozyme, metronidazole, amoxicillin and chlorhexidine exhibited potential synergies against oral bacteria *Streptococcus mutans*, *S. sanguinis*, *S. sobrinus*, *Lactobacillus acidophilus*, *Porphyromonas gingivalis* and *A. actinomycetemcomitans*. This suggests the potential use of AMPs to prevent or treat oral infections, such as dental caries and periodontal disease.

Ruden *et al.* (2009) demonstrated that a combination of silver nanoparticles (an unconventional antibiotic) and the membrane permeabilizing AMP, polymyxin B, exhibited synergism against Gram-negative bacteria. AMPs permeabilize bacterial membranes and might help silver nanoparticles to reach internal target sites.

In addition to antibacterial activity, combination therapy using echinocandins, caspofungin or anidulafungin with a number of structurally diverse AMPs produced a synergistic effect against the fungi *Candida albicans* and *C. glabrata in vitro* in both planktonic and biofilm states (Harris *et al.*, 2010; De Cremer *et al.*, 2015). Tavanti *et al.* (2011) reported that the AMP, hepicidin 20, in combination with amphotericin B, fluconazole, or caspofungin, exhibited a synergistic effect against clinical isolates of *C. glabrata*. Fehri *et al.* (2007) reported that combinations of enrofloxacin and four AMPs (alamethicin, globomycin, gramicidin S and surfactin) produce synergy against *Mycoplasma pulmonis*, a murine pathogen *in vitro*.

11.5 Synergy with AMP Analogues

While the natural forms of the AMPs exhibit potent activity both *in vitro* and *in vivo*, and as described above, often demonstrate synergy with conventional antibiotics, they have several weaknesses as potential therapeutic agents. These include sensitivity to proteases and other inhibitory factors found in the body and toxicity at higher concentrations. In addition, they are much more difficult and expensive to synthesize in the amounts needed as antibiotics. Thus significant effort has been made to create analogues of AMPs that maintain, or enhance their activity, while reducing the weaknesses. These include short, synthetic peptides (Ramesh *et al.*, 2016) or peptide derivatives based on the most active portion of the native peptide, peptoids, β-peptides, γ-AA-peptides and small molecule mimetics (Rotem and Mor, 2009; She *et al.*, 2016).

The activity of a fragment of the sheep myeloid AMP SMAP-29, called novicidin, can be synergized with numerous conventional antibiotics against *Enterobacteriaceae in vitro* (Soren *et al.*, 2015) through a membrane active mechanism. Le *et al.* (2015) demonstrated that five hybrid peptides (DM1–DM5) exhibit potent antipneumococcal activity and produced synergism when used in combination therapy with penicillin.

Peptoids are a class of peptide analogues that are similar to peptides, except their side-chains are attached to the N-terminal region of the amino acid instead of the alpha-carbons, as they are in amino acids. Chongsiriwatana *et al.*, (2011) found strong synergistic interactions between different peptoids, with extremely low FIC indices (as low as 0.16), and between peptoids and AMPs.

Small molecule peptide mimetics such as arylamide foldamers (Tew *et al.*, 2010), and other types of amphipathic molecules exhibit potent antimicrobial activity against a wide variety of microbes (Scott and Tew, 2016). *In vitro* they exhibit synergy against *Candida* with the conventional antifungal agent itraconazole (Hua *et al.*, 2010) and against other oral pathogens with chlorhexidine (Beckloff *et al.*, 2007).

11.6 Conclusion

Combinations of AMPs with each other or with standard antibiotics can produce very effective therapeutic synergy, even overcoming bacterial resistance to antibiotics. Furthermore, it appears that employing mixtures of AMPs, or combinations of AMPs with peptide mimetics or other standard antibiotics, could be the answer to reducing the systemic toxicity of some AMPs while addressing the microbial resistance problem currently seen with standard antibiotics.

The antibiotic efficacy and ease of production of peptide mimetics shows promise in solving the problem of economically feasible AMP production. The examination of synergy with this new class of antibiotics is needed, for the pharmacodynamics of synergy and antagonism between combinations of these agents is complex and varies with the specific combination of agents.

Editor's note

A recent paper also shows the importance of antimicrobial peptides in treating biofilms and emphasizes early treatment for immature biofilms and combined therapy for preformed biofilms of *P. aeruginosa* (Mishra and Wang, 2017).

References

Aoki, W. and Ueda, M. (2013) Characterization of antimicrobial peptides toward the development of novel antibiotics. *Pharmaceuticals* 6, 1055–1081.

Baeder, D.Y., Yu, G., Hoze, N., Rolff, J. and Regoes, R.R. (2015) Antimicrobial combinations: Bliss independence and Loewe additivity derived from mechanistic multi-hit models. *Philosophical Transactions of the Royal Society Series B* 371, 20150294.

Bahar, A.A. and Ren, D. (2013) Antimicrobial peptides. *Pharmaceuticals* 6, 1543–1575.

Beckloff, N., Laube, D., Castro, T., Furgang, D., Park, S., *et al.* (2007) Activity of an antimicrobial peptide mimetic against planktonic and biofilm cultures of oral pathogens. *Antimicrobial Agents and Chemotherapy* 51, 4125–4132.

Bedran, T.B.L., Mayer, M.P.A., Spolidorio, D.P. and Grenier, D. (2014) Synergistic anti-inflammatory activity of the antimicrobial peptides human beta-defensin-3 (hBD-3) and cathelicidin (LL-37) in a three-dimensional co-culture model of gingival epithelial cells and fibroblasts. *PLoS One* 9, 1–10.

Berditsch, M., Strempel, N., Schwartz. T. and Ulrich, A.S. (2015) Synergistic effect of membrane-active peptides polymyxin B and gramicidin S on multidrug-resistant strains and biofilms of *Pseudomonas aeruginosa*. *Antimicrobial Agents and Chemotherapy* 59, 5288–5296.

Bowdish, D.M., Davidson, D.J., Scott, M.G. and Hancock, R.E. (2005) Immunomodulatory activities of small host defense peptides. *Antimicrobial Agents and Chemotherapy* 49, 1727–1732.

Brogden, K.A. (2005) Antimicrobial peptides: pore formers or metabolic inhibitors in bacteria? *Nature Reviews Microbiology* 3, 238–250.

Brogden, N.K. and Brogden, K.A. (2011) Will new generations of modified antimicrobial peptides improve their potential as pharmaceuticals? *International Journal of Antimicrobial Agents* 38, 217–225.

Buyck, J.M., Plesiat, P., Traore, H., Vanderbist, F., Tulkens, P.M. and Van Bambeke, F. (2012) Increased susceptibility of *Pseudomonas aeruginosa* to macrolides and keolides in eukaryotic cell culture media and biological fluids due to decreased expression of *oprM* and increased outer membrane permeability. *Clinical Infectious Diseases* 55, 534–542.

Cassir, N., Rolain, J.M. and Brouqui, P. (2014) A new strategy to fight antimicrobial resistance: the revival of old antibiotics. *Frontiers in Microbiology* 5, 551.

Cassone, M. and Otvos, L., Jr (2010) Synergy among antibacterial peptides and between peptides and small-molecule antibiotics. *Expert Reviews in Anti-Infective Therapy* 8, 703–716.

Casteels, P., Romagnolo, J., Castle, M., Casteels-Josson, K., Erdjument-Bromage, H., and Tempst, P. (1994) Biodiversity of apidaecin-type peptide antibodies. *Journal of Biologial Chemistry* 269, 26107–26115.

Chernysh, S., Gordya, N. and Suborova, T. (2015) Insect antimicrobial peptide complexes prevent resistance development in bacteria. *PLoS One* 10, e0130788.

Cho, Y., Turner, J.S., Dinh, N.N. and Lehrer, R.I. (1998) Activity of protegrins against yeast-phase *Candida albicans. Infection and Immunity* 66, 2486–2493.

Choi, H. and Lee, D.G. (2012) Synergistic effect of antimicrobial peptide arenicin-1 in combination with antibiotics against pathogenic bacteria. *Research in Microbiology* 163, 479–486.

Choi, K.Y., Chow, L.N. and Mookherjee, N. (2012) Cationic host defence peptides: multifaceted role in immune modulation and inflammation. *Journal of Innate Immunity* 4, 361–370.

Chongsiriwatana, N.P., Wetzler, M. and Barron, A.E. (2011) Functional synergy between antimicrobial peptoids and peptides against Gram-negative bacteria. *Antimicrobial Agents and Chemotherapy* 55, 5399–5402.

Cirioni, O., Silvestri, C., Ghiselli, R., Orlando, F., Riva, A., *et al.* (2008) Protective effects of the combination of α-helical antimicrobial peptides and rifampicin in three rat models of *Pseudomonas aeruginosa* infection. *Journal of Antimicrobial Chemotherapy* 62, 1332–1338.

Cirioni, O., Silvestri, C., Pierpaoli, E., Barucca, A., Kamysz, W., *et al.* (2016) IB-367 pre-treatment improves the *in vivo* efficacy of teicoplanin and daptomycin in an animal model of wounds infected with methicillin-resistant *Staphylococcus aureus. Journal of Medical Microbiology* 62, 1552–1558.

Clark, D.P., Durell, S., Maloy, W.L. and Zasloff, M. (1994) Ranalexin: a novel antimicrobial peptide from bullfrog (*Rana catesbeiana*) skin, structurally related to the bacterial antibiotic, polymyxin. *Journal of Biologial Chemistry* 269, 10849–10855.

Climo, M.W., Ehlert, K. and Archer, G.L. (2001) Mechanism and suppression of lysostaphin resistance in oxacillin-resistant *Staphylococcus aureus. Antimicrobial Agents and Chemotherapy* 45,1431–1437.

Cole, A.M., Darouiche, R.O., Legarda, D., Connell, N. and Diamond, G. (2000) Characterization of a fish antimicrobial peptide: gene expression, subcellular localization, and spectrum of activity. *Antimicrobial Agents and Chemotherapy* 44, 2039–2045.

Daniel, A., Euler, C., Collin, M., Chahales, P., Gorelick, K.J. and Fischetti, V.A. (2010) Synergism between a novel chimeric lysin and oxacillin protects against infection by methicillin-resistant *Staphylococcus aureus. Antimicrobial Agents and Chemotherapy* 54, 1603–1612.

Darveau, R.P., Cunningham, M.D., Seachord, C.L., Cassiano-Clough, L., Cosand, W.L., Blake, J. and Watkins, C.S. (1991) β-Lactam antibiotics potentiate magainin 2 antimicrobial activity *in vitro* and *in vivo. Antimicrobial Agents and Chemotherapy* 35, 1153–1159.

De Cremer, K., Staes, I., Delattin, N., Cammue, B., Thevissen, K. and De Brucker, K. (2015) Combinatorial drug approaches to tackle *Candida albicans* biofilms. *Expert Reviews in Anti-infective Therapy* 13 973–984.

Desbois, A.P. and Coote, P.J. (2011) Bactericidal synergy of lysostaphin in combination with antimicrobial peptides. *European Journal of Clinical Microbiology and Infectious Diseases* 30, 1015–1021.

Desbois, A.P., Gemmell, C.G. and Coote, P.J. (2010) *In vivo* efficacy of the antimicrobial peptide ranalexin in combination with the endopeptidase lysostaphin against wound and systemic methicillin-resistant *Staphylococcus aureus* (MRSA) infections. *International Journal of Antimicrobial Agents* 35, 559–565.

Diamond, G., Beckloff, N., Weinberg, A. and Kisich, K.O. (2009) The roles of antimicrobial peptides in innate host defense. *Current Pharmaceutical Design* 15, 2377–2392.

Djurkovic, S., Loeffler, J.M. and Fischetti, V.A. (2005) Synergistic killing of *Streptococcus pneumoniae* with the bacteriophage lytic enzyme Cpl-1 and penicillin or gentamicin depends on the level of penicillin resistance. *Antimicrobial Agents and Chemotherapy* 49, 1225–1228.

Dobson, A.J., Purves, J., Kamysz, W. and Rolff, J. (2013) Comparing selection on *S. aureus* between antimicrobial peptides and common antibiotics. *PLoS One* 8, 3–7.

Fehri, L.F., Wróblewski, H. and Blanchard, A. (2007) Activities of antimicrobial peptides and synergy with enrofloxacin against *Mycoplasma pulmonis. Antimicrobial Agents and Chemotherapy.* 51, 468–474.

Giacometti, A., Cirioni, O., Ghiselli, R., Mocchegiani, F., D'Amato, G., *et al.* (2003) Administration of protegrin peptide IB-367 to prevent endotoxin induced mortality in bile duct ligated rats. *Gut* 52, 874–878.

Giacometti, A., Cirioni, O., Riva, A., Kamysz, W., Silvestri, C., *et al.* (2007) *In vitro* activity of aurein 1.2 alone and in combination with antibiotics against Gram-positive nosocomial cocci. *Antimicrobial Agents and Chemotherapy* 51, 1494–1496.

Graham, S. and Coote, P.J. (2007) Potent, synergistic inhibition of *Staphylococcus aureus* upon exposure to a combination of the endopeptidase lysostaphin and the cationic peptide ranalexin. *Journal of Antimicrobial Chemotherapy* 59, 759–762.

Greco, W.R., Bravo, G. and Parsons, J.C. (1995) The search for synergy: a critical review from a response surface perspective. *Pharmacological Reviews* 47, 331–385.

Guilhelmelli, F., Vilela, N., Albuquerque, P., Derengowski, L. da S., Silva-Pereira, I., and Kyaw, C.M. (2013) Antibiotic development challenges: the various mechanisms of action of antimicrobial peptides and of bacterial resistance. *Frontiers in Microbiology* 4, 353.

Haine, E.R., Moret, Y., Siva-Jothy, M.T. and Rolff, J. (2008) Antimicrobial defense and persistent infection in insects. *Science* 322, 1257–1259.

Hall, M.J., Middleton, R.F. and Westmacott, D. (1983) The fractional inhibitory concentration (FIC) index as a measure of synergy. *Journal of Antimicrobial Chemotherapy* 11, 427–433.

Harris, M.R. and Coote, P.J. (2010) Combination of caspofungin or anidulafungin with antimicrobial peptides results in potent synergistic killing of *Candida albicans* and *Candida glabrata in vitro. International Journal of Antimicrobial Agents* 35, 347–356.

He, J., Eckert, R., Pharm, T., Simanian, M.D., Hu, C., *et al.* (2007) Novel synthetic antimicrobial peptides against *Streptococcus mutans. Antimicrobial Agents and Chemotherapy* 51, 1351–1358.

Hertlein, T., Sturm, V., Lorenz, U., Sumathy, K., Jakob, P. and Ohlsen, K. (2014) Bioluminescence and 19F magnetic resonance imaging visualize the efficacy of lysostaphin alone and in combination with oxacillin against *Staphylococcus aureus* in murine thigh and catheter-associated infection models. *Antimicrobial Agents and Chemotherapy* 58, 1630–1638.

Hu, Y., Shallop, J., Liu, Y. and Coates, A. (2015) Investigation into combination of an antimicrobial peptide with existing antibiotics against antibiotic resistant clinical isolates of *Escherichia coli. Antimicrobial Resistance and Infection Control* 4 (suppl. 1), 15.

Hua, J., Scott, R.W. and Diamond, G. (2010) Activity of antimicrobial peptide mimetics in the oral cavity: II. Activity against periopathogenic biofilms and anti-inflammatory activity. *Molecular Oral Microbiology* 25, 426–432.

Kang, S.J., Park, S.J., Mishig-Ochir, T. and Lee, B.J. (2014) Antimicrobial peptides: therapeutic potentials. *Expert Reviews in Anti-Infective Therapies* 12, 1477–1486.

Keren, I., Wu, Y., Inocencio, J., Mulcahy, L.R. and Lewis, K. (2013) Killing by bactericidal antibiotics does not depend on reactive oxygen species. *Science* 339, 1213–1216.

Kiri, N., Archer, G. and Climo, M.W. (2002) Combinations of lysostaphin with beta-lactams are synergistic against oxacillin-resistant *Staphylococcus epidermidis. Antimicrobial Agents and Chemotherapy* 46, 2017–2020.

Kohanski, M.A., Dwyer, D.J., Hayete, B., Lawrence, C.A. and Collins, J.J. (2007) A common mechanism of cellular death induced by bactericidal antibiotics. *Cell* 130, 797e810.

Kokai-Kun, J.F., Chanturiya, T. and Mond, J.J. (2007) Lysostaphin as a treatment for systemic *Staphylococcus aureus* infection in a mouse model. *Journal of Antimicrobial Chemotherapy* 60, 1051–1059.

Kumaraswamy, M., Lin, L., Olson, J., Sun, C.F., Nonejuei, P., *et al.* (2016) Standard susceptibility testing overlooks potent azithromycin activity and cationic peptide synergy against MDR *Stenotrophomonas maltophilia. Journal of Antimicrobial Chemotherapy* 71, 1264–1269.

Le, C.F., Yusof, M.Y., Hassan, M.A., Lee, V.S., Isa, D.M. and Sekaran, S.D. (2015) *In vivo* efficacy and molecular docking of designed peptide that exhibits potent antipneumococcal activity and synergises in combination with penicillin. *Scientific Reports* 5, 11886.

Lin, L., Nonejuie, P., Munjuia, J., Hollands, A., Olson, J., *et al.* (2015) Azithromycin synergizes with cationic antimicrobial peptides to exert bactericidal and therapeutic activity against highly multidrug-resistant Gram-negative bacterial pathogens. *EBioMedicine* 2, 690–698.

Liu, Y. and Imlay, J.A. (2013) Cell death from antibiotics without the involvement of reactive oxygen species. *Science* 339, 1210–1213.

Lohner, K. (2016) Novel antibiotics based upon the multiple mechanisms of membrane perturbation by antimicrobial peptides. *Current Topics in Medicinal Chemistry.* http://europepmc.org/abstract/med/27411329 (accessed 27 April 2017).

López-Expósito, I., Pellegrini, A., Amigo, L. and Recio, I. (2008) Synergistic effect between different milk-derived peptides and proteins. *Journal of Dairy Science* 91, 2184–2189.

Lyu, W., Curtis, A.R., Sunkara, L.T. and Zhang, G. (2015) Transcriptional regulation of antimicrobial host defense peptides. *Current Protein and Peptide Science* 16, 672–679.

Maisetta, G., Batoni, G., Esin, S., Luperini, F., Pardini, M., *et al.* (2003) Activity of human β-Defensin 3 alone or combined with other antimicrobial agents against oral bacteria activity of human β-defensin 3 alone or combined with other antimicrobial agents against oral bacteria. *Antimicrobial Agents and Chemotherapy* 47, 3349–3351.

Marxer, M., Vollenweider, V. and Schmid-Hempel, P. (2016) Insect antimicrobial peptides act synergistically to inhibit a trypanosome parasite. *Philosophical Transactions of the Royal Society Series B* 282, 20150293.

Matsuzaki, K., Mitani, Y., Akada, K.Y., Murase, O., Yoneyama, S., Zasloff, M. and Miyajima, K. (1998) Mechanism of synergism between antimicrobial peptides magainin 2 and PGLa. *Biochemistry* 37, 15144–15153.

Mishra, B. and Wang, G. (2017) Individual and combined effects of engineered peptides and antibiotics on *Pseudomonas aeruginosa* biofilms. *Pharmaceuticals* 10(3), 58.

Mohamed, M.F., Hamed, M.I., Panitch, A. and Seleem, M.N. (2014) Targeting methicillin-resistant *Staphylococcus aureus* with short salt-resistant synthetic peptides. *Antimicrobial Agents and Chemotherapy* 58, 4113–4122.

Murdock, C.A., Cleveland, J., Matthews, K.R. and Chikindas, M.L. (2007) The synergistic effect of nisin and lactoferrin on the inhibition of *Listeria monocytogenes* and *Escherichia coli* O157:H7. *Letters in Applied Microbiology* 44, 255–261.

Naghmouchi, K., Le Lay, C., Baah, J. and Drider, D. (2012) Antibiotic and antimicrobial peptide combinations: synergistic inhibition of *Pseudomonas fluorescens* and antibiotic-resistant variants. *Research in Microbiology* 163, 101–108.

Otvos, L., De Olivier Inacio, V., Wade, J.D. and Cudic, P. (2006) Prior antibacterial peptide-mediated inhibition of protein folding in bacteria mutes resistance enzymes. *Antimicrobial Agents and Chemotherapy* 50, 3146–3149.

Pino-Angeles, A., Leveritt, J.M. and Lazaridis, T. (2016) Pore structure and synergy in antimicrobial peptides of the magainin family. *PLoS Computational Biology* 12, 1–17.

Polak, J., Della, L.P. and Blackburn, P. (1993) *In vitro* activity of recombinant lysostaphin-antibiotic combinations toward methicillin-resistant *Staphylococcus aureus*. *Diagnostic Microbiology and Infectious Disease* 17, 265–270.

Pöppel, A.K., Vogel, H., Wiesner, J. and Vilcinskas, A. (2015) Antimicrobial peptides expressed in medicinal maggots of the blow fly *Lucilia sericata* show combinatorial activity against bacteria. *Antimicrobial Agents and Chemotherapy* 59, 2508–2514.

Rahnamaeian, M. (2011) Antimicrobial peptides: modes of mechanism, modulation of defense responses. *Plant Signaling and Behavior* 6, 1325–1332.

Rahnamaeian, M., Langen, G., Imani, J., Khalifa, W., Altincicek, B., *et al.* (2009) Insect peptide metchnikowin confers on barley a selective capacity for resistance to fungal ascomycetes pathogens. *Journal of Experimental Botany* 60, 4105–4114.

Rahnamaeian, M., Cytryńska, M., Zdybicka-Barbaras, A., Dobslaff, K., Wiesner, J., *et al.* (2015) Insect antimicrobial peptides show potentiating functional interactions against Gram-negative bacteria. *Proceedings of the Royal Society Series B* 282, 20150293.

Rahnamaeian, M., Cytryńska, M., Zdybicka-Barbaras, A. and Vilcinskas, A. (2016) The functional interaction between abaecin and pore-forming peptides indicates a general mechanism of antibacterial potentiation. *Peptides* 78, 17–23.

Ramesh, S., Govender, T., Kruger, H.G., de la Torre, B.G. and Albercio, F. (2016) Short antimicrobial peptides (SAMPs) as a class of extraordinary promising therapeutics. *Journal of Peptide Science* 22, 438–451.

Rodriguez-Cerrato, V., Garcia, P., Del Prado, G., Garcia, E., Gracia, M., *et al.* (2007) *In vitro* interactions of LytA, the major pneumococcal autolysin, with two bacteriophage lytic enzymes (Cpl-1 and Pal), cefotaxime and moxifloxacin against antibiotic-susceptible and resistant *Streptococcus pneumoniae* strains. *Journal of Antimicrobial Chemotherapy* 60, 1159–1162.

Rotem, S. and Mor, A. (2009) Antimicrobial peptide mimics for improved therapeutic properties. *Biochimica et Biophysica Acta* 1788, 1582–1592.

Ruden, S., Hilpert, K., Berditsch, M., Wadhwani, P. and Ulrich, A.S. (2009) Synergistic interaction between silver nanoparticles and membrane-permeabilizing antimicrobial peptides. *Antimicrobial Agents and Chemotherapy* 53, 3538–3540.

Ryan, L.K., Rhodes, J., Bhat, M. and Diamond, G. (1998) Expression of ß-defensin genes in bovine alveolar macrophages. *Infection and Immunity* 66, 878–881.

Ryan, L.K., Dai, J., Megjugorac, N., Uhlhorn, V., Yim, S., *et al.* (2011) Modulation of human ß-defensin-1 (hBD-1) in plasmacytoid dendritic cells (PDC), monocytes and epithelial cells by influenza virus, Herpes simplex virus and Sendai virus and its possible role in innate immunity. *Journal of Leukocyte Biology* 90, 343–356.

Scott, R.W. and Tew, G.N. (2016) Mimics of host defense proteins: strategies for translation to therapeutic applications. *Current Topics in Medicinal Chemistry* 17(5), 576–589.

Seo, M.D., Won, H.S., Kim, J.H., Mishig-Ochir, T. and Lee, B.J. (2012) Antimicrobial peptides for therapeutic applications: a review. *Molecules* 17, 12276–12286.

She, F., Oyesiku, O., Peiguang, Z., Zhuang, S., Koenig, D.W. and Cai, J. (2016) The development of antimicrobial γ-AA peptides. *Future Medicinal Chemistry* 8, 1101–1110.

Soren, O., Brinch, K.S., Patel, D., Liu, Y., Liu, A., Coates, A. and Hu, Y. (2015) Antimicrobial peptide novicidin synergizes with rifampin, ceftriaxone, and ceftazidime against antibiotic-resistant *Enterobacteriaceae in vitro. Antimicrobial Agents and Chemotherapy* 59, 6233–6240.

Tang, Y.Q., Yeaman, M.R. and Selsted, M.E. (2002) Antimicrobial peptides from human platelets. *Infection and Immunity* 70, 6524–6533.

Tavanti, A., Maisetta, G., Del Gaudio, G., Petruzzelli, R., Sanguinetti, M., Batoni, G. and Senesi, S. (2011) Fungicidal activity of the human peptide hepcidin 20 alone or in combination with other antifungals against *Candida glabrata* isolates. *Peptides* 32, 2484–2487.

Tew, G.N., Scott, R.W., Klein, M.L. and Degrado, W.F. (2010) De novo design of antimicrobial polymers, foldamers, and small molecules: from discovery to practical applications. *Accounts of Chemical Research* 43,30–39.

Ventola, C.L. (2015) The antibiotic resistance crisis: part 1: causes and threats. *Pharmacy and Therapeutics* 40, 277–283.

Vouillamoz, J., Entenza, J.M., Giddey, M., Fischetti, V.A., Moreillon, P. and Resch, G. (2013) Bactericidal synergism between daptomycin and the phage lysin Cpl-1 in a mouse model of pneumococcal bacteraemia. *International Journal of Antimicrobial Agents* 42, 416–421.

Westerhoff, H.V., Zasloff, M., Rosner, J.L., Hedler, R.W., De Waal, A., Vas Gomes, A., Jongsma, P.M., Riethorst, A. and Juretić D. (1995) Functional synergism of the magainins PGLa and magainin-2 in *Escherichia coli*, tumor cells and liposomes. *European Journal of Biochemistry* 228, 257–264.

Wilmes, M., Cammue, B.P., Sahl, H.G. and Thevissen, K. (2011) Antibiotic activities of host defense peptides: more to it than bilayer perturbation. *Natural Products Reports* 28, 1350–1358.

Wittekind, M. and Schuch, R. (2016) Cell wall hydrolases and antibiotics: exploiting synergy to create efficacious new antimicrobial treatments. *Current Opinion in Microbiology* 33, 18–24.

Yan, H. and Hancock, R.E.W. (2001) Synergistic interactions between mammalian antimicrobial defense peptides. *Antimicrobial Agents and Chemotherapy* 45, 1558–1560.

Yeh, P.J., Hegreness, M.J., Aiden, A.P. and Kishony, R. (2009) Drug interactions and the evolution of antibiotic resistance. *Nature Reviews Microbiology* 7, 460–466.

Yenugu, S. and Narmadha, G. (2010) The human male reproductive tract anti-microbial peptides of the HE2 family exhibit potent synergy with standard antibiotics. *Journal of Peptide Science* 16, 337–341.

Yu, G., Baeder, D.Y., Regoes, R.R. and Rolff, J. (2016) Combination effects of antimicrobial peptides. *Antimicrobial Agents and Chemotherapy* 60, 1717–1724.a

12 Surface Immobilization of Antimicrobial Peptides to Prevent Biofilm Formation

Biswajit Mishra*, Scott Reiling and Guangshun Wang*

Department of Pathology and Microbiology, College of Medicine, University of Nebraska Medical Center, Omaha, NE 68198-6495, USA

Abstract

The use of implanted medical devices improves the quality of patients' lives. Both polymers (e.g. polyethylene terephthalate) and metals (e.g. titanium and steel) are used to fabricate these devices. An unwanted accompanying problem with such implants is microbial infection (~3%). Bacteria are able to colonize the surface of implants and form difficult-to-remove polymicrobial biofilms. This chapter reviews an alternative approach, which prevents biofilm formation by immobilization of antimicrobial peptides on biomaterial surfaces. These peptides are usually short, cationic and can rapidly eliminate bacteria, viruses, fungi and parasites. We highlight antimicrobial immobilization methods, physical characterization approaches and biological activity assays for surface-coated peptides, and discuss current achievements as well as existing issues with the development of antibiofilm surfaces.

12.1 Introduction

It is estimated that each person will undergo medical implantation at least once in a lifetime (Gristina, 1987). Examples of medical implant devices are catheters, bone and dental implants, heart valves, stents, shunts and contact lenses. However, the biggest challenge with these medical implants lies in their susceptibility to microbial infection. Implant device infection could result in increased hospital costs, morbidity and mortality. Furthermore, bacteria can adhere to the biomaterial surface to form biofilms, which can be polymicrobial communities enclosed by a matrix of polysaccharides, proteins and extracellular nucleic acids (Thomas *et al.*, 2014). Once established, biofilms could be up to 1000-fold more recalcitrant to conventional antibiotics. Several factors may cause this situation. These include poor diffusion, nutrient limitations, slow growth and an attenuated human immune response. Surprisingly, sub-lethal doses of some currently used antibiotics such as tobramycin and amoxicillin could increase biofilm formation (Hoffman *et al.*, 2005; Mlynek *et al.*, 2016).

Implant-associated infections can be classified into superficial, immediate, deep immediate and deep late infections. While the superficial infections result from normal skin bacteria, which colonize the implant device, deep immediate infections are caused shortly after invasive surgeries, due

---

* Corresponding authors e-mail: gwang@unmc.edu; Biswajit.michra@unmc.edu

to relocation of skin bacteria inside the body. Deep late infections take longer to arise, and can be a result of contaminations during surgery, or migration of bacteria from other infected sites (Dee *et al.*, 2002). Unfortunately, implant-associated infections are generally diagnosed at a late stage, with the presence of damaged surrounding tissues, which frequently leads to replacement of the implant (Darouiche, 2004). Hence, alternative approaches are needed to reduce such device replacements. One appealing approach is to produce a bactericidal layer on implant medical devices to prevent biofilm formation. Recent strategies include (i) creation of a non-fouling (anti-adherent) surface; (ii) coating with bactericidal agents such as antibiotics, polymers, poly-ammonium salts, metal derivatives or antimicrobial peptides (AMPs); and (iii) coating using quorum sensing inhibitors. However, antibiotic coating of biomaterials is also associated with limitations of reduced activity over time, a limited antimicrobial spectrum, the risk of developing bacterial resistance and short-term antimicrobial protection with high cytotoxicity (Willcox *et al.*, 2008; Bagheri *et al.*, 2009).

AMPs are an alternative because they overcome these limitations (Onaizi and Leong, 2011). Such peptides have been discovered in the three life domains: bacteria, archaea and eukarya (Wang, 2015; Wang *et al.*, 2016). These peptides are usually cationic and can rapidly kill a broad spectrum of bacteria, fungi, viruses and parasites, including superbugs (antibiotic-resistant pathogens). There is high interest in developing them into alternative antibiotics to combat superbugs (Zasloff, 2002; Boman, 2003; Wang, 2010; Hancock *et al.*, 2016). In addition, these peptides can be surface-immobilized to prevent bacterial colonization and biofilm formation. These approaches are currently in the development stage and are being actively studied by various laboratories around the world. In this chapter, we summarize strategies for the development of various AMP-based chemical immobilization platforms, which confer antimicrobial

and antibiofilm activity to biomaterial surfaces with potential use in both food and medical industries. In addition, peptide surface immobilization also opens the door to other potential applications such as sensors for bacterial detection. Interested readers can refer to a recent review article (Wang *et al.*, 2015).

12.2 Surface Coating Methods

12.2.1 Non-peptide microbicidal materials

In the 1970s, the first non-leaching surface was reported to have microbicidal action (Battice and Hales, 1985). This surface was composed of 3-(trimethoxysilyl) propyl dimethyl alkyl ammonium chloride, with a 6 to 22 carbon chain attached to silicon. It was found to be anti-algal. In the early 1980s, cationic surfaces were also discovered to possess antimicrobial properties (Speier and Malek, 1982). Immobilized non-natural polycations, such as long-chain alkylated polyvinyl pyridines and poly-ethyl amines, were shown to be active against *S. aureus*, *S. epidermidis*, *P. aeruginosa* and *E. coli* (Tiller *et al.*, 2001; Tiller *et al.*, 2002) over a glass surface without promoting antimicrobial resistance (Klibanov, 2007). Further silanization with quaternary ammonium containing silane-like alkoxy silane octadecyldimethyl (3-trimethoxy silylpropyl)-ammonium chloride, modified with microfibrillated cellulose, was found to be highly active against *S. aureus*, *E. coli* and *P. aeruginosa* (Andresen *et al.*, 2007). Similar studies using triethoxysilane were also reported (Saif *et al.*, 2009).

Natural polycations, like chitosan, have found biomedical applications that include wound dressing (Burkatovskaya *et al.*, 2006) and artery related bio-implants, which have already been approved by the FDA (www.fda.gov). Immobilization of a TiO_2 surface, with a silane glutaraldehyde linker followed by deacetylated chitosan (91%), was found to have cell adhesive characters to mammalian tissues and also possess antimicrobial character (Bumgardner *et al.*, 2003). These surfaces also displayed excellent antibiofilm properties against bacteria and fungi (Carlson *et al.*, 2008). For instance, they reduced the biofilms of *S. aureus*, *S. epidermidis*, *P. aeruginosa*, *K. pneumoniae* and *C. albicans* by 95–99% within 54 hours.

Non-leaching, physically adsorbed polycation chains were also reported (Fuchs and Tiller, 2006). These were synthesized using a dip-coating or painting procedure. Cations were held onto the surface by non-covalent hydrophobic interactions. For example, N-N dodecylmethyl-poly ethylamine painted on a glass surface was found to be highly effective against *S. aureus*, *E. coli* and influenza viruses (Haldar *et al.*, 2006). Water insoluble PS-bP4VMP polymer coatings were active against *S. aureus* (Fuchs and Tiller, 2006).

Extending the physical adsorption method, a layer-by-layer assembly of polycations was also reported to be effective. Here, opposite charge layers are held together by electrostatic attraction. For example, a surface where cationic polyhexamethylene guanidine hydrochloride assembled with acetylated polyvinyl alcohol/sodium acrylate was microbicidal against *S. aureus* and *E. coli* (Pan *et al.*, 2008). However, potential problems with leaching and activity loss of the surface after a single use are major concerns.

12.2.2 Antibiotic immobilized surfaces

Immobilization of commonly used antibiotics conjugated with polymer supports is frequently reported (Aumsuwan *et al.*, 2007). These products are more likely to be approved by the FDA, since the antibiotics have already been approved, and only the polymer part is of concern with regard to safety. Recently, penicillin immobilized on an expanded polytetrafluoroethylene surface (ePTFE) was found to be highly effective against *S. aureus* and *P. aeruginosa*

(Aumsuwan *et al.*, 2007). This study also included a polyethylene glycol (PEG) spacer before attaching the final antibiotic molecule onto the surface. The use of PEG might have facilitated the interaction of the antibiotics with the bacterial surface. A similar platform was also used to immobilize ampicillin, leading to effective surfaces against *S. aureus*, *B. thuringiensis*, *E. faecalis*, *E. coli*, *P. putida* and *S. enterica* (Aumsuwan *et al.*, 2008). Further, gentamicin (sold as Garamycin) attached to a polyethylene terephthalate (PET) surface was also bactericidal against *E. coli*, *P. aeruginosa* and *S. aureus* up to 28 days upon incubation with the prosthetic surface (Ginalska *et al.*, 2005). Covalent immobilization of vancomycin onto the titanium surface for orthopaedic implants was shown to reduce bacterial colonization of *S. aureus* and *S. epidermidis* for up to six weeks (Antoci *et al.*, 2007). This titanium surface was specifically active against Gram-positive bacteria.

Amphogel (dextran hydrogels adsorbed with amphotericin B) showed excellent candidacidal activity (up to 24 h of contact) and lacked haemolysis. Additionally, its antibiofilm nature against *C. albicans* was well established in a mouse model (Zumbuehl *et al.*, 2007). However, the immobilization of the antibiotic was limited by its antimicrobial spectrum, bacterial resistance, the upscaling processes and the complex chemistry.

12.2.3 Antimicrobial peptide immobilization

AMPs can be immobilized either physically or chemically. While the physically immobilized method depends on the adsorption of the peptide onto the biomaterial surface, which is held together by non-covalent interactions, the chemical methods join the AMP molecule via a covalent bond.

Non-covalent immobilization

A simple method using a layer-by-layer approach (Etienne *et al.*, 2004) was adopted in non-covalent immobilization. An AMP-layer is sandwiched between two polyionic polymers on either side. In addition, the number of AMP layers was controllable and this device had the advantage of a high loading capacity. Earlier work of Etienne *et al.* (2004) was successful in immobilizing a defensin from *Anopheles gambiae*. A 10-layer adsorbed surface showed a high efficacy with 98% reduction in *E. coli*. An advanced hydrophobic interaction of AMPs as aggregates on the surface was also developed as a possibility (Duval-Terrié *et al.*, 2003). Poly-electrolyte multilayers using polysaccharides and AMPs, such as modified carboxymethyl pullulans with gramicidin A, was demonstrated to be active against *E. faecalis* for one week (Guyomard *et al.*, 2008). Chrysophsins-1 and -3 were used with acrylate to form self-oriented and self-aggregating layers during resin curing. They prevented the colonization of *S. aureus* and *E. coli* on aluminium foil (Fulmer *et al.*, 2010). A drawback of this approach is that only the superficial layer of coating is in contact with the pathogen. The lower architecture of the bottom layer is so complex that parameters, such as tortuosity, diffusion pathway, assembly thickness and peptide-polymer nature, differ (Ehtezazi and Washington, 2000). However, an excessive loading of AMPs could cause non-selective cell lysis in surrounding tissues. In addition, leaching and long-term stability of the surfaces should also be investigated.

Covalent immobilization

Alternatively, covalent immobilization of AMPs on biomedical surfaces provides a more realistic and promising approach. Peptides immobilized in this manner are unlikely to be leached. Table 12.1 provides a list of important AMP immobilization examples.

Earlier studies on immobilization of antimicrobial peptides date back to the work by Kennedy and Humphreys in 1976, where water insoluble hydroxides of metal ions like zirconium, titanium and iron were used to prepare insoluble derivatives of a cyclic peptide by the facile chelation process (Kennedy and Humphreys, 1976). Also, Haynie *et al.* (1995) succeeded in immobilizing magainin 2 onto ethylene diamine modified polyamide resin (pepsin K). The peptide coated resin was found to be effective against a wide range of bacteria (Table 12.1). Moreover, this study also highlighted the importance of orientation-specific attachment of the peptide. As a milestone, the full length LL-37, an important α-helical peptide from humans (Wang, 2008), was immobilized on the titanium surface using site-directed maleimide chemistry via the N-terminal appended cysteine (Gabriel *et al.*, 2006). This study demonstrated the importance of the PEG linker and N-terminal coupling for LL-37 activity against *E. coli*. Bagheri *et al.* (2009) showed that immobilization of KLAL and MK5E (a magainin-derived peptide) on the resin beads (TentaGel) reduced the activity against *E. coli* and *B. subtilis*. It was demonstrated that melimine (a hybrid peptide of melittin and protamine) attached to contact lenses reduced the biofilm formation of *P. aeruginosa* and *S. aureus* by more than 70% (Willcox *et al.*, 2008). Using a sol-gel technology of silane coating with an epoxide ring exposed, Mohorcic *et al.* (2010) demonstrated that polymyxin B covalently bound to the glass substrate had antimicrobial (5 magnitude order), and antibiofilm characteristics (99% inhibition), against *E. coli* (Mohorcic *et al.*, 2010). In addition, Statz *et al.* (2008) made the first surface immobilized antimicrobial peptoids onto titanium surfaces that damaged the *E. coli* membranes.

Because surface immobilization influences peptide activity, Hilpert *et al.* (2009) screened a library of short peptides tethered to cellulose. They synthesized 122 peptides by using the cellulose-amino-hydroxylpropyl ether linker chemistry, followed by measuring antibacterial and antifungal activity without peptide cleavage. From the identified active peptides with 9 to 13 amino acids, they propose that the positioning of charged and hydrophobic residues affected peptide activity.

Table 12.1. Important surface immobilization chemistry.

Study	Year	Peptide	Chemistry	Organism[a]	Comments
Kennedy and Humphreys	1976	Neomycin, polymyxin B, streptomycin etc.	On metal matrix like zirconium hydroxide for cyclic peptide antibiotic by facile chelation process	EC, SA, PA, SF, SM1, SV	First peptide antibiotic immobilization
Haynie et al.	1995	Magainin 2 and related amphiphilic peptides	Short spacers of 2–6 carbon chain was introduced in between polyamide resin and peptide	EC, SA, KP, BS, PA, Candida albicans, Aspergillus niger	First use of spacers; AMP orientation control via C-terminal coupling; on resin synthesis
Gabriel et al.	2006	LL-37	Maleimide reaction on PEG heterolinker, on a titanium surface	EC	Effects of PEGylated spacers
Statz et al.	2008	PMPI-AMP	Immersion on peptide solution	EC	First peptoid immobilization
Willcox et al.	2008	Melimine	Peptide amine reacts with carboxyl of contact lens activated by EDC	PA, SA and SP	First application to commercial eye lens
Bagheri et al.	2009	KLAL peptide magainin derivative MK5E	Resin beads tentagels (amine) with PEG spacers joined by covalent immobilization	EC and BS	Same activity spectrum after immobilization, but activity decreases
Glinel et al.	2009	Magainin I	Non-fouling copolymer brushes grafted on surface controlled AMP coupling using maleimide chemistry	LI and BC	First polymer brushes; maleimide chemistry
Humblot et al.	2009	Magainin I	Amines of the peptides immobilized onto mixed carboxyl and hydroxyl SAM with the EDC/NHS chemistry	LI, EF and SA	First SAM and the use of EDC/NHS carbodimide coupling
Hilpert et al.	2009	Bac2A variants and indolicidin	AMPs immobilized on cellulose bifunctional resin (CAPE linker) on a microtitre plate via biotin-streptavidin interaction	PA, SA and CA	First large scale library screening of peptides synthesized on cellulose
Gao et al.	2011	Tet-213, 1010cys, Tet-20, Tet21, Tet-26, HH2, MXX226	AMP immobilized via a DMA/APMA brush activated by ATRP and final conjugation through maleimide chemistry	SA	First in vivo test of antimicrobial and antibiofilm titanium implants
Santos et al.	2013	IG-25 (C-terminus of LL-37)	The alkynyl group on contact lens reacts with the azido-OEG tag at the N-terminus	PA	Click chemistry for peptide coupling
Mishra et al.	2014	Lasioglossin LL-III	AGE brush on silicone catheter attached to PEG spacers and conjugated to the peptide via maleimide chemistry	EF and EC	First prototype of AMP coated silicone catheter
Rai et al.	2016	Cecropinmelittin/gold nanoparticles	Standard maleimide chemistry	SA, PA, EC, KP	High-density surface coating 2 at $110\,\mu g/cm^2$ achieved

[a]BC: *Bacillus cereus*; BS: *Bacillus subtilis*; EC: *Escherichia coli*; EF: *Enterococcus faecalis*; LI: *Listeria ivanovii*; LS: *Lactobacillus salivarius*; PA: *Pseudomonas aeruginosa*; SA: *Staphylococcus aureus*; SE: *Staphylococcus epidermidis*; SF: *Streptococcus faecalis*; SG: *Streptococcus gordonii*; SM1: *Serratia marcescens*; SM: *Streptococcus mutans*; SP: *Streptococcus pneumoniae*; SS: *Streptococcus sanguinis*; SV: *Stylidium violacium*.

Activation of the surfaces is made through various chemical and physical methods. For covalent immobilization, one of the convenient methods of AMP functionalization is the use of self-assembled monolayers (SAM) (Gooding *et al.*, 2003). The same layers can be optimized with various functional groups in order to effectively assemble AMPs (Onaizi and Leong, 2011). SAM formed with a mixture of 11-MUA (11-marcaptoundecanoic acid) and 6-marcaptohexanol was used to immobilize magainin I onto a gold surface by Humblot *et al.* (2009). The reaction with peptide was not site-specific. It involved a carboxyl from MUA and an amine from lysine. The platform was very effective in inhibiting *L. ivanovii* by 80% and *E. faecalis* and *S. aureus* by 50 and 60%, respectively. Interestingly, the surface was stable up to 6 months with no peptide detected in the vicinity. A similar chemistry was also applied to immobilizing gramicidin A onto cystamine monolayers. This system was very efficient in inhibiting adhesion of a variety of Gram-positive and Gram-negative bacteria (Yala *et al.*, 2011).

To increase peptide coating density, polymer brushes have been generated on material surfaces. Polymer brushes also provide the following advantages:

1. Increased flexibility to allow the attached peptide to better interact with bacteria.
2. Antifouling properties to keep the material clean by reducing bacterial adhesion.
3. Increased biocompatibility using hydrophilic brushes.

These brushes contain functional groups that enable the peptide to connect with the surface. Glinel *et al.* (2009) developed a polymer brush formed by copolymerization between 2-(2-methoxyethoxy) ethylmethacrylate and hydroxyl terminated oligo (ethylene glycol) methacrylate. A short bifunctional linker was utilized to link the free hydroxyl of the polymer to cysteine-containing magainin I. Final peptide immobilization was achieved through maleimide chemistry. The modified surface was not only antifouling because of the polymer (less than 1% bacterial adhesion), but also antimicrobial against *L. ivanovii* and *B. cereus*. Adherence of AMPs to the polymer brush was also studied by the Jayachandran group (Hadjesfandiari *et al.*, 2014; Yu *et al.*, 2015). The same group also developed polymer brushes on various substrates like silicon wafers, titanium and titanium implants. The brush was made by copolymerization of DMA (N, N-dimethylacrylamide) and APMA (N-(3-aminopropyl) methacrylamide hydrochloride) using an initiator molecule, followed by introduction of a short bifunctional linker like 3-maleimidosuccinic acid ester, which provided a specific functional group for coupling with the cysteine in the peptide. The Tet-20 peptide, immobilized on a titanium implant in this manner, reduced the *P. aeruginosa* colony forming units (CFU) by at least fivefold after one hour post incubation. A correlation was found between the increasing antimicrobial potency of the surface and the more peptide that was coated on the polymer brushes (Vreuls *et al.*, 2010; Godoy-Gallardo *et al.*, 2015). Importantly, Gao *et al.* (2011) demonstrated the antibacterial and antibiofilm property of a hydrophilic N-substituted polyacrylamide brush on a titanium implant *in vivo*. Rats were challenged with 10^8 CFU of *S. aureus*. The implants retained both antimicrobial and antibiofilm properties even after 7 days.

Click chemistry has also found use in immobilizing peptides (Rostovtsev *et al.*, 2002; Costa *et al.*, 2011). Santos *et al.* (2013) succeeded in coating IG-25, a C-terminal fragment corresponding to residues 13–37 of human cathelicidin LL-37 (Li *et al.*, 2006), on the surface of a contact lens. In this coupling, the alkynyl group attached to the contact lens reacted with the azido-OEG tag at the N-terminus of IG-25.

Recently, the Leong group has developed an allyl glycidyl ether (AGE) based chemical platform on silicon and silicone surfaces. They immobilized insect polybia-MPI onto the silicon surface with antimicrobial and antibiofilm properties against *E. coli* (Basu *et al.*, 2013). The same group has also developed a prototype commercial catheter for a urinary tract by employing the AGE polymerization platform coated with lasioglossin LL-III (Mishra *et al.*, 2014). The coated catheter has antibacterial and antibiofilm activity against *E. coli* and *E. faecalis*. In a separate study, they also immobilized lasioglossin LL-III onto a silicon wafer via the PEG linker, effectively reducing the bacterial CFU and adhesion (Mishra *et al.*, 2013).

There have also been efforts in developing surfaces with a combination of antifouling and antimicrobial properties. Laloyaux *et al.* (2010) developed a reversible system that switches between antifouling and antimicrobial natures controlled by temperature. At a lower temperature ~26°C, the surface becomes more antimicrobial against *E. coli* and *L. ivanovii*; at a higher temperature ~38°C, the AMP layers are buried inside the brush, thereby masking the bactericidal components. However, the new surface retains anti-adhesive characteristics against a similar set of microorganisms. Recently, Alves *et al.* (2016) have demonstrated a proof-of-concept study where two antibiofilm agents are coated to handle the bimicrobial infection of *P. aeruginosa* and *S. aureus*. While DNase I conferred the surface with anti-adhesive properties to prevent the attachment of both bacteria, a lipopeptide called PALM inhibited *S. aureus*.

12.3 Chemical and Physical Characterization of Peptide Coated Surfaces

During the establishment of a chemical platform for coating, an easy way of monitoring the progression of the desired reaction is crucial. It is common to utilize chemical methods to verify the presence of certain functional groups (e.g. Kaiser test for free amino group). A quantitative analysis can also be conducted. For example, the use of sulfo-SDTB to react with free amino groups on the material surfaces enables a colorimetric measurement of the coated peptides based on the Beer–Lambert law because of the high molar extinction coefficient of $70,000\,M^{-1}\,cm^{-1}$ of the product (Gaur and Gupta, 1989).

Physical methods, however, are more convenient and convincing. Table 12.2 describes different biophysical techniques for characterization of the peptide immobilized surface. Scanning electron microscopy (SEM) has been utilized to view the morphology of the surface before and after coating. Atomic force microscopy (AFM) and peal force microscopy are used for peptide coverage and surface topology studies by measuring the attachment force with specialized tips. Peptide coating also alters the properties of the surface. A

Table 12.2. Biophysical techniques for surface characterization.

Techniques	Uses
FT-IR, ATRIR and SFG-VS, Raman spectroscopy	Unique peptide amide bands provide definitive evidence for the coupling of the peptide with the linker
XPS	Provide definitive support for the attachment of the peptide to the surface, especially for Cys-containing peptides based on the detection of sulfur
CD	Peptide conformation in immobilized form
Confocal microscopy	Provide a view on dead and live cells
SEM, FESEM, AFM	Surface view of roughness and dead and live cells
Contact angle	Hydrophobicity and hydrophilicity changes of surfaces
Fluorescence reader/dye	Evidence for membrane permeation of the coated peptides
NMR	Component nuclei, structure and dynamics analysis
Ellipsometry, AFM	Thickness of the attached layer on the surface
Surface plasmon resonance (SPR)	Binding behavior of AMP immobilized surfaces with membranes

hydrophilic peptide can facilitate water to spread out on the surface, leading to a smaller contact angle (a solid surface is considered hydrophilic if the contact angle is less than 90°). An excellent example is provided by Alves *et al.* (2016) who nicely illustrated the water contact angle changes with various surface coatings. In addition, ellipsometry is used to obtain the thickness of the attached layer (Basu *et al.*, 2013).

It is important to generate evidence that the changed properties are indeed due to the peptide coating. X-ray photoelectron spectroscopy (XPS) is frequently used to detect the surface elemental composition. For example, the detection of sulfur can provide unambiguous evidence for the coupling of the peptide to the surface if the peptide contains a cysteine. The coupling of the peptide with the surface can be further validated by Fourier transform-infrared spectroscopy (FT-IR) that can detect the characteristic amide bands from the peptide. Circular dichroism (CD) can be used to provide the secondary structural information of immobilized AMPs. Sum frequency generation vibrational spectroscopy (SFG-VS) is also used to deduce structural information. NMR is helpful in analysing the nuclei, structure and dynamics of the peptides. A conformational change of the peptide from random coils to an amphipathic helix provides a basis for targeting bacterial membranes. The damaging effect of the surface-tethered peptide can be viewed by electron microscopy (EM) and FESEM (Field emission–scanning electron microscopy). In addition, there are commercial staining kits to validate live and dead cells (bacteria or host cells) on the surface via fluorescence spectroscopy. Other analytical techniques, including optical wavelength light-mode spectroscopy, quartz crystal microbalance, surface plasmon resonance and Raman spectroscopy, can also be utilized.

The use of multiple physical technologies enables us to better characterize the surface and validate our results. One should avoid potential surface contamination during sample handling or shipment. It is also important to avoid artefacts from physical analysis since it has been reported that strong beams can damage the surface. For example, XPS may damage the surface and generates bromide (Br⁻) from the brominated furanone-coated surface (Al-Bataineh *et al.*, 2006).

12.4 Antimicrobial and Antibiofilm Activities of Peptide Coated Surfaces

Antimicrobial and antibiofilm activities of peptide immobilized surfaces have been tested in a variety of ways. For antimicrobial activity, some researchers have used a luminescence-based assay (e.g. *P. aeruginosa* lux strain) standardized with colony counting techniques (Gao *et al.*, 2011). Others also report assays based on a modified ISO protocol that involves only CFU counting (Kowalczuk *et al.*, 2010). GFP-based quantitation (Santos *et al.*, 2013) and kinetic microplate method of antimicrobial activity determination is also in current practice (Arcidiacono *et al.*, 2011). Although these protocols used different initial bacterial loads, there are clear-cut trends. Similarly, there are different approaches for antibiofilm activity assays. Since biofilms are formed after the initial attachment of bacterial cells onto the substrate, experiments that examine the reduction of initial bacterial colonization and inhibition of biofilm formation on the substrates are critical. However, most of the experiments reported in current literature are anti-adherent, analysing the efficacy of the surfaces in preventing only the preliminary stage in biofilm formation: the adhesion of the bacterial cells to the surface.

Furthermore, these experiments used a high dose of initial bacterial inoculum and tested for a short time up to 4 h (Table 12.3). In an assay to evaluate biofilm formation, however, normally 24 h is used to allow bacteria to grow biofilms. In both experiments, the bacterial counts are done calorimetrically and by CFU counting (Gao *et al.*, 2011; Mishra *et al.*, 2014). Table 12.3 lists

Table 12.3. Select anti-adherent and antibiofilm surfaces immobilized with antimicrobial peptides.

Study	Peptide/surface	Biofilm experiment (time)	Organism[a]	Technology/activity
Qi *et al.*, 2011	Nisin/multi-walled carbon nanotubes	Biofilm formation (18 h)	EC, SA, PA and BS	100-fold higher biofilm inhibition
Peyre *et al.*, 2012	Magainin I/TiO2	Anti-adherence and biofilm formation (3 h)	LI	70% and 90% decrease in adherence and biofilm formation
Xu *et al.*, 2013	Cecropin B/titanium	Anti-adherence and biofilm formation (24 h)	PA and SA	Quantitated by microscopy (SEM and CLSM)
Lim *et al.*, 2013	Arginine-tryptophan rich (CWR11/PDMS)	Biofilm formation (24 h)	PA	~75% inhibition
Chen *et al.*, 2014	GL13K peptide/titanium	Biofilm formation (48 h)	SG	5-fold reduction
Mishra *et al.*, 2014	Lasioglossin-III/commercial silicone catheter	Biofilm formation (24 h)	EC and EF	30 and 60% inhibition for EC and EF respectively
Yu *et al.*, 2015	Covalent DMA-coAPMA brush, ATRP mediated polymer brush conjugated to E6 or Tet-20/Titanium	Anti-adherence (4 h)	SA	~50% reduction in adherence
Shi *et al.*, 2015	Non-covalent, *multilayer coating* using chitosan/ hyaluronic acid and Tet213/ collagen on titanium	Anti-adherence of oral pathogens (1.5 h)	SA, PG	*Sustained bacterial inhibition for a month.* ~50% reduction in adherence
Godoy-Gallardo *et al.*, 2015	Covalent silanization or polymer brushes, hLf1–11 peptides/Titanium	Anti-adherence and biofilm formation (2 h)	SS and LS	~50% reduction in adherence; 50-60% inhibition of biofilm
Lim *et al.*, 2015	Trp-Arg-rich (CWR11)/silicone coated Foley catheters	Anti-adherence (24 h)	PA	92% reduction in adherence
Costa *et al.*, 2015	Dhvar5/titanium	Anti-adherence (2 h)and biofilm formation (24 h)	MRSA	~66% reduction in adhesion in 2h and 50% in 24 h; 50% biofilm inhibition
Song *et al.*, 2016	Cys-KR12/silk fibroin *nanofiber*	Biofilm formation (24 h)	SA and EC	No biofilm observed by FE-SEM
Alves *et al.*, 2016	Lipopeptide palm with DNase1/ PDMS	Anti-adhesion (24 h)	PA and SA	*Co-immobilization;* ~60% reduction in adherence
Yazici *et al.*, 2016	KL rich chimeric peptide/ Titanium	Anti-adherence (2 h)	SM, SE and EC	~95% reduction in adherence
Yeroslavsky *et al.*, 2015	Lysostaphin/polydopamine coated glass slides	Biofilm formation (20 h)	SA	~75% inhibition

[a]Abbreviations used for bacteria: BS: *Bacillus subtilis*; EC: *Escherichia coli*; EF: *Enterococcus faecalis*; LI: *Listeria ivanovii*; LS: *Lactobacillus salivarius*; PA: *Pseudomonas aeruginosa*; PG, *Porphyromonas gingivalis*; SS: *Streptococcus sanguinis*; SA: *Staphylococcus aureus*; SE: *Staphylococcus epidermidis*: SG: *Streptococcus gordonii*; SM: *Streptococcus mutans*.

immobilized peptides with known antibiofilm properties.

The activity of a peptide has been shown to be greatly influenced by immobilization. A good understanding of the parameters will help establish a framework for the development of more potent, efficient, and long-lasting peptide coated biodevices. Their studies have reported sub-optimal activity of immobilized peptide compared to the soluble counterpart (Appendini and Hotchkiss, 2001; Bagheri *et al.*, 2009). There are numerous factors influencing peptide activity. They can be classified into two categories:

1. Physical factors due to peptide immobilization.
2. Parameters regulated in the testing environment.

The physical factors involve surface type, immobilization chemistry, spacers or linkers, and peptide orientation. These factors influence the surface peptide concentration and activity. There appears to be a positive correlation between elevated biological activity and increased surface peptide concentration (Appendini and Hotchkiss, 2001; Chen *et al.*, 2009; Costa *et al.*, 2011). Though not a universal approach, the surfaces are usually initially prepared by creating functional groups on them. Such functional groups can be created either chemically by radical generation, or physically using high-energy plasma and UV. Surface functional groups include the creation of aldehyde, carboxylic acid, epoxide, maleimide, amine, isothiocyanate, thiol, alcohol, etc. (Onaizi and Leong, 2011), which are further linked with the AMPs. For polymer-brush chemistry, the graft density is critical. A recent study demonstrated that an increase in argon plasma and UV time during the radical transfer reaction can increase surface-bound peptide concentration on a silicon surface (Basu *et al.*, 2013).

The requirement of a spacer or linker depends on the peptide and immobilization chemistry. For example, Hilpert *et al.* (2009) have reported activity of a short 9-mer peptide attached to the substrate without any spacers. However, they postulated a different mechanism of action of electrostatic interference and destabilization, but not the peptide penetration based bacterial killing. In other studies, peptides immobilized without a spacer are shown to be active (Willcox *et al.*, 2008; Humblot *et al.*, 2009). However, both nisin and LL-37 lost activity after immobilization on a solid support without a spacer (Lante *et al.*, 1994; Gabriel *et al.*, 2006). Immobilized peptides have been shown to be only active when attached to PEG spacers (Cho *et al.*, 2007; Steven and

Hotchkiss, 2008). Bagheri *et al.* (2009) also reported reduced bactericidal activity of amphipathic model KLAL and magainin derived MK5E peptides with a decrease in PEG spacer length. Similarly, Mishra *et al.* (2013) noted the reduction of bacterial CFU with increase of PEG spacer lengths from 12 to 24 units. These studies establish that the use of a PEG spacer usually offers advantages. In addition, antifouling spacers such as PEG may provide dual characteristics to the peptide-coated surface. Such a surface can reduce initial bacterial colonization because of the spacer's non-adhesive character; it is also bactericidal because of the action of the immobilized peptide. Note that Haynie *et al.* (1995) found no differences in peptide bactericidal activity with the use of a two- or six-carbon chain linker binding magainin onto polyamide resins. Other spacers, like polymethyl methacrylate and polyvinyl chloride, are stiff and restrict lateral mobility of the peptide unless the length is increased. It is postulated that increased spacer length provides ample flexibility for the peptide to penetrate membranes, thereby increasing antimicrobial efficacy (Gabriel *et al.*, 2006; Bagheri *et al.*, 2009).

It has been demonstrated that the orientation of a peptide (i.e. via either N- or C-terminal coupling) in surface coating influences its activity (Bagheri *et al.*, 2009; North and Taitt, 2015). Binding behaviour of the bacteria and magainin I is influenced by immobilized peptide orientation (Kulagina *et al.*, 2005). Steven and Hotchkiss (2008) performed attachment of various N-side-chain reactions and found only the N-terminal attachment active. Some peptides, such as neomycin and polymyxin B, were found to be effective only when coupled via the N-termini to a longer spacer (Kennedy and Humphreys, 1976). Similarly, cecropin P1 attached to a solid support by different immobilization methods was shown to have been modulated by peptide orientation (Strauss *et al.*, 2010). Hence, a controlled or orientation-specific attachment of AMPs to the surface is crucial to antimicrobial efficacy. To achieve orientation-specific coupling, thiol-maleimide, di-thiol, or epoxide-thiol can be used to react with a cysteine added to either terminus of the peptide (Glinel *et al.*, 2009; Guani-Guerra *et al.*, 2010). Additional strategies include the use of click chemistry (Table 12.1). Interestingly, KR-12, the minimal AMP from human cathelicidin LL-37 (Wang, 2008), has been immobilized successfully via the N- and the C-terminus; both orientations have been demonstrated to be antimicrobial (Nie *et al.*, 2016; Song *et al.*, 2016).

Biological factors, such as pH, salt, serum and various blood cells, are known to affect the activity of AMPs and can also influence the antimicrobial efficacy of body-implanted materials (Onaizi and Leong, 2011). Coating of a synthetic AMP 6K8L to the polystyrene resin beads via a PEG linker yielded a surface that was active against *E. coli* O157: H7 at pH 3.5 to 7 (Appendini and Hotchkiss, 2001). The same surface was also resistant to autoclaving at 121°C for 15 min or dry heating at 120 and 200°C for 1 and 0.5 h, respectively. Antoci *et al.* (2007) found that vancomycin-coated titanium surfaces remained active in the presence of serum up to 24 h. Importantly, this vancomycin-coated surface was more potent in preventing *S. aureus* colonization than free vancomycin in solution. A recent study has achieved a very high density of peptide coating on nanoparticles, which appeared to retain activity after pretreatment with serum (Rai *et al.*, 2016).

12.5 Mechanism of Action of Immobilized Peptides

It is important to know whether AMPs work in the same manner before and after surface immobilization. In the free state, many linear membrane-targeting AMPs change their conformation from random coils to a helical structure upon membrane association (Boman, 2003; Zasloff, 2002). Circular dichroism (CD) is a convenient technique to follow this conformational change. Gao *et al.* (2012) immobilized the IDR-1010 peptide on a solid quartz substrate and analysed its interaction with model membranes using CD, which revealed a helical conformation similar to free AMPs. However, the orientation of the peptide on the surface can influence the helix formation. For cecropin A, no helical conformation was detected when coupled via the N-terminus of the peptide (North and Taitt, 2015).

Cho *et al.* (2007) found secondary β-sheet structures were also critical for retaining antimicrobial characteristics. These results suggest that surface immobilization does affect peptide conformations. There is evidence that the conformation of immobilized peptides may not always be identical to those of the free peptides before association with bacteria (Yu *et al.*, 2015). Other biophysical technologies such as chromophore leakage experiments and microscopic analysis can also provide insight into the mechanism of action of immobilized peptides. Rai *et al.* (2016) observed delayed inner membrane permeation by a nanoparticle attached cecropin–melittin hybrid peptide, when compared to the free form. Mishra *et al.* (2017) found that a Trp-rich peptide retained not only antimicrobial and antibiofilm activity, but also the same membrane-permeating mechanism before and after covalent coupling to the PET surface. In particular, the entrance of the propidium iodide dye into bacteria indicates damaged membranes (Gabriel *et al.*, 2006). Therefore, to what extent the mechanism will be similar can depend on the peptide, immobilization chemistry and the nature of the surface.

There are also other potential impacts on bacteria. It is conceivable that at a sub-lethal concentration, the effects of the peptide can differ from those at or above the MIC. In 2009, Hilpert *et al.* postulated that the disturbance in the surface electrostatic interaction might upset the Donnan equilibrium, leading to a variety of abrupt changes inside the cytoplasm, triggering cell autolysis. DNA microarrays have been used to study the changes in gene expression with and without peptide treatment, usually at a sub-MIC (RNA-Seq is now in use as well). For example, our unpublished study reveals that multiple toxin genes of *S. aureus* USA300 are suppressed by 17BIPHE2, a peptide engineered from LL-37 (Wang *et al.*, 2014). Recently, Basu *et al.* (2015) employed this technique to distinguish the differential gene expression patterns of *E. coli* cells in response to insect lasioglossin LL-III, both in its free and immobilized forms on a silicon wafer via a PEG linker. They found that genes responsive to membrane targeting, transport, the LPS layer modification, and an autolysing enzyme are upregulated. These observations suggest that immobilized peptides could affect bacterial cells in a variety of ways, ranging from genome reprogramming to bacterial death.

12.6 Biocompatibility

Ideally, the antimicrobial and antibiofilm surfaces do not exert unwanted toxic effects and can support surrounding human cells. It was found that covalent immobilization could reduce peptide toxicity and increase lifetime compared to release or leaching methods (Costa *et al.*, 2011). In addition, the AMP coating appears to confer other beneficial effects. For instance, a titanium surface functionalized with insect peptide cecropin B improves biocompatibility and inhibits inflammation responses (lower levels of cytokines TNFα and IL-6) of macrophages (Xu *et al.*, 2013). Recently, KR-12 was immobilized onto silk fibroin nanofibers (Song *et al.*, 2016). The immobilized peptide showed various effects on wound healing, including bacterial killing, promotion of cell proliferation and differentiation, and inhibition of inflammatory cytokine expression. In addition, Nie *et al.* (2016) found that the titanium surface coated with KR-12 facilitates adhesion and proliferation of human bone marrow mesenchymal stem cells (hBMSCs). These observations could all result from the parent molecule, human LL-37, which is known to have multiple functional roles (Wang, 2014).

12.7 Conclusions and Future Outlook

AMPs have been immobilized on a variety of surfaces, including metals such as titanium and stainless steel, ceramics, coverslips, model surfaces (SAM), microtitre plates, silicon, polymers like silicone, and various resins. Even commercial substrates have served as immobilization surfaces, including contact lenses and urinary tract catheters (Costa *et al.*, 2011). With increasing instances of infections, biofilm prevention strategies via surface coating is becoming increasingly important (Ferreira and Zumbuehl, 2009; Onaizi and Leong, 2011; Hadjesfandiari *et al.* 2014). The use of polycations and antibiotics have their own restrictions. While polycations present biocompatibility issues, antibiotics have limited activity against biofilms. AMPs are promising candidates for immobilization applications because of their broad-spectrum activity, fast killing, biocompatibility and rare occurrence of bacterial resistance. However, the reduction of peptide activity after immobilization is a common issue. Different strategies have been explored to retain or enhance peptide activity. The use of suitable chemistry could increase peptide concentrations on the surface. Radical generation either chemically (acid or base treatment) or by high energy UV or plasma treatment should be explored for individual surfaces. The use of polymer brushes increases peptide coating density and activity (Yu *et al.*, 2015). Further, bifunctional linkers are also important as they provide flexibility to the bound peptide to help it retain its activity. In addition, a specific orientation of the peptide can also be critical. Peptides in the immobilized form may be optimized to minimize activity loss due to the impact of serum, pH and salts. Short peptides and their analogues are attractive as they can be made cost effectively (Mishra *et al.*, 2017).

In the future, it would be economical to further simplify peptide-coupling chemistry. Other promising strategies include the use of a switchable polymer made of betaine esters (Cheng *et al.*, 2008), which possess both antimicrobial and non-fouling properties, allowing fast killing by the cationic surface, and then release of dead bacteria from the zwitterionic surface. Anti-adhesive and antimicrobial co-immobilization also appears to be a promising way to deal with polymicrobial biofilms (Alves *et al.*, 2016). It is anticipated that extending the lifetime of peptide-coated medical implants to make them more affordable and cost effective will be an important research goal for years to come.

Acknowledgements

The construction of this chapter was supported by the NIH grants R01 AI105147 and R03 AI128230 to GW.

Chapter editor: Monique van Hoek

References

Al-Bataineh, S.A., Britcher, L.G., and Griesser, H.J. (2006) Rapid radiation degradation in the XPS analysis of antibacterial coatings of brominated furanones. *Surface and Interface Analsis* 38, 1512–1518.

Alves, D., Magalhaes, A., Grzywacz, D., Neubauer, D., Kamysz, W. and Pereira, M.O. (2016) Co-immobilization of palm and DNase I for the development of an effective antiinfective coating for catheter surfaces. *Acta Biomaterialia* 44, 313–322.

Andresen, M., Stenstad, P., Moretro, T., Langsrud, S., Syverud, K., Johansson, L.S. and Stenius, P. (2007) Nonleaching antimicrobial films prepared from surface-modified microfibrillated cellulose. *Biomacromolecules* 8, 2149–2155.

Antoci, V., Jr, King, S.B., Jose, B., Parvizi, J., Zeiger, A.R., *et al.* (2007) Vancomycin covalently bonded to titanium alloy prevents bacterial colonization. *Journal of Orthopaedic Research* 25, 858–866.

Appendini, P. and Hotchkiss, J.H. (2001) Surface modification of poly(styrene) by the attachment of an antimicrobial peptide. *Journal of Applied Polymer Science* 81, 609–616.

Arcidiacono, S., Meehan, A.M., Kirby, R. and Soares, J.W. (2011) Kinetic microplate assay for determining immobilized antimicrobial peptide activity. *Analytical Biochemistry* 414, 163–165.

Aumsuwan, N., Heinhorst, S. and Urban, M.W. (2007) The effectiveness of antibiotic activity of penicillin attached to expanded poly(tetrafluoroethylene) (ePTFE) surfaces: a quantitative assessment. *Biomacromolecules* 8, 3525–3530.

Aumsuwan, N., Danyus, R.C., Heinhorst, S. and Urban, M.W. (2008) Attachment of ampicillin to expanded poly(tetrafluoroethylene): surface reactions leading to inhibition of microbial growth. *Biomacromolecules* 9, 1712–1718.

Bagheri, M., Beyermann, M. and Dathe, M. (2009) Immobilization reduces the activity of surface-bound cationic antimicrobial peptides with no influence upon the activity spectrum. *Antimicrobial Agents and Chemotherapy* 53, 1132–1141.

Basu, A., Mishra, B. and Leong, S.S.J. (2013) Immobilization of polybia-MPI by allyl glycidyl ether based brush chemistry to generate a novel antimicrobial surface. *Journal of Materials Chemistry B* 1, 4746–4755.

Basu, A., Mishra, B. and Leong, S.S.J. (2015) Global transcriptome analysis reveals distinct bacterial response towards soluble and surface-immobilized antimicrobial peptide (Lasioglossin-III). *RSC Advances* 5, 78712–78718.

Battice, D.R. and Hales, M.G. (1985) A new technology for producing stabilized foams having antimicrobial activity. *Journal of Cellular Plastics* 21, 332–337.

Boman, H.G. (2003) Antibacterial peptides: basic facts and emerging concepts. *Journal of Internal Medicine* 254, 197–215.

Bumgardner, J.D., Wiser, R., Gerard, P.D., Bergin, P., Chestnutt, B., *et al.* (2003) Chitosan: potential use as a bioactive coating for orthopaedic and craniofacial/dental implants. *Journal of Biomaterials Science. Polymer Edition* 14, 423–438.

Burkatovskaya, M., Tegos, G.P., Swietlik, E., Demidova, T.N., P Castano, A. and Hamblin, M.R. (2006) Use of chitosan bandage to prevent fatal infections developing from highly contaminated wounds in mice. *Biomaterials* 27, 4157–4164.

Carlson, R.P., Taffs, R., Davison, W.M. and Stewart, P.S. (2008) Anti-biofilm properties of chitosan-coated surfaces. *Journal of Biomaterials Science. Polymer Edition* 19, 1035–1046.

Chen, G., Zhou, M., Chen, S., Lv, G. and Yao, J. (2009) Nanolayer biofilm coated on magnetic nanoparticles by using a dielectric barrier discharge glow plasma fluidized bed for immobilizing an antimicrobial peptide. *Nanotechnology* 20, 465706.

Chen, X., Hirt, H., Li, Y., Gorr, S. U. and Aparicio, C. (2014) Antimicrobial GL13K peptide coatings killed and ruptured the wall of *Streptococcus gordonii* and prevented formation and growth of biofilms. *PloS One* 9, e111579.

Cheng, G., Xue, H., Zhang, Z., Chen, S. and Jiang, S. (2008) A switchable biocompatible polymer surface with self-sterilizing and nonfouling capabilities. *Angewandte Chemie International Edition in English* 47, 8831–8834.

Cho, W.M., Joshi, B.P., Cho, H. and Lee, K.H. (2007) Design and synthesis of novel antibacterial peptide-resin conjugates. *Bioorganic & Medicinal Chemistry Letters* 17, 5772–5776.

Costa, F.M., Carvalho, I.F., Montelaro, R.C., Gomes, P. and Martins, M.C. (2011) Covalent immobilization of antimicrobial peptides (AMPs) onto biomaterial surfaces. *Acta Biomaterialia* 7, 1431–1440.

Costa, F.M., Maia, S.R., Gomes, P.A. and Martins, M.C. (2015) Dhvar5 antimicrobial peptide (AMP) chemoselective covalent immobilization results on higher anti-adherence effect than simple physical adsorption. *Biomaterials* 52, 531–538.

Darouiche, R.O. (2004) Treatment of infections associated with surgical implants. *The New England Journal of Medicine* 350, 1422–1429.

Dee, K.C., Puleo, D.A. and Bizios, R. (2002) Biomaterials. In: Dee, K.C., Puleo, D.A. and Bizios, R., *An Introduction to Tissue Biomaterial Interactions*. John Wiley & Sons, Inc. Hoboken, New Jersey, pp. 1–13.

Duval-Terrié, C., Cosette, P., Molle, G., Muller, G. and De, E. (2003) Amphiphilic biopolymers (amphibiopols) as new surfactants for membrane protein solubilization. *Protein Science* 12, 681–689.

Ehtezazi, T. and Washington, C. (2000) Controlled release of macromolecules from PLA microspheres: using porous structure topology. *Journal of Controlled Release* 68, 361–372.

Etienne, O., Picart, C., Taddei, C., Haikel, Y., Dimarcq, J.L., *et al.* (2004) Multilayer polyelectrolyte films functionalized by insertion of defensin: a new approach to protection of implants from bacterial colonization. *Antimicrobial Agents and Chemotherapy* 48, 3662–3669.

Ferreira, L. and Zumbuehl, A. (2009) Non-leaching surfaces capable of killing microorganisms on contact. *Journal of Materials Chemistry* 19, 7796–7806.

Fuchs, A.D. and Tiller, J.C. (2006) Contact-active antimicrobial coatings derived from aqueous suspensions. *Angewandte Chemie International Edition in English* 45, 6759–6762.

Fulmer, P.A., Lundin, J.G. and Wynne, J.H. (2010) Development of antimicrobial peptides (AMPs) for use in self-decontaminating coatings. *ACS Applied Materials & Interfaces* 2, 1266–1270.

Gabriel, M., Nazmi, K., Veerman, E.C., Nieuw Amerongen, A.V. and Zentner, A. (2006) Preparation of LL-37-grafted titanium surfaces with bactericidal activity. *Bioconjugate Chemistry* 17, 548–550.

Gao, G., Lange, D., Hilpert, K., Kindrachuk, J., Zou, Y., *et al.* (2011) The biocompatibility and biofilm resistance of implant coatings based on hydrophilic polymer brushes conjugated with antimicrobial peptides. *Biomaterials* 32, 3899–3909.

Gao, G., Cheng, J.T., Kindrachuk, J., Hancock, R.E., Straus, S.K. and Kizhakkedathu, J.N. (2012) Biomembrane interactions reveal the mechanism of action of surface immobilized host defense IDR-1010 peptide. *Chemistry & Biology* 19, 199–209.

Gaur, R.K., and Gupta, K.C. (1989) A spectrophotometric method for the estimation of amino groups on polymer supports. *Analytical Biochemistry* 180, 253–258.

Ginalska, G., Kowalczuk, D. and Osinska, M. (2005) A chemical method of gentamicin bonding to gelatine-sealed prosthetic vascular grafts. *International Journal of Pharmaceutics* 288, 131–140.

Glinel, K., Jonas, A.M., Jouenne, T., Leprince, J., Galas, L. and Huck, W.T. (2009) Antibacterial and antifouling polymer brushes incorporating antimicrobial peptide. *Bioconjugate Chemistry* 20, 71–77.

Godoy-Gallardo, M., Mas-Moruno, C., Yu, K., Manero, J.M., Gil, F.J., Kizhakkedathu, J.N. and Rodriguez, D. (2015) Antibacterial properties of hLf1-11 peptide onto titanium surfaces: a comparison study between silanization and surface initiated polymerization. *Biomacromolecules* 16, 483–496.

Gooding, J.J., Mearns, F., Yang, W. and Liu, J. (2003) Self-assembled monolayers into the 21st century: recent advances and applications. *Electroanalysis* 15, 81–96.

Gristina, A.G. (1987) Biomaterial-centered infection: microbial adhesion versus tissue integration. *Science* 237, 1588–1595.

Guani-Guerra, E., Santos-Mendoza, T., Lugo-Reyes, S.O. and Teran, L.M. (2010) Antimicrobial peptides: general overview and clinical implications in human health and disease. *Clinical Immunology* 135, 1–11.

Guyomard, A., Dé, E., Jouenne, T., Malandain, J., Muller, G. and Glinel, K. (2008) Incorporation of a hydrophobic antibacterial peptide into amphiphilic polyelectrolyte multilayers: a bioinspired approach to prepare biocidal thin coatings. *Advanced Functional Materials* 18, 758–765.

Hadjesfandiari, N., Yu, K., Meiac, Y. and Kizhakkedathu, J.N. (2014) Polymer brush-based approaches for the development of infection-resistant surfaces. *Journal of Materials Chemistry B* 2, 4968–4978.

Haldar, J., An, D., Alvarez de Cienfuegos, L., Chen, J. and Klibanov, A.M. (2006) Polymeric coatings that inactivate both influenza virus and pathogenic bacteria. *Proceedings of the National Academy of Sciences of the United States of America* 103, 17667–17671.

Hancock, R.E., Haney, E.F. and Gill, E.E. (2016) The immunology of host defence peptides: beyond antimicrobial activity. *Nature Reviews Immunology* 16, 321–334.

Haynie, S. L., Crum, G.A. and Doele, B.A. (1995) Antimicrobial activities of amphiphilic peptides covalently bonded to a water-insoluble resin. *Antimicrobial Agents and Chemotherapy* 39, 301–307.

Hilpert, K., Elliott, M., Jenssen, H., Kindrachuk, J., Fjell, C.D., *et al.* (2009) Screening and characterization of surface-tethered cationic peptides for antimicrobial activity. *Chemistry & Biology* 16, 58–69.

Hoffman, L.R., D'Argenio, D.A., MacCoss, M.J., Zhang, Z., Jones, R.A. and Miller, S.I. (2005) Aminoglycoside antibiotics induce bacterial biofilm formation. *Nature* 436, 1171–1175.

Humblot, V., Yala, J.F., Thebault, P., Boukerma, K., Hequet, A., Berjeaud, J.M. and Pradier, C.M. (2009) The antibacterial activity of magainin I immobilized onto mixed thiols self-assembled monolayers. *Biomaterials* 30, 3503–3512.

Kennedy, J.F. and Humphreys, J.D. (1976) Active immobilized antibiotics based on metal hydroxides. *Antimicrobial Agents and Chemotherapy* 9, 766–770.

Klibanov, A.M. (2007) Permanently microbicidal materials coatings. *Journal of Materials Chemistry* 17, 2479-2482.

Kowalczuk, D., Ginalska, G. and Golus, J. (2010) Characterization of the developed antimicrobial urological catheters. *International Journal of Pharmaceutics* 402, 175–183.

Kulagina, N.V., Lassman, M.E., Ligler, F.S. and Taitt, C.R. (2005) Antimicrobial peptides for detection of bacteria in biosensor assays. *Analytical Chemistry* 77, 6504–6508.

Laloyaux, X., Fautre, E., Blin, T., Purohit, V., Leprince, J., Jouenne, T., Jonas, A.M. and Glinel, K. (2010) Temperature-responsive polymer brushes switching from bactericidal to cell-repellent. *Advanced Materials* 22, 5024–5028.

Lante, A., Crapisi, A., Pasini, G. and Scalabrini, P. (1994) Nisin released from immobilization matrices as antimicrobial agent. *Biotechnology Letters* 16, 293–298.

Li, X., Li, Y., Han, H., Miller, D.W. and Wang, G. (2006) Solution structures of human LL37 fragments and NMR-based identification of a minimal membrane-targeting antimicrobial and anticancer region. *Journal of the American Chemical Society* 128, 5776–5785.

Lim, K., Chua, R.R., Saravanan, R., Basu, A., Mishra, B., Tambyah, P.A., Ho, B. and Leong, S.S. (2013) Immobilization studies of an engineered arginine-tryptophan-rich peptide on a silicone surface with antimicrobial and antibiofilm activity. *ACS Applied Materials & Interfaces* 5, 6412–6422.

Lim, K., Chua, R.R., Bow, H., Tambyah, P.A., Hadinoto, K. and Leong, S.S. (2015) Development of a catheter functionalized by a polydopamine peptide coating with antimicrobial and antibiofilm properties. *Acta Biomaterialia* 15, 127–138.

Mishra, B., Basu, A., Saravanan, R., Xiang, L., Yang, L.K. and Leong S.S.J. (2013) Lasioglossin-III: antimicrobial characterization and feasibility study for immobilization applications. *RSC Advances*, 3, 9534–9543.

Mishra, B., Basu, A., Chua, R.R.Y., Saravanan, R., Tambyah, P.A., *et al.* (2014) Site specific immobilization of a potent antimicrobial peptide onto silicone catheters: evaluation against urinary tract infection pathogens. *Journal of Materials Chemistry B* 2, 1706–1716.

Mishra, B., Lushnikova, T., Golla, R.M., Wang, X., and Wang, G. (2017) Design and surface immobilization of short anti-biofilm peptides. *Acta Biomaterialia* 49, 316–328.

Mlynek, K.D., Callahan, M.T., Shimkevitch, A.V., Farmer, J.T., Endres, J.L., *et al.* (2016) Effects of low-dose amoxicillin on *Staphylococcus aureus* USA300 biofilms. *Antimicrobial Agents and Chemotherapy* 60, 2639–2651.

Mohorcic, M., Jerman, I., Zorko, M., Butinar, L., Orel, B., Jerala, R. and Friedrich, J. (2010) Surface with antimicrobial activity obtained through silane coating with covalently bound polymyxin B. *Journal of Materials Science. Materials in Medicine* 21, 2775–2782.

Nie, B., Ao, H., Chen, C., Xie, K., Zhou, J., *et al.* (2016) Covalent immobilization of KR-12 peptide onto a titanium surface for decreasing infection and promoting osteogenic differentiation. *RSC Advances* 6, 46733–46743.

North, S.H. and Taitt, C.R. (2015) Application of circular dichroism for structural analysis of surface-immobilized cecropin A interacting with lipoteichoic acid. *Langmuir* 31, 10791–10798.

Onaizi, S.A. and Leong, S.S. (2011) Tethering antimicrobial peptides: current status and potential challenges. *Biotechnology Advances* 29, 67–74.

Pan, Y., Xiao, H., Zhao, G. and He, B. (2008) Antimicrobial and thermal-responsive layer-by-layer assembly based on ionic-modified guanidine polymer and PVA. *Polymer Bulletin* 61, 541–551.

Peyre, J., Humblot, V., Methivier, C., Berjeaud, J.M. and Pradier, C.M. (2012) Co-grafting of amino-poly(ethylene glycol) and magainin I on a TiO2 surface: tests of antifouling and antibacterial activities. *The Journal of Physical Chemistry B* 116, 13839–13847.

Qi, X., Poernomo, G., Wang, K., Chen, Y., Chan-Park, M.B., Xu, R. and Chang, M.W. (2011) Covalent immobilization of nisin on multi-walled carbon nanotubes: superior antimicrobial and anti-biofilm properties. *Nanoscale* 3, 1874–1880.

Rai, A., Pinto, S., Evangelista, M.B., Gil, H., Kallip, S., Ferreira, M.G. and Ferreira, L. (2016) High-density antimicrobial peptide coating with broad activity and low cytotoxicity against human cells. *Acta Biomaterialia* 33, 64–77.

Rostovtsev, V.V., Green, L.G., Fokin, V.V. and Sharpless, K.B. (2002) A stepwise huisgen cycloaddition process: copper(I)-catalyzed regioselective 'ligation' of azides and terminal alkynes. *Angewandte Chemie International Edition in English* 41, 2596–2599.

Saif, M.J., Anwar, J. and Munawar, M.A. (2009) A novel application of quaternary ammonium compounds as antibacterial hybrid coating on glass surfaces. *Langmuir: The ACS Journal of Surfaces and Colloids* 25, 377–379.

Santos, C.M., Kumar, A., Kolar, S.S., Contreras-Caceres, R., McDermott, A. and Cai, C. (2013) Immobilization of antimicrobial peptide IG-25 onto fluoropolymers via fluorous interactions and click chemistry. *ACS Applied Materials and Interfaces* 5, 12789–12793.

Shi, J., Liu, Y., Wang, Y., Zhang, J., Zhao, S. and Yang, G. (2015) Biological and immunotoxicity evaluation of antimicrobial peptide-loaded coatings using a layer-bylayer process on titanium. *Scientific Reports* 5, 16336.

Song, D.W., Kim, S.H., Kim, H.H., Lee, K.H., Ki, C.S. and Park, Y.H. (2016) Multibiofunction of antimicrobial peptide-immobilized silk fibroin nanofiber membrane: implications for wound healing. *Acta Biomaterialia* 39, 146–155.

Speier, J.L. and Malek, J.R. (1982) Destruction of microorganisms by contact with solid surfaces. *Journal of Colloid and Interface Science* 89, 68–76.

Statz, A.R., Park, J.P., Chongsiriwatana, N.P., Barron, A.E. and Messersmith, P.B. (2008) Surface-immobilised antimicrobial peptoids. *Biofouling* 24, 439–448.

Steven, M.D. and Hotchkiss, J.H. (2008) Covalent immobilization of an antimicrobial peptide on poly(ethylene) film. *Journal of Applied Polymer Science* 110, 2665–2670.

Strauss, J., Kadilak, A., Cronin, C., Mello, C.M. and Camesano, T.A. (2010) Binding, inactivation, and adhesion forces between antimicrobial peptide cecropin P1 and pathogenic *E. coli*. *Colloids and Surfaces B: Biointerfaces* 75, 156–164.

Thomas, V.C., Sadykov, M.R., Chaudhari, S.S., Jones, J., Endres, J.L., *et al.* (2014) A central role for carbon-overflow pathways in the modulation of bacterial cell death. *PLoS Pathogens* 10, e1004205.

Tiller, J.C., Liao, C.J., Lewis, K. and Klibanov, A.M. (2001) Designing surfaces that kill bacteria on contact. *Proceedings of the National Academy of Sciences of the United States of America* 98, 5981–5985.

Tiller, J.C., Lee, S.B., Lewis, K. and Klibanov, A.M. (2002) Polymer surfaces derivatized with poly(vinyl-N-hexylpyridinium) kill airborne and waterborne bacteria. *Biotechnology and Bioengineering* 79, 465–471.

Vreuls, C., Zocchi, G., Thierry, B., Garitte, G., Griesser, S.S., *et al.* (2010) Prevention of bacterial biofilms by covalent immobilization of peptides onto plasma polymer functionalized substrates. *Journal of Materials Chemistry* 20, 8092–8098.

Wang, G. (2008) Structures of human host defense cathelicidin LL-37 and its smallest antimicrobial peptide KR-12 in lipid micelles. *Journal of Biological Chemistry* 283, 32637–32643.

Wang. G. (ed.) (2010) *Antimicrobial Peptides: Discovery, Design and Novel Therapeutic Strategies* CABI, Wallingford, UK.

Wang, G. (2014) Human antimicrobial peptides and proteins. *Pharmaceuticals* 7, 545–594.

Wang, G. (2015) Improved methods for classification, prediction, and design of antimicrobial peptides. *Methods in Molecular Biology* 1268, 43–66.

Wang, G., Hanke, M.L., Mishra, B., Lushnikova, T., Heim, C.E., *et al.* (2014) Transformation of human cathelicidin LL-37 into selective, stable, and potent antimicrobial compounds. *ACS Chemical Biology* 9, 1997–2002.

Wang, G., Mishra, B., Lau, K., Lushnikova, T., Golla, R. and Wang, X. (2015) Antimicrobial peptides in 2014. *Pharmaceuticals* 8, 123–150.

Wang, G., Li, X. and Wang, G. (2016) APD3: the antimicrobial peptide database as a tool for research and education. *Nucleic Acids Research* 44 (database issue), D1087–D1093.

Willcox, M.D., Hume, E.B., Aliwarga, Y., Kumar, N. and Cole, N. (2008) A novel cationic peptide coating for the prevention of microbial colonization on contact lenses. *Journal of Applied Microbiology* 105, 1817–1825.

Xu, D., Yang, W., Hu, Y., Luo, Z., Li, J., Hou, Y., Liu, Y. and Cai, K. (2013) Surface functionalization of titanium substrates with cecropin B to improve their cytocompatibility and reduce inflammation responses. *Colloids and Surfaces B: Biointerfaces* 110, 225–235.

Yala, J.F., Thebault, P., Hequet, A., Humblot, V., Pradier, C.M. and Berjeaud, J.M. (2011) Elaboration of antibiofilm materials by chemical grafting of an antimicrobial peptide. *Applied Microbiology and Biotechnology* 89, 623–634.

Yazici, H., O'Neill, M.B., Kacar, T., Wilson, B.R., Oren, E.E., Sarikaya, M. and Tamerler, C. (2016) Engineered chimeric peptides as antimicrobial surface coating agents toward infection-free implants. *ACS Applied Materials & Interfaces* 8, 5070–5081.

Yeroslavsky, G., Girshevitz, O., Foster-Frey, J., Donovan, D.M. and Rahimipour, S. (2015) Antibacterial and antibiofilm surfaces through polydopamine-assisted immobilization of lysostaphin as an antibacterial enzyme. *Langmuir: The ACS Journal of Surfaces and Colloids* 31, 1064–1073.

Yu, K., Lo, J.C., Mei, Y., Haney, E.F., Siren, E., Kalathottukaren, M.T., Hancock, R.E., Lange, D. and Kizhakkedathu, J.N. (2015) Toward infection-resistant surfaces: achieving high antimicrobial peptide potency by modulating the functionality of polymer brush and peptide. *ACS Applied Materials & Interfaces* 7, 28591–28605.

Zasloff, M. (2002) Antimicrobial peptides of multicellular organisms. *Nature* 415, 389–395.

Zumbuehl, A., Ferreira, L., Kuhn, D., Astashkina, A., Long, L., *et al.* (2007) Antifungal hydrogels. *Proceedings of the National Academy of Sciences of the United States of America* 104, 12994–12998.

13 Sustained Delivery of Cathelicidin Antimicrobial Peptide-inducing Compounds to Minimize Infection and Enhance Wound Healing

Jingwei Xie[1], Gitali Ganguli-Indra[2,3], Arup K. Indra[2,3,4,5,6,7] and Adrian F. Gombart[4,5,*]

[1]*Department of Surgery-Transplant and Holland Regenerative Medicine Program, University of Nebraska Medical Center, Omaha, NE, USA;* [2]*Department of Pharmaceutical Sciences, College of Pharmacy, OSU-OHSU, Corvallis, OR, USA;* [3]*Molecular Cell Biology Program, OSU, Corvallis, OR, USA;* [4]*Department of Biochemistry and Biophysics, OSU, Corvallis, OR, USA;* [5]*Linus Pauling Science Institute, OSU, Corvallis, OR, USA;* [6]*Department of Dermatology, Oregon Health and Science University, Portland, OR, USA;* [7]*Knight Cancer Institute, OHSU, Portland, OR, USA*

Abstract

The cathelicidin antimicrobial peptide gene is critical for epithelial barrier defence and wound healing. Human cathelicidin expression is induced by various natural compounds including vitamin D, resveratrol and short-chain fatty acids. In this chapter, we review relevant literature regarding the role of cathelicidin in fighting infection, promoting wound healing and its regulation by these natural compounds. Further, we summarize recent findings that support developing strategies for therapeutic anti-infective wound dressings using nanofiber encapsulation technologies. Sustained release of these compounds could modulate the host immune response and greatly reduce rates of hospital-acquired infections following surgery and/or combat injuries. This approach may potentially decrease acquisition of antibiotic resistance.

13.1 Introduction

In the US, over 150,000 surgical site infections (SSIs) occur within 30 days of an operation and kill more than 8000 people each year. These infections account for nearly $10 billion annually in additional healthcare costs (Magill *et al.*, 2014). SSIs comprise 22% of all healthcare-associated infections (HAIs) and represent the most common HAI among surgical patients (Magill *et al.*, 2012). These postsurgical infections increase the length of postoperative hospital stays by 7–10 days, rates of readmission to the hospital, expense and rates of death (Anderson *et al.*, 2008). A patient with an SSI is 2–11 times more likely to die compared to those patients without an SSI (Anderson, 2009) and 75% of SSI-associated deaths are directly attributed to the SSI (Anderson *et al.*, 2008; Awad and Lobo, 2012). In addition, preventing

* Corresponding author e-mail: adrian.gombart@oregonstate.edu

battlefield wound infections enhances resuscitation, salvage and ultimately restoration of function in severely injured service personnel.

Over the course of the US military engagement in the Middle East, opportunistic bacterial infections have emerged as a persistent and significant threat in the care of wounded US military personnel (Brulport *et al.*, 2007). In both civilian and combat settings, interventions that can reduce the rate of infections could save thousands of lives and dramatically decrease healthcare costs. Treatment currently uses wound dressings that deliver antibiotics, but their use can select for survival of drug-resistant pathogens. The majority of HAIs involve the antibiotic-resistant ESKAPE pathogens (*Escherichia coli, Staphylococcus aureus, Klebsiella pneumoniae, Acinetobacter baumannii, Pseudomonas aeruginosa* and *Enterococcus faecalis*) (Pendleton *et al.*, 2013). These bacteria thrive in healthcare settings and traditional antibiotics cannot kill them as they are either multi-drug or extremely drug resistant. The increasing frequency of multidrug-resistant clinical isolates of these bacterial species in the United States underscores the need for novel approaches with modes of action different from current antibiotics to bolster the antimicrobial treatment regimens used to prevent infections of wounds and surgical sites.

In this chapter we review evidence for the importance of vitamin D and the cathelicidin antimicrobial peptide gene in epithelial barrier defence and wound healing. In addition, we propose strategies to develop therapeutic anti-infective wound dressings that modulate the host immune response with the goal of greatly reducing rates of HAIs following surgery and/or combat injuries and potentially decrease the development of antibiotic resistance. By leveraging the knowledge researchers have gained about inducing antimicrobial peptide gene expression and nanofiber encapsulation technologies, we could boost the host immune response to attack the pathogen on numerous fronts rather than a single front like traditional antibiotics, thus limiting the selection of resistant bacteria. In this chapter, we will highlight the rationale for, and the efforts we, and others, are making to increase the levels of the inducible human cathelicidin antimicrobial peptide (*CAMP* or LL-37) at wound sites.

13.2 The Role of the CAMP Gene in Protection against Infection

Mammals possess numerous cathelicidin antimicrobial peptide genes (Zanetti *et al.*, 1995). The encoded proteins are targeted to the endoplasmic reticulum (ER) by an N-terminal signal sequence followed by a highly conserved cathelin domain from which a C-terminal antimicrobial domain is released upon proteolytic cleavage (Zanetti *et al.*, 1995). Larrick and colleagues identified the first mammalian cathelicidin in rabbit bone marrow as an 18-kD protein they named CAP18 (Larrick *et al.*, 1991). Furthermore, they demonstrated that it bound and neutralized lipopolysaccharide (LPS) and that the C-terminal 37 amino acids directly killed both Gram-positive and Gram-negative bacteria (Larrick *et al.*, 1993, Larrick *et al.*, 1994).

Subsequently, three independent groups cloned the human cathelicidin gene from granulocytes (Cowland *et al.*, 1995; Larrick *et al.*, 1995a; Frohm *et al.*, 1997). The C-terminal 37 amino acids of hCAP18 (LL-37) also conferred its bactericidal activity against both Gram-positive and Gram-negative bacteria (Larrick *et al.*, 1995b) by disrupting the bacterial cell membrane (Turner *et al.*, 1998; Oren *et al.*, 1999;). In addition, LL-37 demonstrates effective bactericidal activity against methicillin-resistant *S. aureus* (MRSA) and may effectively fight drug-resistant bacterial infections (Turner *et al.*, 1998; Saiman *et al.*, 2001). *Camp*-deficient mice are susceptible to necrotic skin infections caused by Group A Streptococcus (Nizet *et al.*, 2001), and decreased expression of cathelicidin also allows increased entry of *S. aureus* through the epidermal barrier (Nakatsuji *et al.*, 2016). Furthermore, the cathelicidin is required for permeability barrier homeostasis (Aberg *et al.*, 2008; Martin-Ezquerra *et al.*, 2011).

Interestingly, LL-37 usually inhibits biofilms at sub-microbicidal concentrations. For example, LL-37 prevents *P. aeruginosa* biofilm formation at 0.5 μg/ml, whereas the minimum inhibitory concentration for *P. aeruginosa* is 64 μg/ml (Overhage *et al.*, 2008). Similar findings were reported for inhibition of other biofilms (*Aggregatibacter actinomycetemcomitans* (Vahavihu *et al.*, 2010), uropathogenic *Escherichia coli* (Kai-Larsen *et al.*, 2010)), suggesting that biofilm inhibition might be a more physiologically relevant function of LL-37 rather than direct bacterial killing which usually requires higher concentrations of the peptide. LL-37 also suppresses biofilm formation by *Burkholderia pseudomallei* (Kanthawong *et al.*, 2012), *Francisella novisida* (Amer *et al.*, 2010), *S. aureus* (Dean *et al.*, 2011) and *Stenotrophomonas maltophilia* (Pompilio *et al.*, 2011). LL-37 suppresses the quorum-sensing systems in *P. aeruginosa* by down-regulating *lasI* and *rhlR*. In addition, it inhibits assembly of flagella that are essential for initiating adherence during biofilm formation (Overhage *et al.*, 2008). Finally, LL-37 alters expression of the *rhl*A and *rhl*B genes implicated in biofilm formation by *P. aeruginosa* (Dean *et al.*, 2011). How LL-37 blocks biofilm formation by other bacterial species remains largely unknown, but this property could make it highly effective in treating biofilm-mediated wound infections (Duplantier and van Hoek, 2013).

13.3 LL-37 Modulates the Host Immune Response

In addition to enhancing skin barrier function, blocking biofilm formation and killing microorganisms, LL-37 functions as an 'alarmin'. It alerts the host immune system to the presence of a pathogen and acts as a chemoattractant for monocytes, neutrophils, T cells and mast cells and regulates cytokine production in these cells (Bowdish *et al.*, 2006). It also promotes angiogenesis,

wound healing and apoptosis (Bucki *et al.*, 2010). These biological activities probably occur because of the ability of LL-37 to bind and activate several different transmembrane receptors that include the formyl peptide receptor (FPR2), purinergic receptor P2X7, chemokine receptor 2 (CXCR2), mas-related gene X2 (MrgX2) and epidermal growth factor receptor (EGFR). In addition, LL-37 modulates Toll-like receptor (TLR) signalling through binding to their ligands. As discussed below, the activation of these receptors is important for wound healing and preventing infection.

13.3.1 Formyl peptide receptor 2 (FPR2)

FPR2 is a G protein-coupled transmembrane receptor (Le *et al.*, 2002) that is expressed in neutrophils, monocytes and T cells (Coffelt *et al.*, 2009). Activation of FPR2 by LL-37 mobilizes immune cells to sites of infection to clear invading microbes and/or dead host cells (De *et al.*, 2000). In addition, activation of FPR2 in neutrophils inhibits apoptosis and enables increased production of cytokines and superoxide (Nagaoka *et al.*, 2006; Iaccio *et al.*, 2009). Mice lacking the *Camp* gene exhibit delayed neutrophil infiltration in the lung which results in more severe infections (Kovach *et al.*, 2012). FPR2 is also expressed by endothelial cells and activation by LL-37 promotes proliferation of endothelial progenitor cells and enhanced angiogenesis (Koczulla *et al.*, 2003). Using a series of *in vivo* and *in vitro* approaches, investigators demonstrated that activation of FPR2 on classical macrophages by neutrophil-derived LL-37 induces adhesion of macrophages to endothelial bound LL-37 through activation of integrins (Wantha *et al.*, 2013). Furthermore, in mice, activation of FPR2 by murine cathelicidin promotes dendritic cell maturation (Chen *et al.*, 2014). Interestingly, activation of FPR2 by LL-37 enhances epithelial cells lifespan by suppressing apoptosis and secondly, FPR2 signalling feeds into pathways that up-regulate cell migration and proliferation, both of which are crucial to wound healing (Heilborn *et al.*, 2003; Shaykhiev *et al.*, 2005).

13.3.2 Purinergic receptor P2X7

P2X7 participates in transmembrane signalling of LL-37 (Pochet *et al.*, 2006) and is required for induced IL-1 release from human monocytes (Elssner *et al.*, 2004). In addition, LL-37 activation of P2X7 increases cell migration in intestinal epithelial cells (Otte *et al.*, 2009) and stiffness in endothelial cells (Byfield *et al.*, 2011), as well as IL-8, cyclooxygenase-2 (COX-2) and prostaglandin E2 (PGE2) production in gingival fibroblasts (Montreekachon *et al.*, 2011; Chotjumlong *et al.*, 2013). LL-37 induces a proliferative cell response in P2X7 expressing HEK cells, but not cells that lack P2X7 expression (Tomasinsig *et al.*, 2008). In human skin ultraviolet B (UVB) radiation and LL-37 increases inflammasome activation and subsequent IL-1b expression via the P2X7 receptor. This, in turn, enhances the angiogenic potential of endothelial cells (Salzer *et al.*, 2014). The internalization of LL-37 by macrophages through clathrin-mediated endocytosis requires binding to the P2X7 receptor. LL-37 traffics to endosomes and lysosomes where it enhances clearance of bacteria by macrophages (Tang *et al.*, 2015). Taken together, these biological activities that function via the P2X7 receptor contribute to fighting infection and enhancing the healing of wounds.

13.3.3 Toll-like receptors (TLRs)

LL-37 binds LPS and neutralizes TLR4 signalling in macrophages. This abrogates the release of tumour necrosis factor alpha (TNFα) and NO⁻ production (Turner *et al.*, 1998; Brown *et al.*, 2011; Ciornei *et al.*, 2003), while exogenous LL-37 protects mice and rats from Gram-negative bacterial sepsis (Fukumoto *et al.*, 2005; Cirioni *et al.*, 2006). In addition, LL-37 complexes with negatively charged DNA or RNA molecules.

In psoriatic skin, damaged cells release self-DNA and -RNA molecules that bind LL-37. These complexes deliver the extracellular DNA molecules across the membrane and present them to the intracellular TLR9 and TLR7/8 receptors, respectively (Lande *et al.*, 2007; Ganguly *et al.*, 2009). Their activation enhances type I interferon production by plasmacytoid and myeloid dendritic cells, which contributes to the pathogenesis of psoriasis (Lande *et al.*, 2007; Ganguly *et al.*, 2009,). LL-37 augments TLR9 induced type I interferon production in keratinocytes via the same mechanism (Morizane *et al.*, 2012). Furthermore, LL-37 complexes with polyinosine-polycytidylic acid poly(I:C); however, the effect of LL-37 on TLR3 signalling is cell-type specific. In human fibroblasts, LL-37 suppressed poly(I:C) induced interleukin 6 (IL-6), interleukin 8 (IL-8), and C-X-C motif chemokine 10 (CXCL10) expression (Into *et al.*, 2010). In contrast, IL-6 and IL-8 production was upregulated in human bronchial epithelial cells (Filewod *et al.*, 2009). On the other hand, Hasan *et al.* (2011) showed LL-37 blocked poly(I:C) mediated TLR3 signalling in mouse macrophages, dampening type I interferon production in these cells. The modulation of TLR signalling by LL-37 may be important in regulating the extent of inflammation in the wound during healing.

13.3.4 Other transmembrane receptors

LL-37 stimulates monocyte migration through chemokine (C-X-C motif) receptor 2 (CXCR2) and internalization of CXCR2. Furthermore, it increases calcium mobilization in neutrophils and increases neutrophil migration (Zhang *et al.*, 2009). Mas-related gene X2 (MrgX2) mediates LL-37 induced chemotaxis and degranulation in mast cells (Subramanian *et al.*, 2011). Initially LL-37 was described as a ligand for the epidermal growth factor receptor (EGFR) in airway epithelial cells which activates IL-8 release (Tjabringa *et al.*, 2003). Activation of EGFR by LL-37 in keratinocytes stimulates cell migration and proliferation (Tokumaru *et al.*, 2005; Niyonsaba *et al.*, 2006; Yin and Yu, 2010). The stimulation of these activities induces wound healing in airway epithelial cells, corneas, and tissue granulation in wounds of *ob/ob*-deficient mice that display impaired wound healing (Shaykhiev *et al.*, 2005; Carretero *et al.*, 2008; Gao *et al.*, 2010; Yin and Yu, 2010). Taken together, these data indicate an important role for LL-37 in promoting wound healing during different stages of the process.

13.4 Function of Vitamin D Signalling in Normal Skin Homeostasis

Upon injury or infection, the vitamin D signalling pathway is activated in the skin (Schauber *et al.*, 2007); however, vitamin D also plays a role in normal skin homeostasis. The epidermis of the skin consists of four different layers. The stratum basale being the lowest, followed by stratum spinosum, stratum granulosum, and the uppermost layer is the stratum corneum (Muehleisen *et al.*, 2012). Vitamin D is essential for maintenance of skin homeostasis and its synthesis is initiated in the skin (Bikle, 2011). Humans synthesize vitamin D_3 or calciol from 7-dehydrocholesterol in the skin upon exposure to UVB irradiation from the sun or artificial light. Hydroxylation of vitamin D_3 (calciol) by vitamin D 25-hydroxylase (CYP27A1) in the liver generates 25-hydroxyvitamin D_3 [25(OH)D or calcidiol]; hydroxylation of vitamin D_3 by 25-hydroxyvitamin D_3 1-α-hydroxylase (CYP27B1) in the kidney produces active 1α,25-dihydroxyvitamin D_3 [1α,25(OH)$_2$D$_3$ or calcitriol] (Holick, 2008). Macrophages, keratinocytes and epithelial cells also express CYP27B1 (Jones, 2013); therefore, these cells are capable of synthesizing 1α,25(OH)$_2$D$_3$ independent of other organs (Schuessler *et al.*, 2001).

1α,25(OH)$_2$D$_3$ mediates the majority of its effects through a transcription factor called the vitamin D receptor (VDR), that belongs to the steroid/hormone nuclear receptor family (Mangelsdorf *et al.*, 1995). The VDR forms a heterodimer with the retinoid X receptor (RXR) and binds to vitamin D response elements (VDREs) in the promoters of target genes, and regulates their expression (Christakos *et al.*, 1996). Most cell and tissue types express the VDR and respond to 1α,25(OH)$_2$D$_3$ (Bouillon *et al.*, 1995; James *et al.*, 1999). Recently, Rid and colleagues identified 55 1α,25(OH)$_2$D$_3$ responsive genes that were differentially expressed within human primary keratinocytes; 46 of these genes were novel targets in primary keratinocytes (Rid *et al.*, 2013). Of five enriched clusters, one included genes involved in wounding/inflammatory responses (Rid *et al.*, 2013).

Vitamin D, along with calcium signalling also plays an important role in activation of stem cells in the hair follicle (Oda *et al.*, 2012). These cells play a critical role in wound healing as activated hair follicle stem cells generate the newly formed epidermis in a process called re-epithelialization (Liang *et al.*, 2012). Mice lacking the VDR have growth of a normal first coat hair but display impaired cyclic regeneration of hair follicles leading to development of alopecia due to a defect in the keratinocyte component of the hair follicle (Luderer and Demay, 2010). Overall, there is disrupted function of the keratinocyte stem cells, resulting in deregulated hair follicle cycling and a decrease in bulge keratinocyte stem cells over time. Genetic studies further established ligand independent effects of VDR to maintain hair follicle homeostasis. When VDR or its co-activator levels are reduced, decreased keratinocyte differentiation is observed *in vitro* (Amor *et al.*, 2010).

Keratinocyte proliferation and differentiation is tightly regulated and dictates the amount of 1α,25(OH)$_2$D$_3$ in skin (Piotrowska *et al.*, 2016). Vitamin D signalling also protects melanocytes – the pigment-producing cells in the skin – from the harmful UV irradiation of the sun and regulates their proliferation and survival (Chagani *et al.*, 2016). In the epidermis, calcium forms a gradient with highest amount being in the stratum granulosum and lowest in the stratum basale (Muehleisen *et al.*, 2012). It is known that 1α,25(OH)$_2$D$_3$ initiates calcium induced terminal differentiation leading to increased expression of the early and late differentiation markers such as loricrin, filaggrin, involucrin and transglutaminase (Su *et al.*, 1994). Studies have shown that $1\alpha,25(OH)_2D_3$ may induce formation of intercellular junctions by protein kinase C (PKC) activation (Gniadecki *et al.*, 1997). Vitamin D and the VDR play an important role in tissue barriers in the intestine, lung, kidney and skin (Zhang *et al.*, 2013). $1\alpha,25(OH)_2D_3$ induces the expression of zonula occludens family members, occludin and vinculin, proteins that are key components of tight junctions which seal the space between adjacent epithelial cells (Furuse, 2010). Furthermore, our group and others discovered that $1\alpha,25(OH)_2D_3$ induces *CAMP* expression in human monocytes, macrophages, dendritic cells, keratinocytes and skin (Wang *et al.*, 2004; Gombart *et al.*, 2005; Weber *et al.*, 2005; Lowry *et al.*, 2014). This regulation is conserved only in humans and non-human primates as the VDRE is located on a retrotransposable *Alu*-element or short-interspersed element (SINE) that is specific to primates (Gombart *et al.*, 2005; Gombart *et al.*, 2009). Vitamin D does not induce mouse *Camp* gene expression because a VDRE does not exist in the mouse *Camp* promoter (Gombart *et al.*, 2005). In humans, the regulation of *CAMP* expression could mediate, in part, the important barrier effects attributed to vitamin D.

Psoriasis and atopic dermatitis are two important inflammatory skin conditions that contribute to a breakdown in skin barrier function through disruption of homeostasis. $1\alpha,25(OH)_2D_3$ and its analogues can provide safe and effective treatments for psoriasis because of their anti-proliferative and immunosuppressive properties that decrease proliferation and inflammation in the psoriatic skin (Karthaus *et al.*, 2014; Reichrath *et al.*, 2016; Tremezaygues and Reichrath, 2011). Complete disappearance of psoriatic plaques and restoration of skin barrier function were observed in 20–25% of treated patients (Nagpal *et al.*, 2001). Alleviation of psoriasis after topical treatment with $1\alpha,25(OH)_2D_3$ correlates with

elevated VDR transcripts (Chen *et al.*, 1996). Also, $1\alpha,25(OH)_2D_3$ promotes formation of the cornified envelope by inducing expression of involucrin and transglutaminase (Pillai and Bikle, 1991) and inhibits expression of pro-inflammatory cytokines IL-2, IFN-γ, IL-6 and IL-8 from T-cells that promote skin inflammation (Manolagas *et al.*, 1985). Additionally, $1\alpha,25(OH)_2D_3$ inhibits the transcriptional activity of NFkB, a major inducer of inflammation (Janjetovic *et al.*, 2009). Interestingly, LL-37 is found highly expressed in psoriatic lesions and it was reported that LL-37 contributed to the development of the condition (Ganguly *et al.*, 2009); however, $1\alpha,25(OH)_2D_3$ induces LL-37 expression in the skin. It might seem that this would exacerbate the disease, but $1\alpha,25(OH)_2D_3$ also suppresses inflammation and the combined actions of this compound may restore homeostasis. Interestingly, in a small pilot study in patients with psoriasis, nine out of nine patients showed a significant improvement in their condition after six months of supplementation with 35,000 IU vitamin D_3 daily (Finamor *et al.*, 2013).

Atopic dermatitis (AD), is a chronic inflammatory disease resulting from loss of epidermal barrier function in conjunction with skin inflammation. AD patients are susceptible to colonization by microorganisms, especially *Staphylococcus aureus* and Herpes simplex virus (HSV). This increased susceptibility correlates with reduced expression of LL-37 in the AD skin (Ong *et al.*, 2002). Improvements in disease are noted with vitamin D supplementation in AD children (Sidbury *et al.*, 2008; Di Filippo *et al.*, 2015) and adults and children older than 14 years (Amestejani *et al.*, 2012). Oral administration with 4000 IU/day vitamin D for 21 days, significantly increases expression *CAMP* mRNA in skin lesions from AD patients, but the impact on *S. aureus* colonization was not determined (Hata *et al.*, 2008). In a recent double-blind placebo controlled study, 24 patients with AD were randomly assigned to an arm receiving either 2,000 IU vitamin D per day or matching placebo for four weeks. Significant reductions in disease severity were observed for the vitamin D arm compared with the placebo and an inverse correlation between serum vitamin D levels with *S. aureus* skin colonization and the SCORAD score was observed (Udompataikul *et al.*, 2015). The use of narrow band UVB treatment successfully restored vitamin D levels, increased *CAMP* mRNA levels and reduced inflammation in the skin of both AD and psoriasis patients (Vahavihu *et al.*, 2010). Taken together, these data suggest that vitamin D plays an important role in reducing inflammation and restoring skin barrier function. The use of vitamin D, $1\alpha,25(OH)_2D_3$ or its analogues may provide an important therapeutic approach in treating wounds.

13.5 The Role of Vitamin D and CAMP/LL-37 in Cutaneous Wound Healing

The skin is an important barrier against numerous external assaults. It protects against an arid external environment, pathogenic microorganisms, mechanical stresses, extreme temperatures and solar UV radiation. As with any barrier, it is crucial that damage is efficiently and quickly repaired. Wound healing is a well-orchestrated response to damage or injury of the skin that involves haemostasis, inflammation, proliferation and remodelling. During wound healing, keratinocytes, fibroblasts, endothelial and immune cells communicate with each other to regulate the expression of numerous cytokines, chemokines and growth factors to orchestrate the healing process and prevent infection (Werner and Grose, 2003; Gurtner *et al.*, 2008; Liang *et al.*, 2012).

In the skin, there is constitutive, low expression of *CAMP* in the basal keratinocytes that is upregulated after injury or during inflammation (Frohm Nilsson *et al.*, 1999; Dorschner *et al.*, 2001; Heilborn *et al.*, 2003). After skin injury, TGF-β1 and/or TLR2/6 ligands activate keratinocytes in the skin to express higher CYP27B1 activity. As a result, 25(OH)D is converted into $1\alpha,25(OH)_2D_3$ which activates the VDR and induces expression of *CAMP*, TLR2 and

CD14 (Fig. 13.1) (Schauber *et al.*, 2007). Increased expression of TLR2 and CD14 enhances keratinocyte responses to microbes which further increases expression of the *CAMP* gene and levels of the inactive pro-protein hCAP18. Upon cleavage by serine proteases, the small active cationic helical peptide termed LL-37 is generated (see the book cover illustration). It kills microbes by disrupting their membranes and protects wounds against infection (Schauber *et al.*, 2007; see also Preface). A similar pathway involving TLR activation operates in macrophages, keratinocytes and lung epithelial cells (Hansdottir *et al.*, 2008; Liu *et al.*, 2006). Physiological upregulation of hCAP18/LL-37 expression in normal skin and acute skin wounds is accelerated by topical application of calcipotriol, a $1\alpha,25(OH)_2D_3$ analogue (Weber *et al.*, 2005; Heilborn *et al.*, 2010). Similarly, pattern recognition receptors CD14 and TLR2 mRNA and protein increased in cultured keratinocytes in response to $1\alpha,25(OH)_2D_3$ (Schauber *et al.*, 2007). $1\alpha,25(OH)_2D_3$ has multiple functions in skin and accelerated healing of skin wounds in rats in a dose-dependent manner when applied topically at 5 and 50 ng/day suggesting that it could be a potential compound for accelerating wound healing (Tian *et al.*, 1995). When mice lacking VDR are fed a low calcium diet, they display delayed wound healing because of reduced transcriptional activity of β-catenin that hampers stem cell activation in the hair follicle resulting in reduced proliferation of the cells at the leading edge of the migratory tongue (Oda *et al.*, 2015). *CAMP* has multiple functions and is an important regulator of inflammation and angiogenesis by regulating cytokine production and balancing the immune response during the wound healing phases (Ramos *et al.*, 2011). *CAMP* expression is induced in the keratinocytes following wounding, UVB irradiation, oxidative stress or barrier disruption. In humans, induction of hCAP18/LL-37 mRNA and protein was observed in the epidermis adjacent to the wound and by the second day it was observed in the migratory tongue during the re-epithelialization stage (Heilborn *et al.*,

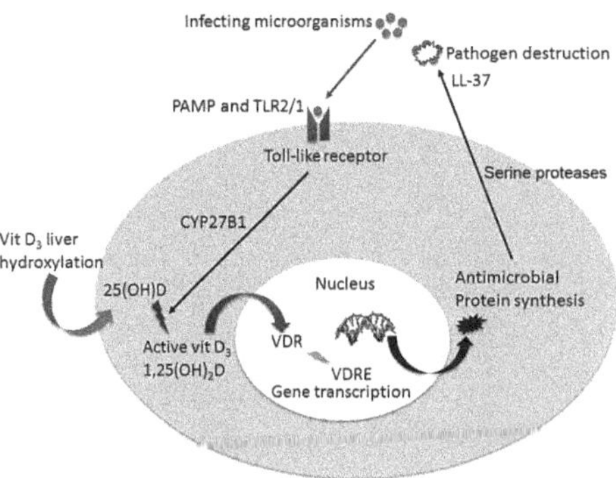

Fig. 13.1. Antimicrobial peptide production is vitamin D-dependent. Specific pathogen associated molecular patterns (PAMPs) are recognized by Toll-like receptors initiating the local intra-cellular conversion of active vitamin D (1,25(OH)$_2$D) from inactive vitamin D (25(OH)D). Active vitamin D$_3$ is bound by the vitamin D receptor (VDR) initiating gene transcription at specific DNA sequences, vitamin D response elements (VDRE). Following protein synthesis of antimicrobial peptides, like cathelicidin (LL-37), pathogen destruction ensues. This intracrine system depends on the local concentration of 25(OH)D.

2003). In the epithelium of hard-to-heal chronic ulcers, hCAP18/LL-37 is absent in the ulcer edge epithelium suggesting that *CAMP* expression is important for proper wound healing (Heilborn *et al.*, 2003).

13.6 Induction of CAMP Gene Expression by Other Natural Compounds

In addition to vitamin D$_3$, we and others discovered that lithocholic acid (LCA), butyrate, phenylbutyrate, resveratrol, nicotinamide and curcumin induce *CAMP* gene expression in different types of immune, skin and epithelial barrier cells (Schauber *et al.*, 2003; Peric *et al.*, 2009; Steinmann *et al.*, 2009; Kyme *et al.*, 2012; Guo *et al.*, 2013; Guo *et al.*, 2014). Furthermore, we, and others, observed synergistic or combinatorial induction of *CAMP* in different cell types by vitamin D$_3$ given together with butyrate, trichostatin A, IL-17, PTH and PTHrP (Peric *et al.*, 2008; Muehleisen *et al.*, 2012). Resveratrol increases cellular

ceramide (Cer) and sphingosine-1-phosphate (S1P) levels and activates an NFκB-C/EBPα-dependent pathway that increases *CAMP*/LL-37 levels (Park *et al.*, 2012; Park *et al.*, 2013). Topical application of resveratrol to murine skin increased *CAMP* mRNA/protein and inhibited invasion by *S. aureus* (Park *et al.*, 2013). Curcumin speeds wound healing by acting on all the stages of the process including inflammation, proliferation, tissue granulation and remodelling (Akbik *et al.*, 2014). Interestingly, Bartik and colleagues reported that VDR is activated by curcumin and induces VDR target genes CYP3A4, CYP24, p21 and TRPV6, suggesting that VDR could be a potential dietary sensor of curcumin (Bartik *et al.*, 2010). On the other hand, we discovered that curcumin induces *CAMP*/LL-37 through a VDR-independent pathway (Guo *et al.*, 2013). The effect of curcumin on *in vivo* *CAMP* expression remains to be tested. Taken together, these findings suggest that curcumin and resveratrol could promote healing by inducing VDR and non-VDR target genes involved in healing. Interestingly, 1α,25(OH)$_2$D$_3$ in combination with resveratrol potentiates VDR signalling and we observed increased *CAMP* expression with a combination of resveratrol and 1α,25(OH)$_2$D$_3$ as compared to either 1α,25(OH)$_2$D$_3$ or resveratrol alone (Guo *et al.*, 2014). Oral resveratrol improved healing of a midline laparotomy in rats by improving collagen deposition, neovascularization and tissue granulation (Yaman *et al.*, 2013). Combinations of these natural compounds could act as potential therapeutics for hard to heal wounds (Guo *et al.*, 2014).

13.7 Preventing Infections and Improving Wound Healing with Vitamin D$_3$ and Other Immune Boosting Compounds

Currently, approaches to increase local concentrations of LL-37 in surgical site incisions or traumatic wounds involves direct peptide application and over-expression via gene therapy, but potential toxicity to host cells and risk of unintended and undesired tissue damage/inflammation hinder these direct approaches (Jiang *et al.*, 2015). We propose to develop electrospun nanofibers that provide sustained local delivery of vitamin D_3 and/or other natural immune-modulating compounds to surgical incision or wound sites and target keratinocytes, monocytes, macrophages and neutrophils that upregulate *CAMP* expression in response to vitamin D_3 treatment. The durable release of these compounds could greatly enhance wound healing and reduce rates of infection. Encapsulating vitamin D_3 alone or in combination with the other natural compounds described above in nanofibers could enhance the production of antimicrobial peptides and other proteins that will speed up the wound-healing process.

The water solubility of vitamin D_3 is very low and it is susceptible to degradation upon exposure to light, heat and oxygen. Encapsulation increases stability and bioactivity, and can control delivery and release (Gonnet *et al.*, 2010). Since the late 1990s, encapsulation of vitamin D_3 for use in nutritional supplementation has been plagued by issues associated with high temperature during preparation, the use of toxic solvents and insufficient loading capacity that have hindered further development in therapeutic delivery of vitamin D_3 (Delaurent and Pepe, 1998; Shi, 2002; Semo *et al.*, 2007). Recent advances in encapsulation technology are promising. Luo *et al.* encapsulated vitamin D_3 (cholecalciferol) in zein nanoparticles using a phase separation method that could encapsulate other hydrophobic immune modulating compounds (Luo *et al.*, 2012). In a separate study, Mohammadi *et al.* (2014) prepared liposomes containing vitamin D_3 using a modified thin-film hydration sonication technique for potential application in beverage fortification. In a different study, Wagner *et al.* (2015) encapsulated vitamin D_3 and ferrous sulfate in niosomes using a novel supercritical CO_2 based method that produced material with good physical stability at 20°C. Vitamin D_3 was also loaded into amphiphilic chitosan derivative-based core-shell micelles (Li *et al.*, 2014). Almouazen *et al.* encapsulated

$1\alpha,25(OH)_2D_3$ in poly(D,L)-lactic acid to form nanoparticles using the nanoprecipitation technique (Almouazen *et al.*, 2013). These nanoparticles showed a high encapsulation efficiency ($\approx$90%) and slow, durable release over 7 days with higher activities on days 7 and 10 after treatment compared to the free, unencapsulated vitamin D_3. Ramalho and colleagues encapsulated $1\alpha,25(OH)_2D_3$ in poly(lactic-co-glycolic acid) (PLGA) nanoparticles using a single emulsion solvent evaporation technique for cancer therapy (Ramalho *et al.*, 2015). The lyophilized nanoparticle formulations were stable under storage conditions for several weeks.

In addition to encapsulation in particles, vitamin D_3 can be incorporated into fibres for topical delivery using electrospinning. A typical electrospinning setup consists of three major components: a high-voltage power supply, a spinneret and an electrically conductive collector (Figure 13.2) (Xie *et al.*, 2008). A hypodermic needle and a piece of aluminium foil serve well as the spinneret and collector, respectively. The liquid (e.g. a polymer solution) for electrospinning is loaded into a syringe and fed at a specific rate set by a syringe pump. The hydrophobic immune modulating agents can be readily encapsulated in nanofibers using a single spinneret during the electrospinning process. Electrospinning is a versatile technique for generating long fibres with nanoscale diameters.

Electrospun nanofiber wound dressings offer significant advantages over hydrogels or sponges for local drug delivery. Collagen, fibrin, poly(ethylene glycol) (PEG) and alginate hydrogels are capable of soft-tissue-like compliance, but are difficult to suture and are often too weak to support physiological loads. In addition, it is difficult to encapsulate hydrophobic molecules inside hydrogels. In sponges, hydrophobic drug molecules are usually crystallized after encapsulation, which slows down the dissolution rate and is unfavourable. On the other hand, electrospun nanofibers serve as ideal materials for topical drug delivery. They offer ease of incorporation of drugs, thanks to the hydrophobic molecules inside

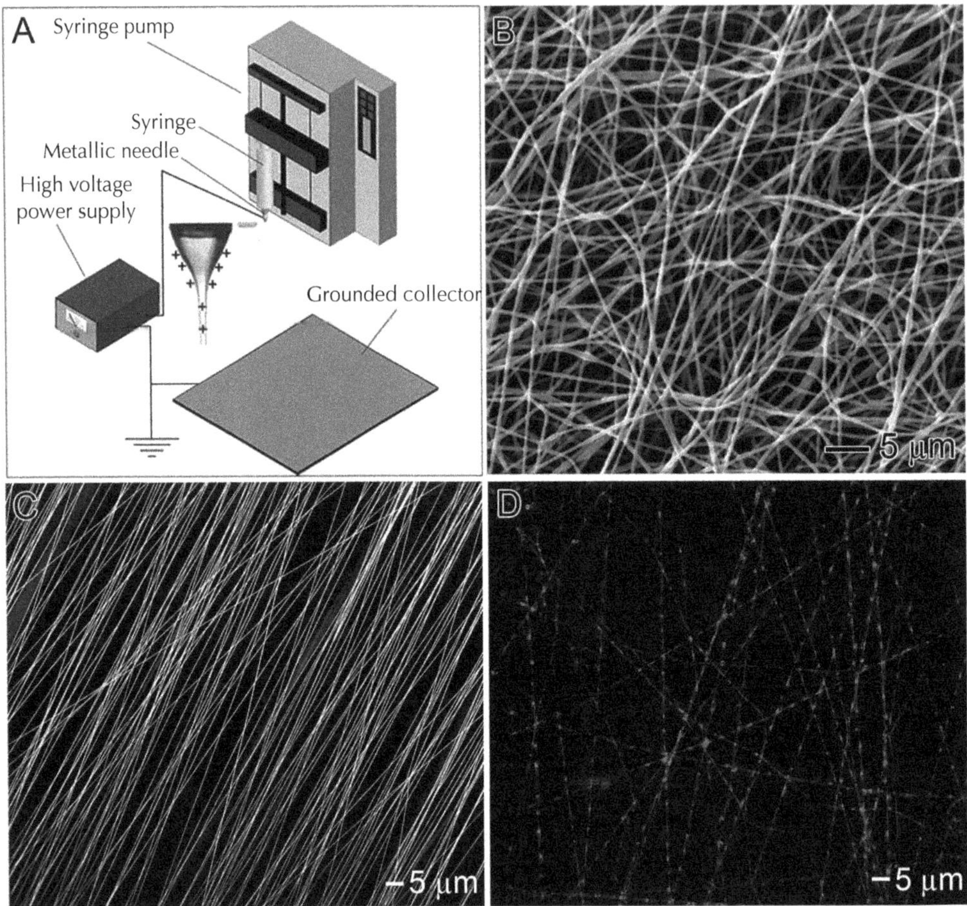

Fig. 13.2. (A) Schematic illustrating typical electrospinning setup; (B) A scanning electron microscopy (SEM) image of PCL nanofibers; (C) Fluorescence micrograph illustrating coumarin 6 (green)-loaded PCL nanofibers; (D) Fluorescence micrograph illustrating Rhodamine B conjugated bovine serum albumin (red)-loaded PCL nanofibers.

the nanofibers. By controlling the nanofiber porosity, it is also easy to control drug release profiles. Moreover, nanofiber degeneration profiles create amorphous states suitable for hydrophobic drug molecules, leading to enhanced drug solubility.

The architecture of electrospun nanofibers mimics the collagen structure of the extracellular matrix (ECM) – a 3D network of collagen fibres 50–500 nm in diameter. Therefore, compared to traditional wound dressings, nanofiber-based wound dressings provide several functional and structural advantages, including haemostasis, high filtration, semi-permeability, conformability and scar-free healing (Xie *et al.*, 2008). Even though electrospun nanofibers offer numerous advantages, their full potential has not yet been realized. Their antimicrobial use is limited to random nanofiber mats, surface modifications with chitosan, Ag and ZnO nanoparticles, and encapsulation of antibiotics and Ag nanoparticles/ions. Furthermore, electrospun nanofibers could serve as sutures, coatings of biomedical devices, or haemostasis materials for reducing healthcare-acquired infections. Peh *et al.* (2015) used bovine serum albumin as a carrier protein to encapsulate fat-soluble $1\alpha,25(OH)_2D_3$ in PLGA-collagen nanofibers. The bioactivity of released vitamin D_3 was verified by transgenic cell reporter assays.

We have encapsulated paclitaxel, cisplatin and proteins in nanofibers and particles using electrospinning (Xie *et al.*, 2008). In addition to solid nanofibers, nanofibers with porous, beaded and core-sheath secondary structures can be fabricated to tailor drug-release rates. Recently, we demonstrated for the first time the encapsulation of $25(OH)D_3$, a hydrophobic compound, in electrospun PCL and PLA nanofibers for induction of *CAMP* gene expression (Jiang *et al.*, 2015). The initial drug loading was 0.1% and we observed durable release for more than 4 weeks in cell culture. Plasma treatment enhanced hydrophilicity of the nanofibers and promoted the release rate of $25(OH)D_3$. Incubation of skin HaCaT and U937 cells with PCL-$25(OH)D_3$ nanofibers induced *CAMP* gene expression as demonstrated by an increasingly intense positive staining for hCAP18/LL-37 at days 1, 3 and 5 post-treatment. Interestingly, for the first 3 days the plasma-treated PCL-$25(OH)D_3$ fibres released $\sim5.0\times10^{-7}$M $25(OH)D_3$ into the culture medium of both cell types and induced hCAP18, but the equivalent concentration of free 25(OH)D did not induce detectable levels of LL-37 (Jiang *et al.*, 2015). The consistent, durable release of 25(OH)D from the nanofibers induced LL-37 more effectively than a single dose of free, unencapsulated 25(OH)D. Further, we found LL-37 protein production in both HaCaT keratinocytes and U937 monocytic cells was significantly higher when incubated with PCL-$25(OH)D_3$ than the free $25(OH)D_3$ for both days 3 and 5 post-treatment. The amount of LL-37 produced by U937 cells increased when treated with 5.0×10^{-6}M $25(OH)D_3$ for 3 days and then decreased sharply after 5 days. Interestingly, PCL-$25(OH)D_3$-treated cell cultures contained $\sim5.0\times10^{-7}$M $25(OH)D_3$ and produced 8–10 times higher levels of LL-37 than the cells treated with 5.0×10^{-6}M unencapsulated, free drug. Increased LL-37 expression coincided with increased antibacterial activity of U937 cell lysates (Jiang *et al.*, 2015). Our findings support the encapsulation of compounds like vitamin D, resveratrol, curcumin and phenylbutyrate to induce *CAMP* expression in wounds as a potential therapy for reducing infection and speeding wound healing.

13.8 Summary

To date, few studies have examined the encapsulation of immune modulating compounds in nanomaterials for inducing antimicrobial peptide production. Going forward it is important that multidisciplinary teams investigate the combination of multiple immune modulating agents on antimicrobial production using *in vitro* and *in vivo* models for preclinical studies. Further work to optimize the encapsulation and release of compounds is needed. For example, co-encapsulated $1\alpha,25(OH)_2D_3$ and resveratrol in nanofibers can be readily realized during electrospinning deposition on the collector. Because phenylbutyrate is soluble in water, a co-axial electrospinning technique could be applied to fabricate core-sheath nanofibers by encapsulating $1\alpha,25(OH)_2D_3$ in the shell and phenylbutyrate in the core for prolonged release. Sustained delivery of these immune modulating compounds could be co-incorporated with traditional antibiotics, silver or antimicrobial peptides using various techniques (Gatti *et al.*, 2013; Annur *et al.*, 2015; Piras *et al.*, 2015a; Piras *et al.*, 2015b; Water *et al.*, 2015; Ron-Doitch *et al.*, 2016) The potential for nanofiber wound dressings to combat HAIs, reduce the selection for antibiotic microbes and enhance wound healing is great.

Acknowledgements

The writing of this chapter was supported in part by the Otis Glebe Medical Research Foundation (to JX), National Institute of Arthritis and Musculoskeletal and Skin Diseases of the National Institutes of Health (NIH 1R15AR06858 to GGI), the National Institute of General Medical Sciences at NIH (IROIGM 123081 to JX) and the National Center for Complementary and Integrative Health at the NIH (5R01AT00916 to AFG).

References

Aberg, K.M., Man, M.Q., Gallo, R.L., Ganz, T., Crumrine, D., *et al.* (2008) Co-regulation and interdependence of the mammalian epidermal permeability and antimicrobial barriers. *Journal of Investigative Dermatology* 128, 917–925.

Akbik, D., Ghadiri, M., Chrzanowski, W. and Rohanizadeh, R. (2014) Curcumin as a wound healing agent. *Life Sciences* 116, 1–7.

Almouazen, E., Bourgeois, S., Jordheim, L.P., Fessi, H. and Briancon, S. (2013) Nano-encapsulation of vitamin D3 active metabolites for application in chemotherapy: formulation study and in vitro evaluation. *Pharmaceutical Research* 30, 1137–1146.

Amer, L.S., Bishop, B.M. and Van Hoek, M.L. (2010) Antimicrobial and antibiofilm activity of cathelicidins and short, synthetic peptides against *Francisella*. *Biochemical and Biophysical Research Communications* 396, 246–251.

Amestejani, M., Salehi, B.S., Vasigh, M., Sobhkhiz, A., Karami, M., *et al.* (2012) Vitamin D supplementation in the treatment of atopic dermatitis: a clinical trial study. *Journal of Drugs in Dermatology* 11, 327–330.

Amor, K.T., Rashid, R.M. and Mirmirani, P. (2010) Does D matter? The role of vitamin D in hair disorders and hair follicle cycling. *Dermatology Online Journal* 16, 3.

Anderson, D.J., Kaye, K.S., Classen, D., Arias, K.M., Podgorny, K., *et al.* (2008) Strategies to prevent surgical site infections in acute care hospitals. *Infection Control and Hospital Epidemiology* 29 Suppl 1, S51–61.

Annur, D., Wang, Z.K., Liao, J.D. and Kuo, C. (2015) Plasma-synthesized silver nanoparticles on electrospun chitosan nanofiber surfaces for antibacterial applications. *Biomacromolecules* 16, 3248–3255.

Awad, S. and Lobo, D.N. (2012) Metabolic conditioning to attenuate the adverse effects of perioperative fasting and improve patient outcomes. *Current Opinion in Clinical Nutrition and Metabolic Care* 15, 194–200.

Bartik, L., Whitfield, G.K., Kaczmarska, M., Lowmiller, C.L., Moffet, E.W., *et al.* (2010) Curcumin: a novel nutritionally derived ligand of the vitamin D receptor with implications for colon cancer chemoprevention. *The Journal of Nutritional Biochemistry* 21, 1153–1161.

Bikle, D.D. (2011) Vitamin D metabolism and function in the skin. *Molecular and Cellular Endocrinology* 347, 80–89.

Bouillon, R., Garmyn, M., Verstuyf, A., Segaert, S., Casteels, K. and Mathieu, C. (1995) Paracrine role for calcitriol in the immune system and skin creates new therapeutic possibilities for vitamin D analogs. *European Journal of Endocrinology* 133, 7–16.

Bowdish, D.M., Davidson, D.J. and Hancock, R.E. (2006) Immunomodulatory properties of defensins and cathelicidins. *Current Topics in Microbiology and Immunology* 306, 27–66.

Brown, K.L., Poon, G.F., Birkenhead, D., Pena, O.M., Falsafi, R., *et al.* (2011) Host defense peptide LL-37 selectively reduces proinflammatory macrophage responses. *Journal of Immunology* 186, 5497–5505.

Brulport, M., Schormann, W., Bauer, A., Hermes, M., Elsner, C., *et al.* (2007) Fate of extrahepatic human stem and precursor cells after transplantation into mouse livers. *Hepatology* 46, 861–870.

Bucki, R., Leszczynska, K., Namiot, A. and Sokolowski, W. (2010) Cathelicidin LL-37: a multitask antimicrobial peptide. *Archivum Immunologiae et Therapiae Experimentalis* 58, 15–25.

Byfield, F.J., Wen, Q., Leszczynska, K., Kulakowska, A., Namiot, Z., Janmey, P.A. and Bucki, R. (2011) Cathelicidin LL-37 peptide regulates endothelial cell stiffness and endothelial barrier permeability. *American Journal of Physiology: Cell Physiology* 300, C105–112.

Carretero, M., Escamez, M.J., Garcia, M., Duarte, B., Holguin, A., *et al.* (2008) In vitro and in vivo wound healing-promoting activities of human cathelicidin LL-37. *Journal of Investigative Dermatology* 128, 223–236.

Chagani, S., Kyryachenko, S., Yamamoto, Y., Kato, S., Ganguli-Indra, G. and Indra, A.K. (2016) In vivo role of vitamin D receptor signaling in UVB-induced DNA damage and melanocyte homeostasis. *Journal of Investigative Dermatology* 136, 2108–2111

Chen, K., Xiang, Y., Huang, J., Gong, W., Yoshimura, T. *et al.* (2014) The formylpeptide receptor 2 (Fpr2) and its endogenous ligand cathelin-related antimicrobial peptide (CRAMP) promote dendritic cell maturation. *Journal of Biological Chemistry* 289, 17553–17563.

Chen, M.L., Perez, A., Sanan, D.K., Heinrich, G., Chen, T.C. and Holick, M.F. (1996) Induction of vitamin D receptor mRNA expression in psoriatic plaques correlates with clinical response to 1,25-dihydroxyvitamin D3. *Journal of Investigative Dermatology* 106, 637–641.

Chotjumlong, P., Bolscher, J.G., Nazmi, K., Reutrakul, V., Supanchart, C., Buranaphatthana, W. and Krisanaprakornkit, S. (2013) Involvement of the P2X7 purinergic receptor and c-Jun N-terminal and extracellular signal-regulated kinases in cyclooxygenase-2 and prostaglandin E2 induction by LL-37. *Journal of Innate Immunity* 5, 72–83.

Christakos, S., Raval-Pandya, M., Wernyj, R.P. and Yang, W. (1996) Genomic mechanisms involved in the pleiotropic actions of 1,25-dihydroxyvitamin D3. *Biochemical Journal* 316 (Pt 2), 361–371.

Ciornei, C.D., Egesten, A. and Bodelsson, M. (2003) Effects of human cathelicidin antimicrobial peptide LL-37 on lipopolysaccharide-induced nitric oxide release from rat aorta in vitro. *Acta Anaesthesiologica Scandinavica* 47, 213–220.

Cirioni, O., Giacometti, A., Ghiselli, R., Bergnach, C., Orlando, F., *et al.* (2006) LL-37 protects rats against lethal sepsis caused by Gram-negative bacteria. *Antimicrobial Agents and Chemotherapy* 50, 1672–1679.

Coffelt, S.B., Tomchuck, S.L., Zwezdaryk, K.J., Danka, E.S. and Scandurro, A.B. (2009) Leucine leucine-37 uses formyl peptide receptor-like 1 to activate signal transduction pathways, stimulate oncogenic gene expression, and enhance the invasiveness of ovarian cancer cells. *Molecular Cancer Research* 7, 907–915.

Cowland, J.B., Johnsen, A.H. and Borregaard, N. (1995) hCAP-18: a cathelin/pro-bactenecin-like protein of human neutrophil specific granules. *FEBS Letters* 368, 173–176.

De, Y., Chen, Q., Schmidt, A.P., Anderson, G.M., Wang, J.M., *et al.* (2000) LL-37: the neutrophil granule- and epithelial cell-derived cathelicidin, utilizes formyl peptide receptor-like 1 (FPRL1) as a receptor to chemoattract human peripheral blood neutrophils, monocytes, and T cells. *Journal of Experimental Medicine* 192, 1069–1074.

Dean, S.N., Bishop, B.M. and Van Hoek, M.L. (2011) Natural and synthetic cathelicidin peptides with anti-microbial and anti-biofilm activity against *Staphylococcus aureus*. *BMC Microbiology* 11, 114.

Delaurent, C.S.A. and Pepe, G. (1998) Cyclodextrin inclusion complexes with vitamin D$_3$: investigation of the solid complex characterization. *Chemia Analityczna* 43, 601–616.

Di Filippo, P., Scaparrotta, A., Rapino, D., Cingolani, A., Attanasi, M., *et al.* (2015) Vitamin D supplementation modulates the immune system and improves atopic dermatitis in children. *International Archives of Allergy and Immunology* 166, 91–96.

Dorschner, R.A., Pestonjamasp, V.K., Tamakuwala, S., Ohtake, T., Rudisill, J., *et al.* (2001) Cutaneous injury induces the release of cathelicidin anti-microbial peptides active against group A Streptococcus. *Journal of Investigative Dermatology* 117, 91–97.

Duplantier, A.J. and Van Hoek, M.L. (2013) The human cathelicidin antimicrobial peptide LL-37 as a potential treatment for polymicrobial infected wounds. *Frontiers in Immunology* 4, 143.

Elssner, A., Duncan, M., Gavrilin, M. and Wewers, M.D. (2004) A novel P2X7 receptor activator, the human cathelicidin-derived peptide LL37, induces IL-1 beta processing and release. *Journal of Immunology* 172, 4987–4994.

Filewod, N.C., Pistolic, J. and Hancock, R.E. (2009) Low concentrations of LL-37 alter IL-8 production by keratinocytes and bronchial epithelial cells in response to proinflammatory stimuli. *FEMS Immunology and Medical Microbiology* 56, 233–240.

Finamor, D.C., Sinigaglia-Coimbra, R., Neves, L.C., Gutierrez, M., Silva, J.J., *et al.* (2013) A pilot study assessing the effect of prolonged administration of high daily doses of vitamin D on the clinical course of vitiligo and psoriasis. *Dermato-Endocrinology* 5, 222–234.

Frohm, M., Agerberth, B., Ahangari, G., Stahle-Backdahl, M., Liden, S., Wigzell, H. and Gudmundsson, G.H. (1997) The expression of the gene coding for the antibacterial peptide LL-37 is induced in human keratinocytes during inflammatory disorders. *Journal of Biological Chemistry* 272, 15258–15263.

Frohm Nilsson, M.B., Sandstedt, B., Sorensen, O., Weber, G., Borregaard, N. and Stahle-Backdahl, M. (1999) The human cationic antimicrobial protein (hCAP18), a peptide antibiotic, is widely expressed in human squamous epithelia and colocalizes with interleukin-6. *Infection and Immunity* 67, 2561–2566.

Fukumoto, K., Nagaoka, I., Yamataka, A., Kobayashi, H., Yanai, T., Kato, Y. and Miyano, T. (2005) Effect of antibacterial cathelicidin peptide CAP18/LL-37 on sepsis in neonatal rats. *Pediatric Surgery International* 21, 20–24.

Furuse, M. (2010) Molecular basis of the core structure of tight junctions. *Cold Spring Harbor Perspectives in Biology* 2, a002907.

Ganguly, D., Chamilos, G., Lande, R., Gregorio, J., Meller, S., *et al.* (2009) Self-RNA-antimicrobial peptide complexes activate human dendritic cells through TLR7 and TLR8. *Journal of Experimental Medicine* 206, 1983–1994.

Gao, N., Kumar, A., Jyot, J. and Yu, F.S. (2010) Flagellin-induced corneal antimicrobial peptide production and wound repair involve a novel NF-kappaB-independent and EGFR-dependent pathway. *PloS One* 5, e9351.

Gatti, J.W., Smithgall, M.C., Paranjape, S.M., Rolfes, R.J. and Paranjape, M. (2013) Using electrospun poly(ethylene-oxide) nanofibers for improved retention and efficacy of bacteriolytic antibiotics. *Biomedical Microdevices* 15, 887–893.

Gniadecki, R., Gajkowska, B. and Hansen, M. (1997) 1,25-dihydroxyvitamin D3 stimulates the assembly of adherens junctions in keratinocytes: involvement of protein kinase C. *Endocrinology* 138, 2241–2248.

Gombart, A., Borregaard, N. and Koeffler, H.P. (2005) Human cathelicidin antimicrobial peptide (*CAMP*) gene is a direct target of the vitamin D receptor and is strongly up-regulated in myeloid cells by 1,25-dihydroxyvitamin D3. *FASEB Journal* 19, 1067–1077.

Gombart, A., Saito, T. and Koeffler, H.P. (2009) Exapation of an ancient Alu short interspersed element provides a highly conserved vitamin D-mediated innate immune response in humans and primates. *BMC Genomics* 10, 321.

Gonnet, M., Lethuaut, L. and Boury, F. (2010) New trends in encapsulation of liposoluble vitamins. *Journal of Controlled Release* 146, 276–290.

Guo, C., Rosoha, E., Lowry, M.B., Borregaard, N. and Gombart, A.F. (2013) Curcumin induces human cathelicidin antimicrobial peptide gene expression through a vitamin D receptor-independent pathway. *The Journal of Nutritional Biochemistry* 24, 754–759.

Guo, C., Sinnott, B., Niu, B., Lowry, M.B., Fantacone, M.L. and Gombart, A.F. (2014) Synergistic induction of human cathelicidin antimicrobial peptide gene expression by vitamin D and stilbenoids. *Molecular Nutrition and Food Research* 58, 528–536.

Gurtner, G.C., Werner, S., Barrandon, Y. and Longaker, M.T. (2008) Wound repair and regeneration. *Nature* 453, 314–321.

Hansdottir, S., Monick, M.M., Hinde, S.L., Lovan, N., Look, D.C. and Hunninghake, G.W. (2008) Respiratory epithelial cells convert inactive vitamin D to its active form: potential effects on host defense. *Journal of Immunology* 181, 7090–7099.

Hasan, M., Ruksznis, C., Wang, Y., and Leifer, C.A. (2011) Antimicrobial peptides inhibit polyinosinic-polycytidylic acid-induced immune responses. *Journal of Immunology* 187, 5653–5659.

Hata, T.R., Kotol, P., Jackson, M., Nguyen, M., Paik, A. (2008) Administration of oral vitamin D induces cathelicidin production in atopic individuals. *Journal of Allergy and Clinical Immunology* 122, 829–831.

Heilborn, J.D., Nilsson, M.F., Kratz, G., Weber, G., Sorensen, O., Borregaard, N. and Stahle-Backdahl, M. (2003) The cathelicidin anti-microbial peptide LL-37 is involved in re-epithelialization of human skin wounds and is lacking in chronic ulcer epithelium. *Journal of Investigative Dermatology* 120, 379–389.

Heilborn, J.D., Weber, G., Gronberg, A., Dieterich, C. and Stahle, M. (2010) Topical treatment with the vitamin D analogue calcipotriol enhances the upregulation of the antimicrobial protein hCAP18/LL-37 during wounding in human skin in vivo. *Experimental Dermatology* 19, 332–338.

Holick, M.F. (2008) Vitamin D: a D-Lightful health perspective. *Nutrition Reviews* 66, S182–S194.

Iaccio, A., Cattanco, F., Mauro, M. and Ammendola, R. (2009) FPRL1-mediated induction of superoxide in LL-37-stimulated IMR90 human fibroblast. *Archives of Biochemistry and Biophysics* 481, 94–100.

Into, T., Inomata, M., Shibata, K. and Murakami, Y. (2010) Effect of the antimicrobial peptide LL-37 on Toll-like receptors 2-, 3- and 4-triggered expression of IL-6, IL-8 and CXCL10 in human gingival fibroblasts. *Cellular Immunology* 264, 104–109.

James, S.Y., Williams, M.A., Newland, A.C. and Colston, K.W. (1999) Leukemia cell differentiation: cellular and molecular interactions of retinoids and vitamin D. *General Pharmacology* 32, 143–154.

Janjetovic, Z., Zmijewski, M.A., Tuckey, R.C., Deleon, D.A., Nguyen, M.N., Pfeffer, L.M. and Slominski, A.T. (2009) 20-hydroxycholecalciferol, product of vitamin D3 hydroxylation by P450scc, decreases NF-kappaB activity by increasing IkappaB alpha levels in human keratinocytes. *PloS One* 4, e5988.

Jiang, J., Chen, G., Shuler, F.D., Wang, C.H. and Xie, J. (2015) Local sustained delivery of 25-hydroxyvitamin D3 for production of antimicrobial peptides. *Pharmaceutical Research* 32, 2851–2862.

Jones, G. (2013) Extrarenal vitamin D activation and interactions between vitamin D(2), vitamin D(3), and vitamin D analogs. *Annual Review of Nutrition* 33, 23–44.

Kai-Larsen, Y., Luthje, P., Chromek, M., Peters, V., Wang, X., *et al.* (2010) Uropathogenic *Escherichia coli* modulates immune responses and its curli fimbriae interact with the antimicrobial peptide LL-37. *PLoS Pathogens* 6, e1001010.

Kanthawong, S., Bolscher, J.G., Veerman, E.C., Van Marle, J., De Soet, H.J., Nazmi, K., Wongratanacheewin, S. and Taweechaisupapong, S. (2012) Antimicrobial and antibiofilm activity of LL-37 and its truncated variants against *Burkholderia pseudomallei*. *International Journal of Antimicrobial Agents* 39, 39–44.

Karthaus, N., Van Spriel, A.B., Looman, M.W., Chen, S., Spilgies, L.M., *et al.* (2014) Vitamin D controls murine and human plasmacytoid dendritic cell function. *Journal of Investigative Dermatology* 134, 1255–1264.

Koczulla, R., Von Degenfeld, G., Kupatt, C., Krotz, F., Zahler, S., *et al.* (2003) An angiogenic role for the human peptide antibiotic LL-37/hCAP-18. *Journal of Clinical Investigation* 111, 1665–1672.

Kovach, M.A., Ballinger, M.N., Newstead, M.W., Zeng, X., Bhan, U., *et al.* (2012) Cathelicidin-related antimicrobial peptide is required for effective lung mucosal immunity in Gram-negative bacterial pneumonia. *Journal of Immunology* 189, 304–311.

Kyme, P., Thoennissen, N. H., Tseng, C.W., Thoennissen, G.B., Wolf, A.J., *et al.* (2012) C/EBPepsilon mediates nicotinamide-enhanced clearance of *Staphylococcus aureus* in mice. *Journal of Clinical Investigation* 122, 3316–3329.

Lande, R., Gregorio, J., Facchinetti, V., Chatterjee, B., Wang, Y.H., *et al.* (2007) Plasmacytoid dendritic cells sense self-DNA coupled with antimicrobial peptide. *Nature* 449, 564–569.

Larrick, J.W., Morgan, J.G., Palings, I., Hirata, M. and Yen, M.H. (1991) Complementary DNA sequence of rabbit CAP18: a unique lipopolysaccharide binding protein. *Biochemical and Biophysical Research Communications* 179, 170–175.

Larrick, J.W., Hirata, M., Shimomoura, Y., Yoshida, M., Zheng, H., Zhong, J. and Wright, S.C. (1993) Antimicrobial activity of rabbit CAP18-derived peptides. *Antimicrobial Agents and Chemotherapy* 37, 2534–2539.

Larrick, J.W., Hirata, M., Shimomoura, Y., Yoshida, M., Zheng, H., Zhong, J. and Wright, S.C. (1994) Rabbit CAP18 derived peptides inhibit Gram negative and Gram positive bacteria. *Progress in Clinical and Biological Research* 388, 125–135.

Larrick, J.W., Hirata, M., Balint, R.F., Lee, J., Zhong, J. and Wright, S.C. (1995a) Human CAP18: a novel antimicrobial lipopolysaccharide-binding protein. *Infection and Immunity* 63, 1291–1297.

Larrick, J.W., Hirata, M., Zhong, J. and Wright, S.C. (1995b) Anti-microbial activity of human CAP18 peptides. *Immunotechnology* 1, 65–72.

Le, Y., Yang, Y., Cui, Y., Yazawa, H., Gong, W., Qiu, C. and Wang, J.M. (2002) Receptors for chemotactic formyl peptides as pharmacological targets. *International Immunopharmacology* 2, 1–13.

Li, W., Peng, H., Ning, F., Yao, L., Luo, M., Zhao, Q., Zhu, X. and Xiong, H. (2014) Amphiphilic chitosan derivative-based core-shell micelles: synthesis, characterisation and properties for sustained release of Vitamin D3. *Food Chemistry* 152, 307–315.

Liang, X., Bhattacharya, S., Bajaj, G., Guha, G., Wang, Z., *et al.* (2012) Delayed cutaneous wound healing and aberrant expression of hair follicle stem cell markers in mice selectively lacking Ctip2 in epidermis. *PloS One* 7, e29999.

Liu, P.T., Stenger, S., Li, H., Wenzel, L., Tan, B.H., *et al.* (2006) Toll-like receptor triggering of a vitamin D-mediated human antimicrobial response. *Science* 311, 1770–1773.

Lowry, M.B., Guo, C., Borregaard, N. and Gombart, A.F. (2014) Regulation of the human cathelicidin antimicrobial peptide gene by 1alpha,25-dihydroxyvitamin D3 in primary immune cells. *Journal of Steroid Biochemistry and Molecular Biology* 143, 183–191.

Luderer, H.F. and Demay, M.B. (2010) The vitamin D receptor, the skin and stem cells. *Journal of Steroid Biochemistry and Molecular Biology* 121, 314–316.

Luo, Y., Teng, Z. and Wang, Q. (2012) Development of zein nanoparticles coated with carboxymethyl chitosan for encapsulation and controlled release of vitamin D3. *Journal of Agricultural and Food Chemistry* 60, 836–843.

Magill, S.S., Hellinger, W., Cohen, J., Kay, R., Bailey, C., *et al.* (2012) Prevalence of healthcare-associated infections in acute care hospitals in Jacksonville, Florida. *Infection Control and Hospital Epidemiology* 33, 283–291.

Magill, S.S., Edwards, J.R. and Fridkin, S.K. (2014) Survey of health care-associated infections. *New England Journal of Medicine* 370, 2542–2543.

Mangelsdorf, D.J., Thummel, C., Beato, M., Herrlich, P., Schutz, G., *et al.* (1995) The nuclear receptor superfamily: the second decade. *Cell* 83, 835–839.

Manolagas, S.C., Provvedini, D.M. and Tsoukas, C.D. (1985) Interactions of 1,25-dihydroxyvitamin D3 and the immune system. *Molecular and Cellular Endocrinology* 43, 113–122.

Martin-Ezquerra, G., Man, M.Q., Hupe, M., Rodriguez-Martin, M., Youm, J.K., *et al.* (2011) Psychological stress regulates antimicrobial peptide expression by both glucocorticoid and beta-adrenergic mechanisms. *European Journal of Dermatology* 21, 48–51.

Mohammadi, M., Ghanbarzadeh, B. and Hamishehkar, H. (2014) Formulation of nanoliposomal vitamin D3 for potential application in beverage fortification. *Advanced Pharmaceutical Bulletin* 4, 569–575.

Montreekachon, P., Chotjumlong, P., Bolscher, J.G., Nazmi, K., Reutrakul, V. and Krisanaprakornkit, S. (2011) Involvement of P2X(7) purinergic receptor and MEK1/2 in interleukin-8 up-regulation by LL-37 in human gingival fibroblasts. *Journal of Periodontal Research* 46, 327–337.

Morizane, S., Yamasaki, K., Muhleisen, B., Kotol, P.F., Murakami, M., *et al.* (2012) Cathelicidin antimicrobial peptide LL-37 in psoriasis enables keratinocyte reactivity against TLR9 ligands. *Journal of Investigative Dermatology* 132, 135–143.

Muehleisen, B., Bikle, D.D., Aguilera, C., Burton, D.W., Sen, G.L., Deftos, L.J. and Gallo, R.L. (2012) PTH/PTHrP and vitamin D control antimicrobial peptide expression and susceptibility to bacterial skin infection. *Science Translational Medicine* 4, 135ra66.

Nagaoka, I., Tamura, H. and Hirata, M. (2006) An antimicrobial cathelicidin peptide, human CAP18/LL-37, suppresses neutrophil apoptosis via the activation of formyl-peptide receptor-like 1 and P2X7. *Journal of Immunology* 176, 3044–3052.

Nagpal, S., Lu, J. and Boehm, M.F. (2001) Vitamin D analogs: mechanism of action and therapeutic applications. *Current Medicinal Chemistry* 8, 1661–1679.

Nakatsuji, T., Chen, T.H., Two, A.M., Chun, K.A., Narala, S., *et al.* (2016) *Staphylococcus aureus* exploits epidermal barrier defects in atopic dermatitis to trigger cytokine expression. *Journal of Investigative Dermatology* 136, 2192–2200.

Niyonsaba, F., Nagaoka, I. and Ogawa, H. (2006) Human defensins and cathelicidins in the skin: beyond direct antimicrobial properties. *Critical Reviews in Immunology* 26, 545–576.

Nizet, V., Ohtake, T., Lauth, X., Trowbridge, J., Rudisill, J., *et al.* (2001) Innate antimicrobial peptide protects the skin from invasive bacterial infection. *Nature* 414, 454–457.

Oda, Y., Hu, L., Bul, V., Elalieh, H., Reddy, J. K. and Bikle, D.D. (2012) Coactivator MED1 ablation in keratinocytes results in hair-cycling defects and epidermal alterations. *Journal of Investigative Dermatology* 132, 1075–1083.

Oda, Y., Tu, C.L., Menendez, A., Nguyen, T. and Bikle, D.D. (2015) Vitamin D and calcium regulation of epidermal wound healing. *Journal of Steroid Biochemistry and Molecular Biology* 164, 379–385.

Ong, P.Y., Ohtake, T., Brandt, C., Strickland, I., Boguniewicz, M., *et al.* (2002) Endogenous antimicrobial peptides and skin infections in atopic dermatitis. *New England Journal of Medicine* 347, 1151–1160.

Oren, Z., Lerman, J.C., Gudmundsson, G.H., Agerberth, B. and Shai, Y. (1999) Structure and organization of the human antimicrobial peptide LL-37 in phospholipid membranes: relevance to the molecular basis for its non-cell-selective activity. *Biochemical Journal* 341, 501–513.

Otte, J.M., Zdebik, A.E., Brand, S., Chromik, A.M., Strauss, S., *et al.* (2009) Effects of the cathelicidin LL-37 on intestinal epithelial barrier integrity. *Regulatory Peptides* 156, 104–117.

Overhage, J., Campisano, A., Bains, M., Torfs, E.C., Rehm, B.H. and Hancock, R.E. (2008) Human host defense peptide LL-37 prevents bacterial biofilm formation. *Infection and Immunity* 76, 4176–4182.

Park, K., Elias, P.M., Hupe, M., Borkowski, A.W., Gallo, R.L., *et al.* (2013) Resveratrol stimulates sphingosine-1-phosphate signaling of cathelicidin production. *Journal of Investigative Dermatology* 133, 1942–1949.

Park, S.J., Ahmad, F., Philp, A., Baar, K., Williams, T., *et al.* (2012) Resveratrol ameliorates aging-related metabolic phenotypes by inhibiting cAMP phosphodiesterases. *Cell* 148, 421–433.

Peh, P., Lim, N.S., Blocki, A., Chee, S.M., Park, H.C., *et al.* (2015) Simultaneous delivery of highly diverse bioactive compounds from blend electrospun fibers for skin wound healing. *Bioconjugate Chemistry* 26, 1348–1358.

Pendleton, J.N., Gorman, S.P. and Gilmore, B.F. (2013) Clinical relevance of the ESKAPE pathogens. *Expert Review of Anti-Infective Therapy* 11, 297–308.

Peric, M., Koglin, S., Kim, S.M., Morizane, S., Besch, R., *et al.* (2008) IL-17A enhances vitamin D3-induced expression of cathelicidin antimicrobial peptide in human keratinocytes. *Journal of Immunology* 181, 8504–8512.

Peric, M., Koglin, S., Dombrowski, Y., Gross, K., Bradac, E., Ruzicka, T. and Schauber, J. (2009) VDR and MEK-ERK dependent induction of the antimicrobial peptide cathelicidin in keratinocytes by lithocholic acid. *Molecular Immunology* 46, 3183–3187.

Pillai, S. and Bikle, D.D. (1991) Role of intracellular-free calcium in the cornified envelope formation of keratinocytes: differences in the mode of action of extracellular calcium and 1,25 dihydroxyvitamin D3. *Journal of Cellular Physiology* 146, 94–100.

Piotrowska, A., Wierzbicka, J. and Zmijewski, M.A. (2016) Vitamin D in the skin physiology and pathology. *Acta Biochimica Polonica* 63, 1104.

Piras, A.M., Maisetta, G., Sandreschi, S., Gazzarri, M., Bartoli, C., *et al.* (2015a) Chitosan nanoparticles loaded with the antimicrobial peptide temporin B exert a long-term antibacterial activity in vitro against clinical isolates of *Staphylococcus epidermidis*. *Frontiers in Microbiology* 6, 372.

Piras, A.M., Sandreschi, S., Maisetta, G., Esin, S., Batoni, G. and Chiellini, F. (2015b) Chitosan nanoparticles for the linear release of model cationic peptide. *Pharmaceutical Research* 32, 2259–2265.

Pochet, S., Tandel, S., Querriere, S., Tre-Hardy, M., Garcia-Marcos, *et al.* (2006) Modulation by LL-37 of the responses of salivary glands to purinergic agonists. *Molecular Pharmacology* 69, 2037–2046.

Pompilio, A., Scocchi, M., Pomponio, S., Guida, F., Di Primio, A., *et al.* (2011) Antibacterial and anti-biofilm effects of cathelicidin peptides against pathogens isolated from cystic fibrosis patients. *Peptides* 32, 1807–1814.

Ramalho, M.J., Loureiro, J.A., Gomes, B., Frasco, M.F., Coelho, M.A. and Pereira, M.C. (2015) PLGA nanoparticles as a platform for vitamin D-based cancer therapy. *Beilstein Journal of Nanotechnology* 6, 1306–1318.

Ramos, R., Silva, J.P., Rodrigues, A.C., Costa, R., Guardao, L., *et al.* (2011) Wound healing activity of the human antimicrobial peptide LL37. *Peptides* 32, 1469–1476.

Reichrath, J., Zouboulis, C.C., Vogt, T. and Holick, M.F. (2016) Targeting the vitamin D endocrine system (VDES) for the management of inflammatory and malignant skin diseases: an historical view and outlook. *Reviews in Endocrine and Metabolic Disorders* 17, 405–417.

Rid, R., Wagner, M., Maier, C.J., Hundsberger, H., Hintner, H., Bauer, J.W. and Onder, K. (2013) Deciphering the calcitriol-induced transcriptomic response in keratinocytes: presentation of novel target genes. *Journal of Molecular Endocrinology* 50, 131–149.

Ron-Doitch, S., Sawodny, B., Kuhbacher, A., David, M.M., Samanta, A., *et al.* (2016) Reduced cytotoxicity and enhanced bioactivity of cationic antimicrobial peptides liposomes in cell cultures and 3D epidermis model against HSV. *Journal of Controlled Release* 229, 163–171.

Saiman, L., Tabibi, S., Starner, T.D., San Gabriel, P., Winokur, P.L., *et al.* (2001) Cathelicidin peptides inhibit multiply antibiotic-resistant pathogens from patients with cystic fibrosis. *Antimicrobial Agents and Chemotherapy* 45, 2838–2844.

Salzer, S., Kresse, S., Hirai, Y., Koglin, S., Reinholz, M., Ruzicka, T. and Schauber, J. (2014) Cathelicidin peptide LL-37 increases UVB-triggered inflammasome activation: possible implications for rosacea. *Journal of Dermatological Science* 76, 173–179.

Schauber, J., Svanholm, C., Termen, S., Iffland, K., Menzel, T., *et al.* (2003). Expression of the cathelicidin LL-37 is modulated by short chain fatty acids in colonocytes: relevance of signalling pathways. *Gut* 52, 735–741.

Schauber, J., Dorschner, R.A., Coda, A.B., Buchau, A.S., Liu, P.T., *et al.* (2007) Injury enhances TLR2 function and antimicrobial peptide expression through a vitamin D-dependent mechanism. *Journal of Clinical Investigation* 117, 803–811.

Schuessler, M., Astecker, N., Herzig, G., Vorisek, G. and Schuster, I. (2001) Skin is an autonomous organ in synthesis, two-step activation and degradation of vitamin D(3): CYP27 in epidermis completes the set of essential vitamin D(3)-hydroxylases. *Steroids* 66, 399–408.

Semo, E., Kesselman, E., Danino, D. and Livney, Y.D. (2007) Casein micelle as a natural nano-capsular vehicle for nutraceutical. *Food Hydrocolloids* 21, 936–942.

Shaykhiev, R., Beisswenger, C., Kandler, K., Senske, J., Puchner, A., *et al.* (2005) Human endogenous antibiotic LL-37 stimulates airway epithelial cell proliferation and wound closure. *American Journal of Physiology: Lung Cellular and Molecular Physiology* 289, L842–L848.

Shi Xy, T.T. (2002) Preparation of chitosan/ethycellulose complex microcapsules and its application in controlled release of vitamin D2. *Biomaterials* 23, 4469–4473.

Sidbury, R., Sullivan, A.F., Thadhani, R.I. and Camargo, C.A., Jr (2008) Randomized controlled trial of vitamin D supplementation for winter-related atopic dermatitis in Boston: a pilot study. *British Journal of Dermatology* 159, 245–247.

Steinmann, J., Halldorsson, S., Agerberth, B. and Gudmundsson, G.H. (2009) Phenylbutyrate induces antimicrobial peptide expression. *Antimicrobial Agents and Chemotherapy* 53, 5127–5133.

Su, M.J., Bikle, D.D., Mancianti, M.L. and Pillai, S. (1994) 1,25-Dihydroxyvitamin D3 potentiates the keratinocyte response to calcium. *Journal of Biological Chemistry* 269, 14723–14729.

Subramanian, H., Gupta, K., Guo, Q., Price, R. and Ali, H. (2011) Mas-related gene X2 (MrgX2) is a novel G protein-coupled receptor for the antimicrobial peptide LL-37 in human mast cells: resistance to receptor phosphorylation, desensitization, and internalization. *Journal of Biological Chemistry* 286, 44739–44749.

Tang, X., Basavarajappa, D., Haeggstrom, J.Z. and Wan, M. (2015) P2X7 receptor regulates internalization of antimicrobial peptide LL-37 by human macrophages that promotes intracellular pathogen clearance. *Journal of Immunology* 195, 1191–1201.

Tian, X.Q., Chen, T.C. and Holick, M.F. (1995) 1,25-dihydroxyvitamin D3: a novel agent for enhancing wound healing. *Journal of Cellular Biochemistry* 59, 53–56.

Tjabringa, G.S., Aarbiou, J., Ninaber, D.K., Drijfhout, J.W., Sorensen, O.E., *et al.* (2003) The antimicrobial peptide LL-37 activates innate immunity at the airway epithelial surface by transactivation of the epidermal growth factor receptor. *Journal of Immunology* 171, 6690–6696.

Tokumaru, S., Sayama, K., Shirakata, Y., Komatsuzawa, H., Ouhara, K., *et al.* (2005) Induction of keratinocyte migration via transactivation of the epidermal growth factor receptor by the antimicrobial peptide LL-37. *Journal of Immunology* 175, 4662–4668.

Tomasinsig, L., Pizzirani, C., Skerlavaj, B., Pellegatti, P., Gulinelli, S., *et al.* (2008) The human cathelicidin LL-37 modulates the activities of the P2X7 receptor in a structure-dependent manner. *Journal of Biological Chemistry* 283, 30471–30481.

Tremezaygues, L. and Reichrath, J. (2011) Vitamin D analogs in the treatment of psoriasis: Where are we standing and where will we be going? *Dermato-Endocrinology* 3, 180–186.

Turner, J., Cho, Y., Dinh, N.N., Waring, A.J. and Lehrer, R.I. (1998) Activities of LL-37, a cathelin-associated antimicrobial peptide of human neutrophils. *Antimicrobial Agents and Chemotherapy* 42, 2206–2214.

Udompataikul, M., Huajai, S., Chalermchai, T., Taweechotipatr, M. and Kamanamool, N. (2015) The effects of oral vitamin D supplement on atopic dermatitis: a clinical trial with *Staphylococcus aureus* colonization determination. *Journal of the Medical Association of Thailand* 98, Suppl 9, S23–S30.

Vahavihu, K., Ala-Houhala, M., Peric, M., Karisola, P., Kautiainen, H., *et al.* (2010) Narrowband ultraviolet B treatment improves vitamin D balance and alters antimicrobial peptide expression in skin lesions of psoriasis and atopic dermatitis. *British Journal of Dermatology* 163, 321–328.

Wagner, M.E., Spoth, K.A., Kourkoutis, L.F. and Rizvi, S.S. (2015) Stability of niosomes with encapsulated vitamin D3 and ferrous sulfate generated using a novel supercritical carbon dioxide method. *Journal of Liposome Research* 26, 261–268.

Wang, T.T., Nestel, F.P., Bourdeau, V., Nagai, Y., Wang, Q., *et al.* (2004) Cutting edge: 1,25-dihydroxyvitamin D3 is a direct inducer of antimicrobial peptide gene expression. *Journal of Immunology* 173, 2909–2912.

Wantha, S., Alard, J.E., Megens, R.T., Van Der Does, A.M., Doring, Y., *et al.* (2013) Neutrophil-derived cathelicidin promotes adhesion of classical monocytes. *Circulation Research* 112, 792–801.

Water, J.J., Smart, S., Franzyk, H., Foged, C. and Nielsen, H.M. (2015) Nanoparticle-mediated delivery of the antimicrobial peptide plectasin against *Staphylococcus aureus* in infected epithelial cells. *European Journal of Pharmaceutics and Biopharmaceutics* 92, 65–73.

Weber, G., Heilborn, J.D., Chamorro Jimenez, C.I., Hammarsjo, A., Torma, H. and Stahle, M. (2005) Vitamin D induces the antimicrobial protein hCAP18 in human skin. *Journal of Investigative Dermatology* 124, 1080–1082.

Werner, S. and Grose, R. (2003) Regulation of wound healing by growth factors and cytokines. *Physiological Reviews* 83, 835–870.

Xie, J., Li, X. and Xia, Y. (2008) Putting electrospun nanofibers to work for biomedical research. *Macromolecular Rapid Communications* 29, 1775–1792.

Yaman, I., Derici, H., Kara, C., Kamer, E., Diniz, G., Ortac, R. and Sayin, O. (2013) Effects of resveratrol on incisional wound healing in rats. *Surgery Today* 43, 1433–1438.

Yin, J. and Yu, F.S. (2010) LL-37 via EGFR transactivation to promote high glucose-attenuated epithelial wound healing in organ-cultured corneas. *Investigative Ophthalmology and Visual Science* 51, 1891–1897.

Zanetti, M., Gennaro, R. and Romeo, D. (1995) Cathelicidins: a novel protein family with a common proregion and a variable C-terminal antimicrobial domain. *FEBS Letters* 374, 1–5.

Zhang, Y.G., Wu, S. and Sun, J. (2013) Vitamin D, vitamin D receptor, and tissue barriers. *Tissue Barriers* 1, e23118.

Zhang, Z., Cherryholmes, G., Chang, F., Rose, D.M., Schraufstatter, I. and Shively, J.E. (2009) Evidence that cathelicidin peptide LL-37 may act as a functional ligand for CXCR2 on human neutrophils. *European Journal of Immunology* 39, 3181–3194.

14 Immunomodulatory Activities of Cationic Host Defence Peptides and Novel Therapeutic Strategies

Kelli C. Wuerth and Robert E.W. Hancock*

Centre for Microbial Diseases and Immunity Research, Department of Microbiology and Immunology, University of British Columbia, Vancouver, Canada

Abstract

Cationic host defence peptides (HDPs), or antimicrobial peptides (AMPs), are seemingly ubiquitous and thousands have been discovered. Once regarded as only direct antimicrobials, their additional functions as immunomodulators in host defence have been emerging over the past two decades, with roles in the control of microbial infections and inflammation, in wound healing and angiogenesis, as anticancer agents and in many other functions. In this chapter, we discuss the classes of HDPs and their roles in immunity and host defence, then examine the applications of HDPs in recent clinical trials and their potential in treating human diseases and medical conditions.

Host defence peptides (HDPs) are small (10–50 amino acids in length), amphipathic and generally have an abundance of hydrophobic residues (Jenssen *et al.*, 2006). While anionic HDPs exist, most are cationic, with a net +2 to +9 charge, and thus the focus of this chapter will be on cationic HDPs from humans (Jenssen *et al.*, 2006).

Traditionally, many of the peptides now called HDPs were studied only for their direct antimicrobial properties and were thus called antimicrobial peptides (AMPs). However, while many of the AMPs were bactericidal in traditional laboratory media, when they were studied in conditions representative of those found *in vivo*, such as at higher salt concentrations, the bactericidal effects were severely dampened or completely antagonized (Turner *et al.*, 1998; Jenssen *et al.*, 2006). Other studies emerged showing that the AMPs cause a variety of changes in the immune system to combat not only infections but also to increase wound healing, angiogenesis, cell recruitment and other functions, and that these occur under physiological conditions such as those found in tissue culture or *in vivo* (Hilchie *et al.*, 2013). Thus, the term 'host defence peptides' (HDPs) was coined to reflect that most of these peptides contribute to immunity in ways other than direct antimicrobial killing. Using this definition of HDP also means that other host-derived cationic peptides, such as cationic neuropeptides and peptide hormones, can also be classified as HDPs. However, the term AMP is still used when discussing the direct antimicrobial activities of peptides.

In this chapter, we review classes of cationic HDPs and their activities, discuss

---

* Corresponding author e-mail: bob@hancocklab.com

their potential clinical applications and then consider the peptides currently being examined in clinical trials.

14.1 Classical AMPs and HDPs

More than 7000 peptides have been described, and almost 3000 peptides have been classified as AMPs, isolated from Eukarya, Prokarya, and even Archaea (Wuerth *et al.*, 2013; Fosgerau and Hoffmann, 2015; Wang *et al.*, 2016). While many have been investigated for their antimicrobial activities, studies are now revealing that most of those tested also possess immunomodulatory activity, defined as changes to the immune response that tend to restore homeostasis and prevent either an excessive or insufficient immune response. Immunomodulation may include altering cell recruitment; affecting the release of cytokines, chemokines, metabolites and other mediators; or modifying tissue repair such as wound healing and angiogenesis. We have proposed that these activities might be the most predominant natural role for such HDPs (Hilchie *et al.*, 2013).

HDPs have often been classified on the basis of structure, with generally four described categories: (i) α-helical; (ii) β-sheet; (iii) cyclic and (iv) unstructured linear with repeating motifs or rich in certain amino acids, such as proline or tryptophan (Hancock, 1997; Jenssen *et al.*, 2006). These structures, along with common motifs and peptide locations, have been used to separate HDPs into generalized families, such as cathelicidins (synthesized with a cathelin prosequence domain), defensins (β-sheets with multiple disulfide bonds) and histatins (histidine-rich; located in the oral cavity) (Zanetti, 2004; Jenssen *et al.*, 2006; Wilmes and Sahl, 2014; Melino *et al.*, 2014). Several human HDPs are discussed below and in Table 14.1. Please note that there are dozens of genes for defensins and defensin-like entities that are not listed since their equivalent protein products have not been well characterized or even investigated.

14.1.1 Defensins

The defensins are found in eukaryotes, are well conserved in vertebrates, and can be divided into three subfamilies based on the pairings of the cysteines used for the three disulfide bonds (Ganz, 2003; Wilmes and Sahl, 2014). In humans, there are proteins from two of the subfamilies, α- and β-defensins (Ganz, 2003; Wilmes and Sahl, 2014). The third category, the cyclic θ-defensins, are found in some non-human primates but in humans the six pseudogenes do not create functional proteins due to premature stop codons (Nguyen *et al.*, 2003).

The α-defensins include human neutrophil peptides (HNP) 1–4 and HD5 and HD6. As the name suggests, the main source of HNP-1 to -4 is the azurophilic (primary) granules in neutrophils, while HD5 and HD6 are found largely in the intestinal Paneth cells (Ganz, 2003). Humans have four major β-defensins, hBD-1 to -4. They are produced by epithelial cells in the skin and the gastrointestinal, urinary and respiratory tracts, along with many other locations (Bowdish *et al.*, 2005; Ganz, 2003). Both α- and β-defensins have been found in eye tissues and in tears (Kolar and McDermott, 2011).

Defensins are expressed as a prepropeptide form, with post-translational processing occurring to remove the signal peptide and propeptide sequence by signal peptidases and proteases respectively. Additionally, the organization of defensin genes in the human genome is complex, with defensin copy numbers having a role in several diseases including psoriasis and Crohn's disease (Wehkamp *et al.*, 2005; Hollox *et al.*, 2008). Numerous additional defensin genes have also been annotated, although only a few, such as β-defensins 118, 123 and 131, have been studied at the protein level (Yenugu *et al.*, 2004; Motzkus *et al.*, 2006; Kim *et al.*, 2015).

14.1.2 Cathelicidins

Humans have a single cathelicidin, LL-37, that is synthesized as a 170 residue

Table 14.1. Classical examples of human HDPs and synthetic peptides.

Name and number of amino acids in mature peptide	Locations and cells	Functions in host defence	Further reading
α-defensins HNP-1: 30 HNP-2: 29 HNP-3: 30 HNP-4: 33 HD5: 32 HD6: 32	Plasma; eyes Cells: Paneth cells, neutrophils, some macrophages	Anti-infective; chemoattractant; affect chemokine release; promote wound healing	(Ganz, 2003; Aarbiou et al., 2004; Kolar and McDermott, 2011; Wilmes and Sahl, 2014)
β-defensins hBD-1: 36 hBD-2: 41 hBD-3: 45 hBD-4: 37	Multiple locations, including skin; eyes; GI tract; urinary tract; respiratory tract Cells: epithelial cells	Anti-infective; chemoattractant; affect chemokine release; promote wound healing	(Yang et al., 1999; Garcia et al., 2001; Ganz, 2003; Niyonsaba et al., 2007; Hirsch et al., 2009; Kolar and McDermott, 2011; Wilmes and Sahl, 2014)
LL-37: 37	Multiple locations, including skin; respiratory tract; GI tract; eyes; sweat; breast milk; saliva; plasma. Cells: multiple cell types, including epithelial cells, keratinocytes, neutrophils, dendritic cells (DCs), lymphocytes and monocytes/macrophages.	Anti-infective; promotes chemotaxis: chemoattractant and induces chemokines; binds to LPS; pro-angiogenic; promotes wound healing; anti-inflammatory	(Turner et al., 1998; Yang et al., 2000; Sorensen et al., 2001; Koczulla et al., 2003; Zanetti, 2004; Dürr et al., 2006; Mookherjee et al., 2006; Nijnik and Hancock, 2009; Vandamme et al., 2012; Fabisiak et al., 2016)
Histatins His-1: 38 His-3: 32 His-5: 24	Saliva	Anti-infective; anti-candidiasis; promote wound healing	(Gusman et al., 2001; Oudhoff et al., 2008; Melino et al., 2014)
Hepcidin (LEAP-1): 25	Liver. Cells: hepatocytes, monocytes	Anti-infective through iron regulation	(Huang et al., 2012; Michels et al., 2015)
LEAP-2: 40	Liver	Proposed directly antimicrobial	(Krause et al., 2003)
IDRs IDR-1: 12 IDR-1002: 12 IDR-1018: 12	Synthetic	Anti-infective; antibiofilm; chemoattractant; induce chemokines; promote wound healing; anti-inflammatory	(Nijnik et al., 2010; Steinstraesser et al., 2012; Hilchie et al., 2013)

prepropeptide. The signalling peptide is then removed and the remaining sequence stored as the propeptide form (Zanetti, 2004). It contains a conserved cathelin domain in the prosequence, which is then cleaved by proteinase 3 to the final 37 residue α-helical peptide (Sorensen et al., 2001, Zanetti, 2004). LL-37 is found in multiple body locations including the skin, eyes, respiratory tract and gastrointestinal tract, and in fluids such as sweat, breast milk, saliva, plasma and airway surface liquid (Zanetti, 2004; Murakami et al., 2005; Dürr et al., 2006; Kolar and McDermott, 2011; Vandamme et al., 2012). It is produced by numerous cell types including epithelial cells, keratinocytes and many leukocytes including neutrophils, dendritic cells (DCs), lymphocytes and monocytes/macrophages (Dürr et al., 2006; Vandamme et al., 2012). In neutrophils, the propeptide is stored in the secondary granules, while in keratinocytes it is stored in lamellar bodies (Cowland et al., 1995; Sorensen et al., 1997; Braff et al.,

2005). The role of LL-37 has been studied in numerous diseases. In particular, its expression is altered in skin conditions such as psoriasis, atopic dermatitis and rosacea, and LL-37 expression can also be induced by vitamin D_3, a link that seems to play a key role in an effective immune response to *Mycobacterium tuberculosis* (Wang *et al.*, 2004; Liu *et al.*, 2006; Liu *et al.*, 2007; Nijnik and Hancock, 2009; Vandamme *et al.*, 2012).

14.1.3 Histatins and liver-expressed antimicrobial peptides (LEAPs)

There are 12 histatins (His-1-12), which are produced by salivary glands, although most appear to be fragments and only His-1, His-3 and His-5 are considered to be key populations in saliva (Melino *et al.*, 2014). Histatins are histidine-rich (thus only positively charged at acidic pH) and are reported to have both antibacterial and antifungal activity, although these tend to occur under non-physiological conditions. Studies are emerging that demonstrate immunomodulatory effects such as wound healing and proteolytic enzyme inhibition (Gusman *et al.*, 2001; Oudhoff *et al.*, 2008; Oudhoff *et al.*, 2010).

LEAP-1, now known as hepcidin, and LEAP-2, are both highly expressed in the liver but their functions differ. Hepcidin is a key iron regulator, mostly produced by hepatocytes, that binds the membrane protein ferroportin to prevent the extracellular release of stored iron (Michels *et al.*, 2015). While LEAP-2 was reported to show weak direct antimicrobial effects *in vitro* (Krause *et al.*, 2003), this has not been thoroughly studied and it may have additional roles in human defences.

14.1.4 Modified and synthetic HDPs

Many synthetic HDPs have also been produced (Fjell *et al.*, 2011). These are often created by using the sequence of a naturally occurring HDP and substituting amino acids and/or truncating the sequence of peptides or even large proteins, or through semi-random design. For example, the synthetic innate defence regulators (IDRs) were designed in our laboratory by an amino acid substitution array of a linear form of the bovine HDP bactenecin (Hilpert *et al.*, 2005), although the IDR label can be applied to any synthetic cationic peptide, including derivatives of natural HDPs, that possesses immunomodulatory activity at concentrations lower than that at which other functions (e.g. antimicrobial, antibiofilm) are observed. Other examples of synthetic HDPs include truncated forms of lactoferrin, an 80 kDa protein that has antimicrobial properties, such as hLF1-11 (Nibbering *et al.*, 2001). Additional HDP variants include exchanging the naturally occurring L-amino acids for D-amino acids, using non-natural amino acids, or creating peptoids by moving the amino acid side chains from the α-carbon to the nitrogen in the peptide backbone.

14.2 Hormones and Neuropeptides: The New HDPs

While the HDPs have often been limited to the families discussed above, there are numerous cationic peptide hormones and neuropeptides that also have emerging roles in host defence. Interestingly, some of these non-traditional HDPs have also shown direct antimicrobial effects (Krause *et al.*, 2001; Charnley *et al.*, 2008), albeit under *in vitro* settings that may not be relevant to physiological conditions. Table 14.2 lists a selection of these peptides, with highlights discussed below.

14.2.1 Natriuretic peptides

Three natriuretic (aiding sodium excretion into the urine) peptides (NPs), atrial NP (ANP), B-type NP (BNP; also called brain-type NP), and C-type NP (CNP) have been found in humans. The NPs share a common 17-amino acid loop sequence formed by a disulfide bond, and this loop also shows homology with osteocrin (also called musclin), a recently discovered peptide found in osteoblasts, muscle and white

Table 14.2. Examples of small, cationic peptides found in humans that have traditionally been regarded as hormones and/or neuropeptides, but also have emerging roles in human defences. For some peptides, multiple isoforms exist; for these, only the key isoform(s) responsible for biological activity have been included. The UniProt accession number for the peptide or its unprocessed parent protein has been provided for additional information on sequences and processing.

Name and number of amino acids in mature peptide	Locations and cells	Functions	Further reading
Apelin (UniProt Q9ULZ1) Apelin-13: 13 Apelin-28: 28 Apelin-31: 31 Apelin-36: 36	CNS, peripheral blood vessels Cells: neurons, endothelial cells	Cardiovascular and angiogenic effects; stress response	(Lee *et al.*, 2006; Kidoya *et al.*, 2012)
Calcitonin family IAPP (amylin): 37 (UniProt P10997) CGRP-1: 37 (UniProt P06881) CGRP-2: 37 (UniProt P10092)	CNS, PNS, pancreas Cells: β cells, monocytes/macrophages, keratinocytes	Metabolism and glucose response; pain response; pro- and anti-inflammatory; pro-angiogenic	(Wang and Fiscus, 1989; Liu *et al.*, 2000; Ding *et al.*, 2007; Mikami *et al.*, 2012; Granstein *et al.*, 2015; Walsh *et al.*, 2015; Akter *et al.*, 2016)
Catestatin: 21 (UniProt P10645)	Brain, skin Cells: PBMCs, enteroendocrine cells, neurons	Pro-angiogenic; anti-infective; cardiovascular effects; pro-chemotactic; chemokine release effects	(Theurl *et al.*, 2010; Helle and Corti, 2015)
Corticotropin releasing factor family: Urocortin-2: 41 (UniProt Q96RP3) Urocortin-3: 38 (UniProt Q969E3)	Multiple locations including brain, cardiovascular system, GI tract	Anti-infective; vasodilation and other cardiovascular effects; appetite and metabolism regulation; stress response	(Stengel and Tache, 2014)
GRP: 27 (UniProt P07492)	CNS, GI tract Cells: multiple immune cells	Pro-chemotactic; pro-angiogenic	(Jensen *et al.*, 2008; Czepielewski *et al.*, 2012)
Ghrelin: 27 or 28 (UniProt Q9UBU3)	Multiple locations including CNS, pancreas, GI tract Cells: lymphocytes, neutrophils, endocrine cells	Both pro- and anti-inflammatory effects	(Li *et al.*, 2004; Eissa and Ghia, 2015; Xu *et al.*, 2015)
Natriuretic peptides ANP (ANF): 28 (UniProt P01160) BNP: 32 (UniProt P16860) CNP: 22 (UniProt P23582) Osteocrin: 50 (UniProt P61366)	Cardiovascular system, GI tract, CNS, liver Cells: multiple cells depending on the NP, including vascular smooth muscle cells, endothelial cells, leukocytes, chondrocytes, cardiomyocytes, osteoblasts, etc.	Diuretics; natriuretics; cardiovascular effects; long bone growth effects; phagocytosis promotion; anti-inflammatory; anti-cancer; chemotaxis effects	(Vollmar *et al.*, 1997; Krause *et al.*, 2001; Tsukagoshi *et al.*, 2001; Scotland *et al.*, 2005; Moffatt *et al.*, 2007; Potter *et al.*, 2009; Moffatt and Thomas, 2009; De Vito, 2014)

Peptide	Location/Cells	Functions	References
Neuropeptide B and neuropeptide W family Neuropeptide B: 23 or 29 (UniProt Q8NG41) Neuropeptide W: 23 or 30 (UniProt Q8N729)	CNS, genitourinary system, stomach, respiratory tract	Pain and stress responses	(Hondo et al., 2008)
Neurotensin : 13 (UniProt P30990)	CNS, PNS, cardiovascular system, GI tract	Cardiovascular effects; pro-angiogenic	(Osadchii, 2015)
Nociceptin: 17 (UniProt Q13519)	CNS, PNS Cells: lymphocytes, monocytes	Pro-chemotactic; chemokine release effects	(Serhan et al., 2001; Gavioli et al., 2015)
Orexin (hypocretin) (UniProt O43612) Orexin-A: 33 Orexin-B: 28	Brain Cells: only produced by hypothalamus neurons	Cardiovascular effects; stress response	(Grimaldi et al., 2014)
Oxyntomodulin: 37 (UniProt P01275)	GI tract	Metabolic regulation; anti-gastric emptying	(Bataille and Dalle, 2014)
POMC derivatives (UniProt P01189) α-melanotropin (α-MSH): 13 γ-melanotropin (γ-MSH): 11 β-endorphin: 31	CNS, pituitary, skin, GI tract	Metabolism and appetite response effects; analgesics; anti-inflammatory	(Taylor and Namba, 2001; Charnley et al., 2008; Catania et al., 2010; Min et al., 2011; Mountjoy, 2015)
Secretin family VIP: 28 (UniProt P01282) PACAP: 27 or 38 (UniProt P18509) Somatoliberin (GHRH): 44 (UniProt P01286)	CNS, PNS, GI tract, pancreas, etc. Cells: neurons, lymphocytes, neutrophils, monocytes, endocrine cells	Hormone release effects; pain and stress response; cardiovascular effects; homeostasis maintenance; anti-inflammatory; chemotaxis effects; wound healing promotion	(Leceta et al., 2000; Delgado et al., 2004; Harmar et al., 2012; Waschek, 2013; Ganea et al., 2015; Granata, 2016)
Somatostatin family Somatostatin: 14 or 28 (UniProt P61278) Cortistatin: 17 or 29 (UniProt O00230)	CNS, PNS, GI tract, pancreas Cells: endothelial cells, monocytes/macrophages, lymphocytes, etc.	Hormone release regulation; chemotaxis effects; anti-angiogenic	(van Hagen et al., 2008; Rai et al., 2015)
Substance P: 11 (UniProt P20366)	CNS Cells: multiple cells, including neurons, epithelial cells, macrophages, T cells, DCs	Stress and pain responses; vasodilation; cytokine release; pro-angiogenic; chemotactic; phagocytosis promotion	(Cunin et al., 2011, Mashaghi et al., 2016)

Abbreviations: IAPP: islet amyloid polypeptide; CGRP: calcitonin gene-related peptide; GRP: gastrin-releasing peptide; ANP: atrial natriuretic peptide, also called ANF (atrial natriuretic factor); BNP: B-type natriuretic peptide or brain-type natriuretic peptide; CNP: C-type natriuretic peptide; POMC: pro-opiomelanocortin; MSH: melanocyte-stimulating hormone; VIP: vasoactive intestinal peptide; PACAP: pituitary adenylate cyclase-activating polypeptide; GHRH: growth hormone-releasing hormone

abdominal fat (Moffatt *et al.*, 2007; Moffatt and Thomas, 2009).

ANP is produced by vascular smooth muscle and endothelial cells mainly in the atrium of the heart, where the propeptide is stored in atrium granules, although its mRNA has also been detected in other locations including the brain, gastrointestinal and respiratory tracts, and the liver (Potter *et al.*, 2009; De Vito, 2014). ANP can also be produced by leukocytes (De Vito, 2014). BNP and CNP are found in the brain, and BNP is also produced by cardiomyocytes in the ventricles of the heart, while CNP is also produced by chondrocytes in the cartilage as well as endothelial cells (Potter *et al.*, 2009). NPs can produce diuretic and natriuretic effects, with ANP having the most notable role in maintaining homeostasis of the blood pressure, whereas CNP and osteocrin both influence long bone growth (Moffatt and Thomas, 2009; Potter *et al.*, 2009; De Vito, 2014). Evidence is mounting that the NPs also have an immunomodulatory role in host defences, with much of the research focused on ANP, although additional immunomodulatory roles for BNP and CNP are also emerging (Vollmar *et al.*, 1997; Scotland *et al.*, 2005 Potter *et al.*, 2009; De Vito, 2014).

14.2.2 Secretin family

The secretin family includes three members that are cationic peptides: vasoactive intestinal peptide (VIP), pituitary adenylate cyclase-activating polypeptide (PACAP), and growth-hormone releasing hormone (GHRH, also called somatoliberin).

GHRH is produced in the brain, specifically the hypothalamus, along with numerous other tissues. It can also be produced by lymphocytes (Granata, 2016). It is best known for stimulating the pituitary gland to release growth hormone.

VIP is found in multiple locations including the gastrointestinal tract, peripheral nervous system (PNS), and the central nervous system (CNS), and can be released by many cells such as activated T cells, neutrophils, monocytes, neurons and endocrine cells (Delgado *et al.*, 2004; Harmar *et al.*, 2012; Ganea *et al.*, 2015). VIP can stimulate the release of hormones or neurotransmitters such as prolactin and the catecholamines, and is also involved in circadian rhythms and other homeostasis mechanisms (Harmar *et al.*, 2012).

PACAP is found as a 38 amino acid peptide or a shortened 27 amino acid form. It is found in several tissues including the brain and the gastrointestinal tract (Harmar *et al.*, 2012). Similar to VIP, it seems to have roles in catecholamine release and circadian rhythm (Harmar *et al.*, 2012).

Both VIP and PACAP are also involved in insulin secretion in the pancreas, which has made them potential targets for diabetes treatments.

14.2.3 Calcitonin family

Amylin, also called islet amyloid polypeptide (IAPP), is produced by β cells in the pancreas and is involved in glucose regulation through the inhibition of gastric emptying, or release of food from the stomach (Akter *et al.*, 2016). It is stored in β cell secretory granules and released along with insulin (Akter *et al.*, 2016). Due to its activities, amylin is a target for the treatment of diabetes.

Calcitonin gene-related peptide (CGRP) is produced in the CNS and the PNS, as well as by cells such as monocytes/macrophages and keratinocytes (Granstein *et al.*, 2015). It has two versions, CGRP1 and CGRP2, which are both 37 amino acids in length. CGRP is involved in the nociceptive pain response and seems to have a role in migraines, arthritis and psoriasis (Granstein *et al.*, 2015; Walsh *et al.*, 2015).

14.2.4 Somatostatin family

The two members of the somatostatin family, cortistatin and somatostatin itself, are cyclic peptides due to a disulfide bond. Cortistatin is found in two isoforms, cortistatin-17 and a seemingly inactive form called cortistatin-29. It can be produced by numerous leukocytes including monocytes/macrophages and lymphocytes, and can be found in the CNS and pancreas (van Hagen *et al.*, 2008).

Similarly, somatostatin is found in two isoforms, somatostatin-14 and -28, but both are active. Somatostatin is released by neurons in the CNS and PNS, and also by δ cells in the gastrointestinal tract and pancreas (Rai *et al.*, 2015).

Both peptides are involved in regulating neuronal activity, such as inhibiting the release of growth hormone, and are also involved in regulating gastrointestinal peptide and insulin release (van Hagen *et al.*, 2008; Rai *et al.*, 2015).

14.2.5 Pro-opiomelanocortin derivatives

Pro-opiomelanocortin (POMC) is a peptide found in the pituitary, brain and skin that undergoes a series of cleavage events to create several peptides, including the cationic peptides α-melanocyte stimulating hormone (MSH), γ-MSH, and β-endorphin (Mountjoy, 2015). γ-MSH has not been widely studied, but α-MSH, a 13 amino acid derivative of POMC, is involved in numerous regulatory functions in the brain and gastrointestinal tract and has roles in skin pigmentation and in obesity (Catania *et al.*, 2010; Mountjoy, 2015). As with other endorphins, β-endorphin is an endogenous opioid and is involved in analgesia. Interestingly, hBD-3 has been shown to utilize one of the MSH receptors (Nix *et al.*, 2013), demonstrating overlap between the immune and neuroendocrine systems.

14.3 Activities of HDPs

14.3.1 Anti-infective/immunomodulatory

Although they often lose their direct antimicrobial effects under high salt conditions (Turner *et al.*, 1998; Garcia *et al.*, 2001) that reflect the physiological conditions found *in*

vivo, HDPs still possess anti-infective properties through their immunomodulatory activities (Hilchie *et al.*, 2013). One such activity is the inhibition of pro-inflammatory cytokine production, which is often achieved by inhibiting NF-κB activation or affecting the production of cyclic adenosine monophosphate (cAMP). There are five NF-κB transcription factors in humans that are activated by multiple signals including bacterial signatures such as lipopolysaccharide (LPS), viral nucleic acid, and other markers of infection and inflammation such as reactive oxygen species (ROS) or TNF-α (Oeckinghaus *et al.*, 2011). NF-κB activation results in the transcription of numerous pro-inflammatory cytokines, including TNF-α and IL-6. The binding of a G-protein coupled receptor (GPCR) to its ligand often leads to the conversion of ATP to cAMP. The release of cAMP prompts the activation of protein kinase A (PKA), which in turn phosphorylates, and thus activates, numerous transcription factors, such as CREB, as well as affecting other processes such as metabolism, all of which can have a major impact on host defence (Skalhegg and Tasken, 2000).

Several HDPs have been shown to inhibit NF-κB activation, including LL-37, α-MSH, ANP, VIP, PACAP, ghrelin and CGRP, thus limiting inflammation (Manna and Aggarwal, 1998; Leceta *et al.*, 2000; Tsukagoshi *et al.*, 2001; Li *et al.*, 2004; Mookherjee *et al.*, 2006; Ding *et al.*, 2007; Catania *et al.*, 2010; Waschek, 2013). Intriguingly, the effects of LL-37 on the response to bacterial LPS are quite complex and reflect more than just simple binding to and neutralization of LPS. For example, LL-37 inhibits TNF-α protein expression and the translocation and activation of NF-κB p50, p65, and to a lesser extent RelB, after cells are exposed to LPS, but does not affect the other two NF-κB family members, p52 or cRel, and the transcription of several LPS-induced genes is affected (or not) to varying degrees by LL-37 rather than it causing complete inhibition (Mookherjee *et al.*, 2006). Additionally, LL-37 and defensins as well as many of the neuropeptides and hormones, including α-MSH and CGRP, bind to and activate GPCRs (Wang and Fiscus, 1989; Manna and Aggarwal, 1998; Liu *et al.*, 2000; Yang *et al.*, 2000; Yu *et al.*, 2007; Mookherjee *et al.*, 2009; Subramanian *et al.*, 2011; Subramanian *et al.*, 2013). This can lead to an activation of downstream pathways including MAP kinases and possibly an increase in cAMP. The release of pro-inflammatory cytokines can also be suppressed through a variety of other mechanisms, which are likely to occur in parallel rather than independently, by VIP, PACAP, cortistatin, LL-37, defensins and IDR peptides (Delgado and Ganea, 2000; Leceta *et al.*, 2000; Delgado *et al.*, 2004; Gonzalez-Rey *et al.*, 2006; Hilchie *et al.*, 2013; Waschek, 2013).

Some peptides have also been shown to, at least transiently, activate NF-κB, and their immunomodulatory action is dependent on this activation. For example, LL-37 activates NF-κB in human airway epithelial cells, leading to the production of IL-6 and IL-8 but not TNF-α or IL-1β, indicating both a pro- and anti-inflammatory effect for this human cathelicidin (Pistolic *et al.*, 2009). In fact, many HDPs besides LL-37 show a mix of effects including defensins, nociceptin, CGRP and the synthetic IDR peptides. For instance, CGRP is associated with increased inflammation and pain in migraines and arthritis, but it showed protection in a mouse model of endotoxaemia by inhibiting TNF-α production and neutrophil chemotaxis (Gomes *et al.*, 2005; Granstein *et al.*, 2015; Walsh *et al.*, 2015). Similarly, IDR-1002 has an action that is dependent on NF-κB activation *in vitro*, and it is able to protect mice against infections while suppressing pro-inflammatory cytokines (Nijnik *et al.*, 2010).

This combination of anti-inflammatory and pro-inflammatory effects, even by the same peptide, differs from the response to an infection which is primarily pro-inflammatory in the acute phase and then dampens down during the convalescent phase. Thus, these peptides uniquely suppress the production of pro-inflammatory cytokines while enabling the maintenance and/or enhancement of protective mechanisms that are traditionally considered

pro-inflammatory (e.g. chemokine induction and cellular recruitment). This ability of HDPs/IDRs to modulate the immune response, rather than completely activate or suppress it, is one of their appealing features for use as anti-infective agents. For example, LL-37, IDR-1002, hBD-1-4, HNP-1-3, gastrin releasing peptide (GRP), catestatin, and nociceptin increase cell migration; somatostatin and CNP dampen chemotaxis, while VIP shows both pro- and anti-chemotaxis effects (Yang *et al.*, 1999; Yang *et al.*, 2000; Serhan *et al.*, 2001; Aarbiou *et al.*, 2004; Delgado *et al.*, 2004; Scotland *et al.*, 2005; Trombella *et al.*, 2005; Niyonsaba *et al.*, 2007; Theurl *et al.*, 2010; Czepielewski *et al.*, 2012; Madera and Hancock, 2012). Similarly, contributions of HDPs to cell activation and differentiation also vary. For example, LL-37 causes polarization of macrophages, DCs and T cells, and also induces granzyme-mediated apoptosis in regulatory T cells (Davidson *et al.*, 2004; Pena *et al.*, 2013; Mader *et al.*, 2011). α-MSH can decrease T cell proliferation and TNF-α-induced DC maturation, but also promotes the production of regulatory T cells and polarizes to a Th1 response (Taylor and Namba, 2001; Chang *et al.*, 2008; Min *et al.*, 2011; Janelsins *et al.*, 2013). Substance P and CGRP can promote a Th17 response (Cunin *et al.*, 2011; Mikami *et al.*, 2012), while ghrelin suppresses Th17-cell differentiation (Xu *et al.*, 2015). Many of these responses are also affected by the location, cells and stimulus used.

When the balance between pro- and anti-inflammatory responses is perturbed during an infection it can lead to sepsis. Perhaps not surprisingly, several HDPs have been effective in models of sepsis, including LL-37, PACAP, CGRP, α-MSH and hepcidin (Lipton *et al.*, 1994; Gomes *et al.*, 2005; Torossian *et al.*, 2007; Tang *et al.*, 2008; Huang *et al.*, 2012).

HDPs have many additional effects during infection, such as hepcidin limiting iron availability in the blood and thus limiting its accessibility for bacteria (Michels *et al.*, 2015); ANP and substance P enhancing phagocytosis by macrophages (Vollmar *et al.*, 1997; Mashaghi *et al.*, 2016);

IDR-1002 and IDR-1018 improving neutrophil killing of *Escherichia coli* (Niyonsaba *et al.*, 2013); LL-37 binding directly to LPS (Turner *et al.*, 1998; Nagaoka *et al.*, 2001; Molhoek *et al.*, 2009); and α-MSH and cortistatin limiting the release of inflammatory nitric oxide (Catania *et al.*, 2010; Gonzalez-Rey *et al.*, 2006).

14.3.2 Antibiofilm

Bacterial biofilms are a distinct growth state of bacteria on surfaces including body sites. They comprise complex structured micro-colonies enclosed in a matrix that can involve polysaccharides, proteins and extracellular DNA. This growth adaptation protects the bacteria from stresses including those provided by the host and conventional antibiotics, making the bacteria extremely difficult to treat and eradicate. Biofilms are a frequent cause of nosocomial infections and are commonly found on devices such as implants and catheters, in lung, bladder and intestinal infections, and in burn or wound infections. Antibiofilm activity represents the direct action of HDPs on bacterial communities and is included here due to the overlap between antibiofilm and immunomodulatory action and a lesser overlap with direct antibiotic activity (Haney *et al.*, 2015). LL-37, at concentrations one sixteenth of those required to eliminate free-swimming bacteria, prevents the formation of biofilms by *Pseudomonas aeruginosa* (Overhage *et al.*, 2008). Further studies on synthetic antibiofilm peptides showed that IDR-1018 and the D-enantiomeric peptides DJK-5 and DJK-6 prevented and eradicated biofilms produced by *P. aeruginosa*, *E. coli*, *Staphylococcus aureus* and many other multi-drug resistant bacteria (de la Fuente-Nunez *et al.*, 2014; Reffuveille *et al.*, 2014; de la Fuente-Nunez *et al.*, 2015). These peptides worked by targeting the universal bacterial intracellular stringent response mediated by the nucleotide signal ppGpp to mediate their antibiofilm effects (de la Fuente-Nunez *et al.*, 2014).

14.3.3 Anticancer

Some HDPs have demonstrated activity against tumour cells at concentrations that leave non-cancerous cells intact, however, the ratio of these two activities, termed the therapeutic index, can vary widely. While the exact mechanisms behind this distinction are not well understood, it is believed to be due to differences in the composition and charge of membranes in cancer cells *versus* normal cells (Hoskin and Ramamoorthy, 2008). Examples of anticancer peptides include the bovine cathelicidins BMAP-27 and BMAP-28, which demonstrate anticancer effects through direct membrane permeabilization and induction of apoptosis in cancer cells (Hoskin and Ramamoorthy, 2008). However, they also show some toxicity in non-cancerous cells, thus limiting their potential. On the other hand, ANP causes moderate toxicity in pancreatic adenocarcinoma and prostate cancer cells, but not in non-cancerous ones (Skelton *et al.*, 2011). ANP also eliminated 80% of the tumour in a pancreatic adenocarcinoma mouse model (Vesely *et al.*, 2007).

Another method of targeting cancer is by limiting angiogenesis. Somatostatin is anti-angiogenic, inhibiting the release of the growth factor VEGF to limit endothelial cell proliferation and migration (Rai *et al.*, 2015). Additionally, it can also target tumour cells directly through the induction of apoptosis via the somatostatin receptors (Sun and Coy, 2011). Somatostatin analogues, most notably the octameric peptide octreotide, are used in the treatment of neuroendocrine tumours, although this is largely to limit the release of growth hormones rather than to directly target the tumour (Rai *et al.*, 2015).

Due to its angiogenic effects, LL-37 would seem to be a poor option to treat cancer, and indeed it has been shown to promote the growth of several cancers including ovarian and breast cancers (Coffelt *et al.*, 2009; Weber *et al.*, 2009). However, it has also shown anticancer effects, including against colon cancer (Ren *et al.*, 2012), and has recently been approved for a phase I/II clinical trial for intratumuoral injections into melanoma (NCT02225366).

14.3.4 Wound healing and angiogenesis

While there is a desire to limit angiogenesis in cancer, the formation of new blood vessels is a key component in wound healing. LL-37, Substance P, CGRP, GRP and catestatin all show pro-angiogenic effects (Jensen *et al.*, 2008; Theurl *et al.*, 2010; Zheng *et al.*, 2010; Vandamme *et al.*, 2012; Hilchie *et al.*, 2013; Mashaghi *et al.*, 2016). LL-37 has been shown to improve wound healing in a human skin model and a rabbit hind-limb injury model (Heilborn *et al.*, 2003; Koczulla *et al.*, 2003), while mice lacking cathelin-related antimicrobial peptide (CRAMP), the mouse homologue of LL-37, have decreased vascularization during wound healing (Koczulla *et al.*, 2003). GHRH was effective in a wound healing model in mice (Dioufa *et al.*, 2010), hNP-1-3 increased lung epithelial cell wound closure *in vitro* (Aarbiou *et al.*, 2004), and histatin 1 and histatin 2 improve wound healing in the oral environment (Oudhoff *et al.*, 2008).

Diabetic wounds are also a potential area for HDP therapy. Defensin hBD-3 improved wound healing and decreased *S. aureus* bacterial load in a porcine diabetic wound model (Hirsch *et al.*, 2009). In contrast, IDR-1018 worked in non-diabetic *S. aureus*-infected wound models in pigs and mice, but did not show enhanced healing in diabetic mice (Steinstraesser *et al.*, 2012). The mechanism of action in this model was ascribed to enhancement of metabolism, while enhanced recruitment of cells to the wounded site is another prospective wound healing mechanism for these peptides.

14.3.5 Cardiovascular disease and metabolism

Cardiovascular disease (CVD) and obesity are intertwined and represent a major health crisis worldwide, and the emerging field of immunometabolism reflects the involvement of the immune system in these conditions (Mathis and Shoelson, 2011). A guide to immunometabolism has been provided by O'Neill *et al.* (2016). Many of the small cationic peptide hormones are also involved in the regulation of cardiovascular function and metabolism, including the NPs, catestatin, GHRH and α-MSH. In particular, the NPs have been studied extensively in CVD, with elevated BNP a marker of heart failure and both ANP and BNP linked to obesity (Khush *et al.*, 2006). A recombinant form of BNP, called nesiritide, was approved for use in the treatment of heart failure in the US in 2001. However, a 2011 study found it did not significantly improve the rates of death and rehospitalization and it is no longer recommended as a treatment (O'Connor *et al.*, 2011). Despite this setback, the use of HDPs for CVD and/or obesity is a promising area of research. In this regard, short cationic amphipathic apolipoprotein A-I (apoA-I) peptide mimetics (Navab *et al.*, 2005; Kingwell *et al.*, 2014), that have been designed largely on the structural and physical properties thought to confer the ability of apoA-I to induce cholesterol efflux, are undergoing clinical trials as prospective cholesterol-reducing drugs (Navab *et al.*, 2005). They are known to be immunomodulatory with potential against other inflammatory diseases, as seen with the reductions of TNF-α-induced ROS production and asthma-induced airway inflammation by the cationic peptide apoA-I mimetic 5A (Tabet *et al.*, 2010; Yao *et al.*, 2011).

14.3.6 Adjuvants

HDPs have also been tested as adjuvants for vaccines, and LL-37 and defensins have been shown to enhance immune responses (Tani *et al.*, 2000; Kurosaka *et al.*, 2005). An adjuvant with the IDR peptide HH2 added to a CpG oligodeoxynucleotide (ODN) dramatically improved the response in mice to pertussis toxoid compared to the toxoid alone, as indicated by improved IgG and IgA titres (Kindrachuk *et al.*, 2009). Similar effects were seen when using a combination adjuvant comprising the bovine HDP indolicidin, CpG ODN, and polyphosphazene, used in combination with ovalbumin (OVA) (Kovacs-Nolan *et al.*, 2009). Analogous combination adjuvants, in which peptides IDR-1002 or IDR-HH2 were substituted for indolicidin, had the remarkable features of high protective titres (for pertussis and respiratory syncytial virus) with a single dose, mixed Th1/Th2 responses, efficacy in neonatal pigs and mice, protection with multiple targets, and no maternal interference (Gracia *et al.*, 2011; Garlapati *et al.*, 2012; Polewicz *et al.*, 2013). CRAMP also acted as an adjuvant when injected with OVA into mice (Kurosaka *et al.*, 2005). These results indicate that peptides are likely to be useful in vaccine adjuvant formulations.

14.4 HDPs as Therapeutics: Peptides in Clinical Trials

Multiple cationic HDPs have entered clinical trials in humans (Table 14.3). Some of these HDPs are being used as AMPs, while others are taking advantage of immunomodulatory effects. The most successful drugs have been hormones or hormone analogues, and have been used largely to impact on cardiovascular disease and metabolism. For example, a GHRH analogue marketed as Egrifta (tesamorelin) is used for the treatment of lipodystrophy in HIV patients (Sekhar, 2015). GHRH and other analogues are also being examined for use in other metabolic or cardiovascular disorders, such as diabetes and congestive heart failure (NCT00791843, NCT01264497). The NPs have been investigated in multiple conditions, notably the use of BNP (nesiritide), ANP (carperitide), and the chimeric CD-NP (cenderitide) in heart failure and metabolic disorders such as obesity (see Table 14.3). However, as mentioned above, nesiritide is no longer recommended for treating heart failure, and ANP, which is approved for heart failure in Japan, was recently linked to increased mortality (Matsue *et al.*, 2015),

although additional studies must be completed. Cenderitide is still being evaluated, and is currently in a phase II trial in patients with chronic stable heart failure (NCT02359227). Not all of the drugs are used for metabolic or hormone-related disorders. For instance, aviptadil, an analogue of VIP, has been used for pulmonary arterial hypertension and sarcoidosis (Ganea *et al.*, 2015).

The classical HDPs and synthetic versions are also being assessed for use in humans. Many of the peptides are being used for topical wound treatments that can combine both direct antimicrobial and immunomodulatory activities. ACT1, a synthetic peptide designed based on the carboxy-terminus of the gap junction protein connexin-43, was effective as a treatment of chronic venous leg ulcers (Ghatnekar *et al.*, 2015). It is now being evaluated in additional phase I and phase III trials for diabetic foot and venous leg ulcers (Table 14.3). Pexiganan, marketed as Locilex, is a synthetic version of magainin, a peptide isolated from the African clawed frog *Xenopus laevis*. It has undergone clinical trials for the treatment of infected diabetic foot ulcers, but has had difficulty gaining FDA approval. However, as of this review, Dipexium was recruiting participants for additional phase III trials using pexiganan/locilex for mildly infected diabetic foot ulcers (NCT01594762). Omiganan, a synthetic derivative of indolicidin, also faced difficulties in reaching the market, although it has been tested in phase II studies for the prevention of catheter-related infections where it was shown to be safe and significantly decreased microbiologically-confirmed infections and catheter colonization, but missed its primary target (Table 14.3). It was also used as a topical antimicrobial agent and for the treatment of atopic dermatitis (NCT00608959, NCT02456480). It is currently being investigated in advanced clinical trials for the treatment of rosacea, acne, genital warts and vulval epithelial neoplasia (Table 14.3). Another HDP, called C16G2, has been evaluated for use as an oral gel in phase I/II trials (NCT02044081). It specifically targets *Streptococcus mutans*, the major cause of

Table 14.3. Select cationic HDPs in clinical trials or approved for use in humans.

Name and number of amino acids	Functions	Status of select trials
ACT-1: 25	Formulated as granexin gel for use as wound healing agent in diabetic foot ulcers and venous leg ulcers	Currently in phase I (NCT02652572) and phase III (NCT02667327)
ANP: 28 BNP: 32 CD-NP: 37	In multiple trials for treatment of cardiovascular disease and metabolic disorders	Multiple trials, including ones for BNP (NCT00475852, NCT02608996), ANP (NCT00212056), and CD-NP (NCT02071602, NCT02359227)
C16G2 Gel: 36	Antimicrobial peptide specific for *Streptococcus mutans*. Used for oral hygiene and prevention of cavities	Completed phase II (NCT02044081), additional phase II ongoing (NCT02594254)
GHRH (somatoliberin): 44	Used for diagnosis and treatment of growth hormone deficiency	FDA approved
IAPP Chimeric (pramlintide): 37	Treatment of type 1 and 2 diabetes	FDA approved
Lactoferrin-1-11 (hLF-1-11): 11	Used in trial for safety assessment in stem cell transplant recipients. Studies for efficacy against *Staphylococcus epidermis* and candidaemia were withdrawn	Completed phase I (NCT00509938), phase I/II withdrawn (NCT00509847, NCT00509834)
Lanreotide and pasireotide (somatostatin analogues): 6-8	Used for Cushing's disease, acromegaly	FDA approved
LL-37: 37	Anticancer via direct injection into melanoma tumour Used for treatment of venous leg ulcers	Currently recruiting for study (NCT02225366); Venous leg ulcer trial completed (EudraCT 2012-002100-41)
Lucinactant: 21	Surfactant formulation that contains a cationic peptide. Used for preventing respiratory distress syndrome	FDA approved
NA-1 (TAT-NR2B9c): 20	Used as neuroprotective agent for ischaemic brain damage caused by strokes	Completed phase II (NCT00728182), recruiting for phase III (NCT02315443)
Omiganan (MBI 226): 12	Used in trials for the treatment of several conditions including rosacea, atopic dermatitis, catheter infections, acne, genital warts and vulval intraepithelial neoplasia	Currently recruiting for phase II (NCT02596074, NCT02571998, NCT02849262) and phase III (NCT02576847, NCT02576860) trials; has also completed multiple phase II (NCT01784133, NCT02456480) and phase III (NCT00608959, NCT00231153) trials
PAC-113 (P-113): 13	Histatin 5 derivative used for oral candidiasis treatment in HIV+ patients	Completed phase II (NCT00659971)
Pexiganan (Locilex, MSI-78): 22	Used as wound healing and anti-infective agent in mildly infected diabetic foot ulcers	Completed phase II (NCT00563433), recruiting for phase III (NCT01594762)
SGX942: 5	Used for the treatment of oral mucositis in head and neck cancer patients	Currently in phase II trial (NCT02013050)
Substance P: 11	Substance P is being tested in multiple conditions including Type 1 diabetes, allergy treatment, and pain management in cancer patients	Multiple trials (NCT02820558, NCT01280149, NCT02036281, etc.)

Continued

Table 14.3.   Continued.

Name and number of amino acids	Functions	Status of select trials
VIP: 28	Aviptadil, an analogue of VIP, has been used for pulmonary arterial hypertension, sarcoidosis, and erectile dysfunction	FDA approved (aviptadil)
Xenin-25: 25	Used for treatment of type 2 diabetes	Completed phase I (NCT00949663), additional phase I trials ongoing
Ziconotide (Prialt, SNX-111): 25	Pain relief	FDA approved

dental cavities. SGX942, a five amino acid derivative of IDR-1, is completing a phase II trial for oral mucositis in cancer patients, with preliminary data showing encouraging results (NCT02013050). Finally, LL-37 has been used successfully in the treatment of venous leg ulcers (Gronberg *et al.*, 2014), and a trial evaluating the injection of LL-37 directly into melanomas as an anticancer agent is currently recruiting patients (NCT02225366).

Lastly, the antibiotics polymyxin B and gramicidin S that have been marketed for decades, and the former especially is seen as a drug of last choice in the antibiotic resistance era. Both of these molecules are cationic amphipathic peptides produced by bacteria.

14.4.1 Challenges

Despite cationic peptides progressing in commercial development, there are still issues to be addressed. One of the largest drawbacks with the development of peptide drugs is the high cost of synthesis through traditional methods such as fluorenylmethyloxycarbonyl (Fmoc) chemistry, with peptides in modest amounts costing from $100–$600 per gram based on the sequence length and/or the need for inclusion of more difficult chemistry such as disulfide bonds (Hancock and Sahl, 2006), although this cost might be considerably reduced at the kilogram scale. However, alternative synthesis methods may help alleviate some of these costs. For example, production of a

recombinant peptide in bacterial cells has been limited due to the direct antimicrobial nature of many peptides, meaning that successful formation of the peptide would lead to the death of the bacteria producing the peptide. Additionally, as with eukaryotes, prokaryotes produce proteases that could potentially destroy the end product. Several recombinant systems have been developed to overcome these limitations, such as fusing the HDP to a larger protein, for example glutathione transferase, to protect both the peptide and the bacterial host during synthesis, then cleaving the fusion product to give the HDP (Li, 2011; Piers *et al.*, 1993).

The short sequence length of HDPs and ability to readily penetrate cells (analogous to the cell penetrating peptides that can include cationic amphipathic peptides) means they could enter cells and interact with multiple cytoplasmic as well as cell surface receptors, possibly leading to side effects and toxicity. However, many of the licensed neuropeptides and hormones also have multiple effects and targets, so this feature does not inherently prevent the use of peptide drugs and generally speaking no chemical-class-related major toxicities have been revealed in many clinical trials to date. The cationic lipopeptide antibiotic polymyxin is known to be quite toxic, but in this case toxicity has been ameliorated by creating a methanesulfonate prodrug.

Another downside is the short half-life of HDPs. Using D-amino acids and non-natural amino acids is known to limit the effects of proteases, but another option is improved formulations to enhance drug delivery. This can be achieved by packaging the drug into nanoparticles or formulating the drug with chemicals such as polymers to limit degradation. All of these methods can greatly increase HDP half-life.

Despite these issues, protein or peptide drugs already account for more than $40 billion in sales annually (Craik *et al.*, 2013), and small cationic HDPs will undoubtedly continue to be a factor in this growing market.

14.5 Conclusions

While the existence of HDPs has been known for decades, new roles in host defence and uses in the treatment of human disease are continually emerging. Although some challenges remain in using HDPs in humans, such as cost and toxicity, these issues are being overcome and many HDPs have been used in clinical trials or are approved for use in humans. Further study in exciting new areas such as wound healing or anticancer therapeutics, along with the vast amount of research demonstrating their potential as anti-infective agents, will hopefully provide new drugs for a variety of human diseases.

Acknowledgements

R.E.W.H.'s peptide research is supported by a Canadian Institutes for Health Research grant MOP-74493 and by the National Institute of Allergy and Infectious Diseases of the National Institutes of Health under Award Number R33AI098701. The content is solely the responsibility of the authors and does not necessarily represent the official views of the National Institutes of Health. R.E.W.H. holds a Canada Research Chair in Health and Genomics and is also the recipient of a UBC Killam Professorship. K.C. Wuerth was supported by a Cystic Fibrosis Canada doctoral studentship.

References

Aarbiou, J., Verhoosel, R.M., Van Wetering, S., De Boer, W.I., Van Krieken, J.H., *et al.* (2004) Neutrophil defensins enhance lung epithelial wound closure and mucin gene expression *in vitro*. *American Journal of Respiratory Cell and Molecular Biology* 30, 193–201.

Akter, R., Cao, P., Noor, H., Ridgway, Z., Tu, L.H., *et al.* (2016) Islet amyloid polypeptide: structure, function, and pathophysiology. *Journal of Diabetes Research* 2016, 2798269.

Bataille, D. and Dalle, S. (2014) The forgotten members of the glucagon family. *Diabetes Research and Clinical Practice* 106, 1–10.

Bowdish, D.M., Davidson, D.J. and Hancock, R.E.W. (2005) A re-evaluation of the role of host defence peptides in mammalian immunity. *Current Protein and Peptide Science* 6, 35–51.

Braff, M.H., Di Nardo, A. and Gallo, R.L. (2005) Keratinocytes store the antimicrobial peptide cathelicidin in lamellar bodies. *Journal of Investigative Dermatology* 124, 394–400.

Catania, A., Lonati, C., Sordi, A., Carlin, A., Leonardi, P., *et al.* (2010) The melanocortin system in control of inflammation. *Scientific World Journal* 10, 1840–1853.

Chang, S.H., Jung, E.J., Lim, D.G., Park, Y.H., Wee, Y.M., *et al.* (2008) Anti-inflammatory action of alpha-melanocyte stimulating hormone (alpha-MSH) in anti-CD3/CD28-mediated spleen and CD4(+)CD25(-) T cells and a partial participation of IL-10. *Immunology Letters* 118, 44–48.

Charnley, M., Moir, A.J., Douglas, C.W. and Haycock, J.W. (2008) Anti-microbial action of melanocortin peptides and identification of a novel X-Pro-D/L-Val sequence in Gram-positive and Gram-negative bacteria. *Peptides* 29, 1004–1009.

Coffelt, S.B., Marini, F.C., Watson, K., Zwezdaryk, K.J., Dembinski, J.L., *et al.* (2009) The pro-inflammatory peptide LL-37 promotes ovarian tumor progression through recruitment of multipotent mesenchymal stromal cells. *Proceedings of the National Academy of Sciences of the United States of America* 106, 3806–3811.

Cowland, J.B., Johnsen, A.H. and Borregaard, N. (1995) hCAP-18, a cathelin/pro-bactenecin-like protein of human neutrophil specific granules. *FEBS Letters* 368, 173–176.

Craik, D.J., Fairlie, D.P., Liras, S. and Price, D. (2013) The future of peptide-based drugs. *Chemical Biology and Drug Design* 81, 136–147.

Cunin, P., Caillon, A., Corvaisier, M., Garo, E., Scotet, M., *et al.* (2011) The tachykinins substance P and hemokinin-1 favor the generation of human memory Th17 cells by inducing IL-1beta, IL-23, and TNF-like 1A expression by monocytes. *Journal of Immunology* 186, 4175–4182.

Czepielewski, R.S., Porto, B.N., Rizzo, L.B., Roesler, R., Abujamra, A.L., *et al.* (2012) Gastrin-releasing peptide receptor (GRPR) mediates chemotaxis in neutrophils. *Proceedings of the National Academy of Sciences of The United States of America* 109, 547–552.

Davidson, D.J., Currie, A.J., Reid, G.S., Bowdish, D.M., MacDonald, K.L., *et al.* (2004) The cationic antimicrobial peptide LL-37 modulates dendritic cell differentiation and dendritic cell-induced T cell polarization. *Journal of Immunology* 172, 1146–1156.

de la Fuente-Nunez, C., Reffuveille, F., Haney, E.F., Straus, S.K. and Hancock, R.E.W. (2014) Broad-spectrum anti-biofilm peptide that targets a cellular stress response. *PLoS Pathogens* 10, e1004152.

de la Fuente-Nunez, C., Reffuveille, F., Mansour, S.C., Reckseidler-Zenteno, S.L., Hernandez, D., *et al.* (2015) D-enantiomeric peptides that eradicate wild-type and multidrug-resistant biofilms and protect against lethal *Pseudomonas aeruginosa* infections. *Chemistry and Biology* 22, 196–205.

De Vito, P. (2014) Atrial natriuretic peptide: an old hormone or a new cytokine? *Peptides* 58, 108–116.

Delgado, M. and Ganea, D. (2000) Inhibition of IFN-gamma-induced janus kinase-1-STAT1 activation in macrophages by vasoactive intestinal peptide and pituitary adenylate cyclase-activating polypeptide. *Journal of Immunology* 165, 3051–3057.

Delgado, M., Pozo, D. and Ganea, D. (2004) The significance of vasoactive intestinal peptide in immunomodulation. *Pharmacological Reviews* 56, 249–290.

Ding, W., Wagner, J.A. and Granstein, R.D. (2007) CGRP, PACAP, and VIP modulate Langerhans cell function by inhibiting NF-kappaB activation. *Journal of Investigative Dermatology* 127, 2357–2367.

Dioufa, N., Schally, A.V., Chatzistamou, I., Moustou, E., Block, N.L., *et al.* (2010) Acceleration of wound healing by growth hormone-releasing hormone and its agonists. *Proceedings of the National Academy of Sciences of the United States of America* 107, 18611–18615.

Dürr, U.H.N., Sudheendra, U.S. and Ramamoorthy, A. (2006) LL-37, the only human member of the cathelicidin family of antimicrobial peptides. *Biochimica et Biophysica Acta* 1758, 1408–1425.

Eissa, N. and Ghia, J.E. (2015) Immunomodulatory effect of ghrelin in the intestinal mucosa. *Neurogastroenterology and Motility* 27, 1519–1527.

Fabisiak, A., Murawska, N. and Fichna, J. (2016) LL-37: Cathelicidin-related antimicrobial peptide with pleiotropic activity. *Pharmacological Reports* 68, 802–808.

Fjell, C.D., Hiss, J.A., Hancock, R.E.W. and Schneider, G. (2011) Designing antimicrobial peptides: form follows function. *Nature Reviews Drug Discovery* 11, 37–51.

Fosgerau, K. and Hoffmann, T. (2015) Peptide therapeutics: current status and future directions. *Drug Discovery Today* 20, 122–128.

Ganea, D., Hooper, K.M. and Kong, W. (2015) The neuropeptide vasoactive intestinal peptide: direct effects on immune cells and involvement in inflammatory and autoimmune diseases. *Acta Physiologica (Oxford)* 213, 442–452.

Ganz, T. (2003) Defensins: antimicrobial peptides of innate immunity. *Nature Reviews Immunology* 3, 710–720.

Garcia, J.R., Krause, A., Schulz, S., Rodriguez-Jimenez, F.J., Kluver, E., *et al.* (2001) Human beta-defensin 4: a novel inducible peptide with a specific salt-sensitive spectrum of antimicrobial activity. *FASEB Journal* 15, 1819–1821.

Garlapati, S., Garg, R., Brownlie, R., Latimer, L., Simko, E., *et al.* (2012) Enhanced immune responses and protection by vaccination with respiratory syncytial virus fusion protein formulated with CpG oligodeoxynucleotide and innate defense regulator peptide in polyphosphazene microparticles. *Vaccine* 30, 5206–5214.

Gavioli, E.C., de Medeiros, I.U., Monteiro, M.C., Calo, G. and Romao, P.R. (2015) Nociceptin/orphanin FQ-NOP receptor system in inflammatory and immune-mediated diseases. *Vitamins and Hormones* 97, 241–266.

Ghatnekar, G.S., Grek, C.L., Armstrong, D.G., Desai, S.C. and Gourdie, R.G. (2015) The effect of a connexin43-based peptide on the healing of chronic venous leg ulcers: a multicenter, randomized trial. *Journal of Investigative Dermatology* 135, 289–298.

Gomes, R.N., Castro-Faria-Neto, H.C., Bozza, P.T., Soares, M.B., Shoemaker, C.B., *et al.* (2005) Calcitonin gene-related peptide inhibits local acute inflammation and protects mice against lethal endotoxemia. *Shock* 24, 590–594.

Gonzalez-Rey, E., Varela, N., Sheibanie, A.F., Chorny, A., Ganea, D., *et al.* (2006) Cortistatin, an anti-inflammatory peptide with therapeutic action in inflammatory bowel disease. *Proceedings of the National Academy of Sciences of the United States of America* 103, 4228–4233.

Gracia, A., Polewicz, M., Halperin, S.A., Hancock, R.E.W., Potter, A.A., *et al.* (2011) Antibody responses in adult and neonatal BALB/c mice to immunization with novel *Bordetella pertussis* vaccine formulations. *Vaccine* 29, 1595–1604.

Granata, R. (2016) Peripheral activities of growth hormone-releasing hormone. *Journal of Endocrinological Investigation* 39, 721–727.

Granstein, R.D., Wagner, J.A., Stohl, L.L. and Ding, W. (2015) Calcitonin gene-related peptide: key regulator of cutaneous immunity. *Acta Physiologica (Oxford)* 213, 580–594.

Grimaldi, D., Silvani, A., Benarroch, E.E. and Cortelli, P. (2014) Orexin/hypocretin system and autonomic control: new insights and clinical correlations. *Neurology* 82, 271–278.

Gronberg, A., Mahlapuu, M., Stahle, M., Whately-Smith, C. and Rollman, O. (2014) Treatment with LL-37 is safe and effective in enhancing healing of hard-to-heal venous leg ulcers: a randomized, placebo-controlled clinical trial. *Wound Repair and Regeneration* 22, 613–621.

Gusman, H., Travis, J., Helmerhorst, E.J., Potempa, J., Troxler, R.F., *et al.* (2001) Salivary histatin 5 is an inhibitor of both host and bacterial enzymes implicated in periodontal disease. *Infection and Immunity* 69, 1402–1408.

Hancock, R.E.W. (1997) Peptide antibiotics. *Lancet* 349, 418–422.

Hancock, R.E.W. and Sahl, H.-G. (2006) Antimicrobial and host-defense peptides as new anti-infective therapeutic strategies. *Nature Biotechnology* 24, 1551–1557.

Haney, E.F., Mansour, S.C., Hilchie, A.L., de la Fuente-Nunez, C. and Hancock, R.E.W. (2015) High throughput screening methods for assessing antibiofilm and immunomodulatory activities of synthetic peptides. *Peptides* 71, 276–285.

Harmar, A.J., Fahrenkrug, J., Gozes, I., Laburthe, M., May, V., *et al.* (2012) Pharmacology and functions of receptors for vasoactive intestinal peptide and pituitary adenylate cyclase-activating polypeptide: IUPHAR review 1. *British Journal of Pharmacology* 166, 4–17.

Heilborn, J.D., Nilsson, M.F., Kratz, G., Weber, G., Sorensen, O., *et al.* (2003) The cathelicidin antimicrobial peptide LL-37 is involved in re-epithelialization of human skin wounds and is lacking in chronic ulcer epithelium. *Journal of Investigative Dermatology* 120, 379–389.

Helle, K.B. and Corti, A. (2015) Chromogranin A: a paradoxical player in angiogenesis and vascular biology. *Cellular and Molecular Life Sciences* 72, 339–348.

Hilchie, A.L., Wuerth, K. and Hancock, R.E.W. (2013) Immune modulation by multifaceted cationic host defense (antimicrobial) peptides. *Nature Chemical Biology* 9, 761–768.

Hilpert, K., Volkmer-Engert, R., Walter, T. and Hancock, R.E.W. (2005) High-throughput generation of small antibacterial peptides with improved activity. *Nature Biotechnology* 23, 1008–1012.

Hirsch, T., Spielmann, M., Zuhaili, B., Fossum, M., Metzig, M., *et al.* (2009) Human beta-defensin-3 promotes wound healing in infected diabetic wounds. *Journal of Gene Medicine* 11, 220–228.

Hollox, E.J., Huffmeier, U., Zeeuwen, P.L., Palla, R., Lascorz, J., *et al.* (2008) Psoriasis is associated with increased beta-defensin genomic copy number. *Nature Genetics* 40, 23–25.

Hondo, M., Ishii, M. and Sakurai, T. (2008) The NPB/NPW neuropeptide system and its role in regulating energy homeostasis, pain, and emotion. *Results and Problems in Cellular Differentiation* 46, 239–256.

Hoskin, D.W. and Ramamoorthy, A. (2008) Studies on anticancer activities of antimicrobial peptides. *Biochimica et Biophysica Acta* 1778, 357–375.

Huang, Y.H., Yang, Y.L., Tiao, M.M., Kuo, H.C., Huang, L.T., *et al.* (2012) Hepcidin protects against lipopolysaccharide-induced liver injury in a mouse model of obstructive jaundice. *Peptides* 35, 212–217.

Janelsins, B.M., Sumpter, T.L., Tkacheva, O.A., Rojas-Canales, D.M., Erdos, G., *et al.* (2013) Neurokinin-1 receptor agonists bias therapeutic dendritic cells to induce type 1 immunity by licensing host dendritic cells to produce IL-12. *Blood* 121, 2923–2933.

Jensen, R.T., Battey, J.F., Spindel, E.R. and Benya, R.V. (2008) International Union of Pharmacology. LXVIII. Mammalian bombesin receptors: nomenclature, distribution, pharmacology, signaling, and functions in normal and disease states. *Pharmacological Reviews* 60, 1-42.

Jenssen, H., Hamill, P. and Hancock, R.E.W. (2006) Peptide antimicrobial agents. *Clinical Microbiology Reviews* 19, 49–51.

Khush, K.K., Gerber, I.L., McKeown, B., Marcus, G., Vessey, J., *et al.* (2006) Obese patients have lower B-type and atrial natriuretic peptide levels compared with nonobese. *Congestive Heart Failure* 12, 85–90.

Kidoya, H., Kunii, N., Naito, H., Muramatsu, F., Okamoto, Y., *et al.* (2012) The apelin/APJ system induces maturation of the tumor vasculature and improves the efficiency of immune therapy. *Oncogene* 31, 3254–3264.

Kim, J.H., Kim, K.H., Kim, H.J., Lee, J. and Myung, S.C. (2015) Expression of beta-defensin 131 promotes an innate immune response in human prostate epithelial cells. *PLoS One* 10, e0144776.

Kindrachuk, J., Jenssen, H., Elliott, M., Townsend, R., Nijnik, A., *et al.* (2009) A novel vaccine adjuvant comprised of a synthetic innate defence regulator peptide and CpG oligonucleotide links innate and adaptive immunity. *Vaccine* 27, 4662–4671.

Kingwell, B.A., Chapman, M.J., Kontush, A., and Miller, N.E. (2014) HDL-targeted therapies: progress, failures and future. *Nature Reviews Drug Discovery* 13, 445–464.

Koczulla, R., von Degenfeld, G., Kupatt, C., Krötz, F., Zahler, S., *et al.* (2003) An angiogenic role for the human peptide antibiotic LL-37/hCAP-18. *Journal of Clinical Investigation* 111, 1665–1672.

Kolar, S.S. and McDermott, A.M. (2011) Role of host-defence peptides in eye diseases. *Cellular and Molecular Life Sciences* 68, 2201–2213.

Kovacs-Nolan, J., Latimer, L., Landi, A., Jenssen, H., Hancock, R.E.W., *et al.* (2009) The novel adjuvant combination of CpG ODN, indolicidin and polyphosphazene induces potent antibody- and cell-mediated immune responses in mice. *Vaccine* 27, 2055–2064.

Krause, A., Liepke, C., Meyer, M., Adermann, K., Forssmann, W.G., *et al.* (2001) Human natriuretic peptides exhibit antimicrobial activity. *European Journal of Medical Research* 6, 215–218.

Krause, A., Sillard, R., Kleemeier, B., Kluver, E., Maronde, E., *et al.* (2003) Isolation and biochemical characterization of LEAP-2: a novel blood peptide expressed in the liver. *Protein Science* 12, 143–152.

Kurosaka, K., Chen, Q., Yarovinsky, F., Oppenheim, J.J. and Yang, D. (2005) Mouse cathelin-related antimicrobial pepide chemoattracts leukocytes using formyl peptide receptor-like 1/mouse formyl peptide receptor-like 2 as the receptor and acts as an immune adjuvant. *Journal of Immunology* 174, 6257–6265.

Leceta, J., Gomariz, R.P., Martinez, C., Abad, C., Ganea, D., *et al.* (2000) Receptors and transcriptional factors involved in the anti-inflammatory activity of VIP and PACAP. *Annals of the New York Academy of Sciences* 921, 92–102.

Lee, D.K., George, S.R. and O'Dowd, B.F. (2006) Unravelling the roles of the apelin system: prospective therapeutic applications in heart failure and obesity. *Trends in Pharmacological Sciences* 27, 190–194.

Li, W.G., Gavrila, D., Liu, X., Wang, L., Gunnlaugsson, S., *et al.* (2004) Ghrelin inhibits proinflammatory responses and nuclear factor-kappaB activation in human endothelial cells. *Circulation* 109, 2221–2226.

Li, Y. (2011) Recombinant production of antimicrobial peptides in *Escherichia coli*: a review. *Protein Expression and Purification* 80, 260–267.

Lipton, J.M., Ceriani, G., Macaluso, A., McCoy, D., Carnes, K., *et al.* (1994) Antiinflammatory effects of the neuropeptide alpha-MSH in acute, chronic, and systemic inflammation. *Annals of the New York Academy of Sciences* 741, 137–148.

Liu, J., Chen, M. and Wang, X. (2000) Calcitonin gene-related peptide inhibits lipopolysaccharide-induced interleukin-12 release from mouse peritoneal macrophages, mediated by the cAMP pathway. *Immunology* 101, 61–67.

Liu, P.T., Stenger, S., Li, H., Wenzel, L., Tan, B.H., *et al.* (2006) Toll-like receptor triggering of a vitamin D-mediated human antimicrobial response. *Science* 311, 1770–1773.

Liu, P.T., Stenger, S., Tang, D.H. and Modlin, R.L. (2007) Cutting edge: vitamin D-mediated human antimicrobial activity against *Mycobacterium tuberculosis* is dependent on the induction of cathelicidin. *Journal of Immunology* 179, 2060–2063.

Mader, J.S., Ewen, C., Hancock, R.E.W. and Bleackley, R.C. (2011) The human cathelicidin, LL-37, induces granzyme-mediated apoptosis in regulatory T cells. *Journal of Immunotherapy* 34, 229–235.

Madera, L. and Hancock, R.E.W. (2012) Synthetic immunomodulatory peptide IDR-1002 enhances monocyte migration and adhesion on fibronectin. *Journal of Innate Immunity* 4, 553–568.

Manna, S.K. and Aggarwal, B.B. (1998) Alpha-melanocyte-stimulating hormone inhibits the nuclear transcription factor NF-kappa B activation induced by various inflammatory agents. *Journal of Immunology* 161, 2873–2880.

Mashaghi, A., Marmalidou, A., Tehrani, M., Grace, P.M., Pothoulakis, C., *et al.* (2016) Neuropeptide substance P and the immune response. *Cellular and Molecular Life Sciences* 73, 4249–4264.

Mathis, D. and Shoelson, S.E. (2011) Immunometabolism: an emerging frontier. *Nature Reviews Immunology* 11, 81–83.

Matsue, Y., Kagiyama, N., Yoshida, K., Kume, T., Okura, H., *et al.* (2015) Carperitide is associated with increased in-hospital mortality in acute heart failure: a propensity score-matched analysis. *Journal of Cardiac Failure* 21, 859–864.

Melino, S., Santone, C., Di Nardo, P. and Sarkar, B. (2014) Histatins: salivary peptides with copper(II)- and zinc(II)-binding motifs: perspectives for biomedical applications. *FEBS Journal* 281, 657–672.

Michels, K., Nemeth, E., Ganz, T. and Mehrad, B. (2015) Hepcidin and host defense against infectious diseases. *PLoS Pathogens* 11, e1004998.

Mikami, N., Watanabe, K., Hashimoto, N., Miyagi, Y., Sueda, K., *et al.* (2012) Calcitonin gene-related peptide enhances experimental autoimmune encephalomyelitis by promoting Th17-cell functions. *International Immunology* 24, 681–691.

Min, Y., Han, D., Fu, Z., Wang, H., Liu, L., *et al.* (2011) Alpha-MSH inhibits TNF-alpha-induced maturation of human dendritic cells *in vitro* through the up-regulation of ANXA1. *Acta Biochimica et Biophysica Sinica (Shanghai)* 43, 61–68.

Moffatt, P. and Thomas, G. P. (2009) Osteocrin: beyond just another bone protein? *Cellular and Molecular Life Sciences* 66, 1135–1139.

Moffatt, P., Thomas, G.P., Sellin, K., Bessette, M.C., Lafreniere, F., *et al.* (2007) Osteocrin is a specific ligand of the natriuretic peptide clearance receptor that modulates bone growth. *Journal of Biological Chemistry* 282, 36454–36462.

Molhoek, E.M., den Hertog, A.L., de Vries, A.M., Nazmi, K., Veerman, E.C., *et al.* (2009) Structure–function relationship of the human antimicrobial peptide LL-37 and LL-37 fragments in the modulation of TLR responses. *Biological Chemistry* 390, 295–303.

Mookherjee, N., Brown, K.L., Bowdish, D.M., Doria, S., Falsafi, R., *et al.* (2006) Modulation of the TLR-mediated inflammatory response by the endogenous human host defense peptide LL-37. *Journal of Immunology* 176, 2455–2464.

Mookherjee, N., Hamill, P., Gardy, J., Blimkie, D., Falsafi, R., *et al.* (2009) Systems biology evaluation of immune responses induced by human host defence peptide LL-37 in mononuclear cells. *Molecular BioSystems* 5, 483–496.

Motzkus, D., Schulz-Maronde, S., Heitland, A., Schulz, A., Forssmann, W.G., *et al.* (2006) The novel beta-defensin DEFB123 prevents lipopolysaccharide-mediated effects *in vitro* and *in vivo*. *FASEB Journal* 20, 1701–1702.

Mountjoy, K.G. (2015) Pro-opiomelanocortin (POMC) neurones, POMC-derived peptides, melanocortin receptors and obesity: how understanding of this system has changed over the last decade. *Journal of Neuroendocrinology* 27, 406–418.

Murakami, M., Dorschner, R.A., Stern, L.J., Lin, K.H. and Gallo, R.L. (2005) Expression and secretion of cathelicidin antimicrobial peptides in murine mammary glands and human milk. *Pediatric Research* 57, 10–15.

Nagaoka, I., Hirota, S., Niyonsaba, F., Hirata, M., Adachi, Y., *et al.* (2001) Cathelicidin family of antibacterial peptides CAP18 and CAP11 inhibit the expression of TNF-alpha by blocking the binding of LPS to CD14(+) cells. *Journal of Immunology* 167, 3329–3338.

Navab, M., Anantharamaiah, G.M., Reddy, S.T., Hama, S., Hough, G., *et al.* (2005) Apolipoprotein A-I mimetic peptides. *Arteriosclerosis Thrombosis and Vascular Biology* 25, 1325–1331.

Nguyen, T.X., Cole, A.M. and Lehrer, R.I. (2003) Evolution of primate theta-defensins: a serpentine path to a sweet tooth. *Peptides* 24, 1647–1654.

Nibbering, P.H., Ravensbergen, E., Welling, M.M., van Berkel, L.A., van Berkel, P.H., *et al.* (2001) Human lactoferrin and peptides derived from its N terminus are highly effective against infections with antibiotic-resistant bacteria. *Infection and Immunity* 69, 1469–1476.

Nijnik, A. and Hancock, R.E.W. (2009) The roles of cathelicidin LL-37 in immune defences and novel clinical applications. *Current Opinion in Hematology* 16, 41–47.

Nijnik, A., Madera, L., Ma, S., Waldbrook, M., Elliot, M.R., *et al.* (2010) Synthetic cationic peptide IDR-1002 provides protection against bacterial infections through chemokine induction and enhanced leukocyte recruitment. *Journal of Immunology* 184, 2539–2550.

Nix, M.A., Kaelin, C.B., Ta, T., Weis, A., Morton, G.J., *et al.* (2013) Molecular and functional analysis of human beta-defensin 3 action at melanocortin receptors. *Chemistry and Biology* 20, 784–795.

Niyonsaba, F., Ushio, H., Nakano, N., Ng, W., Sayama, K., *et al.* (2007) Antimicrobial peptides human beta-defensins stimulate epidermal keratinocyte migration, proliferation and production of pro-inflammatory cytokines and chemokines. *Journal of Investigative Dermatology* 127, 594–604.

Niyonsaba, F., Madera, L., Afacan, N., Okumura, K., Ogawa, H., *et al.* (2013) The innate defense regulator peptides IDR-HH2, IDR-1002, and IDR-1018 modulate human neutrophil functions. *Journal of Leukocyte Biology* 94, 159–170.

O'Connor, C.M., Starling, R.C., Hernandez, A.F., Armstrong, P.W., Dickstein, K., *et al.* (2011) Effect of nesiritide in patients with acute decompensated heart failure. *New England Journal of Medicine* 365, 32–43.

Oeckinghaus, A., Hayden, M.S. and Ghosh, S. (2011) Crosstalk in NF-kappaB signaling pathways. *Nature Immunology* 12, 695–708.

O'Neill, L.A., Kishton, R.J. and Rathmell, J. (2016) A guide to immunometabolism for immunologists. *Nature Reviews Immunology* 16, 553–565.

Osadchii, O.E. (2015) Emerging role of neurotensin in regulation of the cardiovascular system. *European Journal of Pharmacology* 762, 184–192.

Oudhoff, M.J., Bolscher, J.G., Nazmi, K., Kalay, H., van 't Hof, W., *et al.* (2008) Histatins are the major wound-closure stimulating factors in human saliva as identified in a cell culture assay. *FASEB Journal* 22, 3805–3812.

Oudhoff, M.J., Blaauboer, M.E., Nazmi, K., Scheres, N., Bolscher, J.G., *et al.* (2010) The role of salivary histatin and the human cathelicidin LL-37 in wound healing and innate immunity. *Biological Chemistry* 391, 541–548.

Overhage, J., Campisano, A., Bains, M., Torfs, E.C.W., Rehm, B.H.A., *et al.* (2008) Human host defense peptide LL-37 prevents bacterial biofilm formation. *Infection and Immunity* 76, 4176–4182.

Pena, O.M., Afacan, N., Pistolic, J., Chen, C., Madera, L., *et al.* (2013) Synthetic cationic peptide IDR-1018 modulates human macrophage differentiation. *PLoS One* 8, e52449.

Piers, K.L., Brown, M.H. and Hancock, R.E.W. (1993) Recombinant DNA procedures for producing small antimicrobial cationic peptides in bacteria. *Gene* 134, 7–13.

Pistolic, J., Cosseau, C., Li, Y., Yu, J.J., Filewod, N.C., *et al.* (2009) Host defence peptide LL-37 induces IL-6 expression in human bronchial epithelial cells by activation of the NF-kappaB signaling pathway. *Journal of Innate Immunity* 1, 254–267.

Polewicz, M., Gracia, A., Garlapati, S., van Kessel, J., Strom, S., *et al.* (2013) Novel vaccine formulations against pertussis offer earlier onset of immunity and provide protection in the presence of maternal antibodies. *Vaccine* 31, 3148–3155.

Potter, L.R., Yoder, A.R., Flora, D.R., Antos, L.K. and Dickey, D.M. (2009) Natriuretic peptides: their structures, receptors, physiologic functions and therapeutic applications. *Handbook of Experimental Pharmacology* 2009, 341–366.

Rai, U., Thrimawithana, T.R., Valery, C. and Young, S.A. (2015) Therapeutic uses of somatostatin and its analogues: current view and potential applications. *Pharmacology and Therapeutics* 152, 98–110.

Reffuveille, F., de la Fuente-Nunez, C., Mansour, S. and Hancock, R.E.W. (2014) A broad-spectrum antibiofilm peptide enhances antibiotic action against bacterial biofilms. *Antimicrobial Agents and Chemotherapy* 58, 5363–5371.

Ren, S.X., Cheng, A.S., To, K.F., Tong, J.H., Li, M.S., *et al.* (2012) Host immune defense peptide LL-37 activates caspase-independent apoptosis and suppresses colon cancer. *Cancer Research* 72, 6512–6523.

Scotland, R.S., Cohen, M., Foster, P., Lovell, M., Mathur, A., *et al.* (2005) C-type natriuretic peptide inhibits leukocyte recruitment and platelet-leukocyte interactions via suppression of P-selectin expression. *Proceedings of the National Academy of Sciences of the United States of America* 102, 14452–14457.

Sekhar, R.V. (2015) Treatment of dyslipidemia in HIV. *Current Atherosclerosis Reports* 17, 493.

Serhan, C.N., Fierro, I.M., Chiang, N. and Pouliot, M. (2001) Cutting edge: nociceptin stimulates neutrophil chemotaxis and recruitment: inhibition by aspirin-triggered-15-epi-lipoxin A4. *Journal of Immunology* 166, 3650–3654.

Skalhegg, B.S. and Tasken, K. (2000) Specificity in the cAMP/PKA signaling pathway: differential expression, regulation, and subcellular localization of subunits of PKA. *Frontiers in Bioscience* 5, D678–D693.

Skelton, W.P.T., Pi, G.E. and Vesely, D.L. (2011) Four cardiac hormones cause death of human cancer cells but not of healthy cells. *Anticancer Research* 31, 395–402.

Sorensen, O.E., Arnljots, K., Cowland, J.B., Bainton, D.F. and Borregaard, N. (1997) The human antibacterial cathelicidin, hCAP-18, is synthesized in myelocytes and metamyelocytes and localized to specific granules in neutrophils. *Blood* 90, 2796–2803.

Sorensen, O.E., Follin, P., Johnsen, A.H., Calafat, J., Tjabringa, G.S., *et al.* (2001) Human cathelicidin, hCAP-18, is processed to the antimicrobial peptide LL-37 by extracellular cleavage with proteinase 3. *Blood* 97, 3951–3959.

Steinstraesser, L., Hirsch, T., Schulte, M., Kueckelhaus, M., Jacobsen, F., *et al.* (2012) Innate defense regulator peptide 1018 in wound healing and wound infection. *PLoS One* 7, e39373.

Stengel, A. and Tache, Y. (2014) CRF and urocortin peptides as modulators of energy balance and feeding behavior during stress. *Frontiers in Neuroscience* 8, 52.

Subramanian, H., Gupta, K., Guo, Q., Price, R. and Ali, H. (2011) Mas-related gene X2 (MrgX2) is a novel G protein-coupled receptor for the antimicrobial peptide LL-37 in human mast cells: resistance to receptor phosphorylation, desensitization, and internalization. *Journal of Biological Chemistry* 286, 44739–44749.

Subramanian, H., Gupta, K., Lee, D., Bayir, A.K., Ahn, H., *et al.* (2013) beta-Defensins activate human mast cells via Mas-related gene X2. *Journal of Immunology* 191, 345–352.

Sun, L.C. and Coy, D.H. (2011) Somatostatin receptor-targeted anti-cancer therapy. *Current Drug Delivery* 8, 2–10.

Tabet, F., Remaley, A.T., Segaliny, A.I., Millet, J., Yan, L., *et al.* (2010) The 5A apolipoprotein A-I mimetic peptide displays antiinflammatory and antioxidant properties *in vivo* and *in vitro*. *Arteriosclerosis Thrombosis and Vascular Biology* 30, 246–252.

Tang, Y., Lv, B., Wang, H., Xiao, X. and Zuo, X. (2008) PACAP inhibit the release and cytokine activity of HMGB1 and improve the survival during lethal endotoxemia. *International Immunopharmacology* 8, 1646–1651.

Tani, K., Murphy, W.J., Chertov, O., Salcedo, R., Koh, C.Y., *et al.* (2000) Defensins act as potent adjuvants that promote cellular and humoral immune responses in mice to a lymphoma idiotype and carrier antigens. *International Immunology* 12, 691–700.

Taylor, A. and Namba, K. (2001) In vitro induction of CD25+ CD4+ regulatory T cells by the neuropeptide alpha-melanocyte stimulating hormone (alpha-MSH). *Immunology and Cell Biology* 79, 358–367.

Theurl, M., Schgoer, W., Albrecht, K., Jeschke, J., Egger, M., *et al.* (2010) The neuropeptide catestatin acts as a novel angiogenic cytokine via a basic fibroblast growth factor-dependent mechanism. *Circulation Research* 107, 1326–1335.

Torossian, A., Gurschi, E., Bals, R., Vassiliou, T., Wulf, H.F., *et al.* (2007) Effects of the antimicrobial peptide LL-37 and hyperthermic preconditioning in septic rats. *Anesthesiology* 107, 437–441.

Trombella, S., Vergura, R., Falzarano, S., Guerrini, R., Calo, G., *et al.* (2005) Nociceptin/orphanin FQ stimulates human monocyte chemotaxis via NOP receptor activation. *Peptides* 26, 1497–1502.

Tsukagoshi, H., Shimizu, Y., Kawata, T., Hisada, T., Iwamae, S., *et al.* (2001) Atrial natriuretic peptide inhibits tumor necrosis factor-alpha production by interferon-gamma-activated macrophages via suppression of p38 mitogen-activated protein kinase and nuclear factor-kappa B activation. *Regulatory Peptides* 99, 21–29.

Turner, J., Cho, Y., Dinh, N.N., Waring, A.J. and Lehrer, R.I. (1998) Activities of LL-37, a cathelin-associated antimicrobial peptide of human neutrophils. *Antimicrobial Agents and Chemotherapy* 42, 2206–2214.

van Hagen, P.M., Dalm, V.A., Staal, F. and Hofland, L.J. (2008) The role of cortistatin in the human immune system. *Molecular and Cellular Endocrinology* 286, 141–147.

Vandamme, D., Landuyt, B., Luyten, W. and Schoofs, L. (2012) A comprehensive summary of LL-37, the factotum human cathelicidin peptide. *Cellular Immunology* 280, 22–35.

Vesely, D.L., Eichelbaum, E.J., Sun, Y., Alli, A.A., Vesely, B.A., *et al.* (2007) Elimination of up to 80% of human pancreatic adenocarcinomas in athymic mice by cardiac hormones. *In Vivo* 21, 445–451.

Vollmar, A.M., Forster, R. and Schulz, R. (1997) Effects of atrial natriuretic peptide on phagocytosis and respiratory burst in murine macrophages. *European Journal of Pharmacology* 319, 279–285.

Walsh, D.A., Mapp, P.I. and Kelly, S. (2015) Calcitonin gene-related peptide in the joint: contributions to pain and inflammation. *British Journal of Clinical Pharmacology* 80, 965–978.

Wang, G., Li, X. and Wang, Z. (2016) APD3: the antimicrobial peptide database as a tool for research and education. *Nucleic Acids Research* 44, D1087–D1093.

Wang, T.T., Nestel, F.P., Bourdeau, V., Nagai, Y., Wang, Q., *et al.* (2004) Cutting edge: 1,25-dihydroxyvitamin D3 is a direct inducer of antimicrobial peptide gene expression. *Journal of Immunology* 173, 2909–2912.

Wang, X. and Fiscus, R.R. (1989) Calcitonin gene-related peptide increases cAMP, tension, and rate in rat atria. *American Journal of Physiology* 256, R421–R428.

Waschek, J.A. (2013) VIP and PACAP: neuropeptide modulators of CNS inflammation, injury, and repair. *British Journal of Pharmacology* 169, 512–523.

Weber, G., Chamorro, C.I., Granath, F., Liljegren, A., Zreika, S., *et al.* (2009) Human antimicrobial protein hCAP18/LL-37 promotes a metastatic phenotype in breast cancer. *Breast Cancer Research* 11, R6.

Wehkamp, J., Salzman, N.H., Porter, E., Nuding, S., Weichenthal, M., *et al.* (2005) Reduced paneth cell alpha-defensins in ileal Crohn's disease. *Proceedings of the National Academy of Sciences USA* 102, 18129–18134.

Wilmes, M. and Sahl, H.G. (2014) Defensin-based anti-infective strategies. *International Journal of Medical Microbiology* 304, 93–99.

Wuerth, K.C., Hilchie, A.L., Brown, K.L. and Hancock, R.E.W. (2013) Host defence (antimicrobial) peptides and proteins. *eLS*, 77–84. DOI: 10.1002/9780470015902.90001212.pub3

Xu, Y., Li, Z., Yin, Y., Lan, H., Wang, J., *et al.* (2015) Ghrelin inhibits the differentiation of T helper 17 cells through mTOR/STAT3 signaling pathway. *PLoS One* 10, e0117081.

Yang, D., Chertov, O., Bykovskaia, S.N., Chen, Q., Buffo, M.J., *et al.* (1999) Beta-defensins: linking innate and adaptive immunity through dendritic and T cell CCR6. *Science* 286, 525–528.

Yang, D., Chen, Q., Schmidt, A.P., Anderson, G.M., Wang, J.M., *et al.* (2000) LL-37, the neutrophil granule- and epithelial cell-derived cathelicidin, utilizes formyl peptide receptor-like 1 (FPRL1) as a receptor to chemoattract human peripheral blood neutrophils, monocytes, and T cells. *Journal of Experimental Medicine* 192, 1069–1074.

Yao, X., Dai, C., Fredriksson, K., Dagur, P.K., McCoy, J.P., *et al.* (2011) 5A, an apolipoprotein A-I mimetic peptide, attenuates the induction of house dust mite-induced asthma. *Journal of Immunology* 186, 576–583.

Yenugu, S., Hamil, K.G., Radhakrishnan, Y., French, F.S. and Hall, S.H. (2004) The androgen-regulated epididymal sperm-binding protein, human beta-defensin 118 (DEFB118) (formerly ESC42), is an antimicrobial beta-defensin. *Endocrinology*, 145, 3165–3173.

Yu, J., Mookherjee, N., Wee, K., Bowdish, D.M., Pistolic, J., *et al.* (2007) Host defense peptide LL-37, in synergy with inflammatory mediator IL-1beta, augments immune responses by multiple pathways. *Journal of Immunology* 179, 7684–7691.

Zanetti, M. (2004) Cathelicidins, multifunctional peptides of the innate immunity. *Journal of Leukocyte Biology* 75, 39–48.

Zheng, S., Li, W., Xu, M., Bai, X., Zhou, Z., *et al.* (2010) Calcitonin gene-related peptide promotes angiogenesis via AMP-activated protein kinase. *American Journal of Physiology – Cell Physiology* 299, C1485–C1492.

Index

Page numbers in *italics* indicate figures.